WK 835
02/13

Diabetes

Chronic Complications

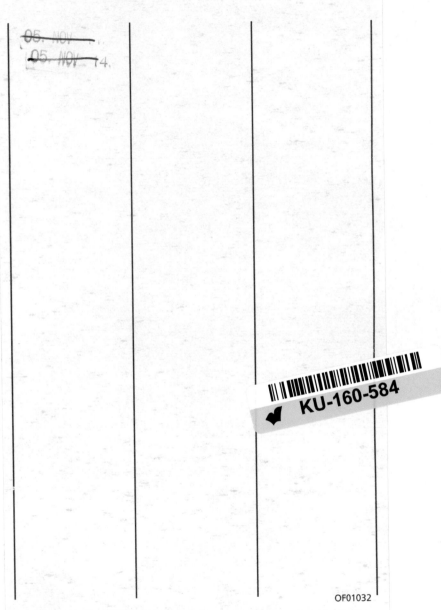

Books should be returned to the SDH Library on or before
the date stamped above unless a renewal has been arranged

Salisbury District Hospital Library

Telephone: Salisbury (01722) 336262 extn. 4432 / 33
Out of hours answer machine in operation

Diabetes
Chronic Complications

EDITED BY

Kenneth M. Shaw MD, FRCP

Honorary Consultant Physician, Queen Alexandra Hospital, Portsmouth Hospitals NHS Trust;
Emeritus Professor of Medicine, University of Portsmouth, Portsmouth, UK

Michael H. Cummings MD, FRCP

Professor of Diabetes and Endocrinology, Academic Department of Diabetes and Endocrinology,
Portsmouth NHS Trust, Queen Alexandra Hospital, Portsmouth, UK

THIRD EDITION

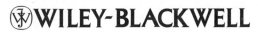
WILEY-BLACKWELL

A John Wiley & Sons, Ltd., Publication

Library of Congress Cataloging-in-Publication Data

Diabetes : chronic complications / edited by Kenneth M. Shaw, Michael H. Cummings. – 3rd ed.
       p. ; cm.
   Includes bibliographical references and index.
   ISBN 978-0-470-65618-1 (hard cover : alk. paper)
   I. Shaw, K. (Kenneth)   II. Cummings, Michael H.
   [DNLM: 1. Diabetes Complications.   WK 835]
   616.4'62–dc23
                         2011035461

A catalogue record for this book is available from the British Library.

Wiley also publishes its books in a variety of electronic formats. Some content that appears in print may not be available in electronic books.

Set in 9.5/13 pt Meridien by Toppan Best-set Premedia Limited

Printed in Singapore by Ho Printing Singapore Pte Ltd

1   2012

Contents

Contributors

Amita Bansal MBBS, MD
Clinical Fellow, Department of Dermatology, St Mary's Hospital, Portsmouth, UK

Stratos Christianakis MD
Assistant Professor of Clinical Medicine, Division of Rheumatology, Department of Medicine, Keck School of Medicine, University of Southern California, Los Angeles, CA, USA

Hywel L Cooper BM BMedSci MRCP Int Dip Acu
Consultant Dermatologist, Department of Dermatology, St Mary's Hospital, Portsmouth, UK

Steven S Coughlin PhD
Senior Epidemiologist, Epidemiology Program, Office of Public Health, Department of Veterans Affairs, Washington, DC; Adjunct Professor, Department of Epidemiology, Rollins School of Public Health Emory University, Atlanta, GA, USA

Iain Cranston FRCP
Consultant Physician (Diabetes and Endocrinology), Academic Department of Diabetes and Endocrinology, Portsmouth NHS Trust, Queen Alexandra Hospital, Portsmouth, UK

Michael H Cummings MD, FRCP
Professor of Diabetes and Endocrinology, Academic Department of Diabetes and Endocrinology, Portsmouth NHS Trust, Queen Alexandra Hospital, Portsmouth, UK

Nigel Davies MA, PhD, FRCOphth
Consultant Ophthalmologist, Chelsea and Westminster Hospital, London, UK

Anna Mae Diehl MD
Chief, Division of Gastroenterology, Duke University Hospital, Durham, NC, USA

Miles Fisher MD, FRCP
Consultant Physician, Glasgow Royal Infirmary; Honorary Professor, University of Glasgow, Glasgow, UK

Edward L Giovannucci MD, PhD
Professor of Epidemiology, Department of Epidemiology, Harvard School of Public Health, Boston, MA, USA

Adam E Haworth MB BChir, MRCPI, FRCP
Consultant Dermatologist, Department of Dermatology, St Mary's Hospital, Portsmouth, UK

Richard IG Holt MA, MB BChir, PhD, FRCP, FHEA
Professor in Diabetes and Endocrinology, Human Development and Health Academic Unit, Faculty of Medicine, University of Southampton, Southampton, UK

George Jerums MD, FRACP
Endocrinologist and Professorial Fellow, Endocrine Centre, Austin Health and University of Melbourne, Melbourne, Victoria, Australia

Lisa Jones MD, MPH
Gastroenterology Fellow, Duke University Hospital, Durham, NC, USA

Richard J MacIsaac BSc(Hons), PhD, MBBS, FRACP
Director and Professorial Fellow, Department of Endocrinology and Diabetes, St Vincent's Hospital and University of Melbourne, Melbourne, Victoria, Australia

Andrew F Macleod MA, MD, FRCP
Consultant Endocrinologist, Royal Shrewsbury Hospital, Shrewsbury, UK

Kate Marsden RGN, BSc
Diabetes Specialist Nurse, Academic Department of Diabetes and Endocrinology, Queen Alexandra Hospital, Portsmouth, UK

Darryl Meeking MB, ChB, MRCP
Senior Lecturer, University of Portsmouth; Senior Lecturer, University of Southampton; Academic Department of Diabetes and Endocrinology, Portsmouth Hospitals NHS Trust, Portsmouth, UK

Minh Chau Nguyen MD
Post-doctoral Fellow, Division of Rheumatology, Department of Medicine, Keck School of Medicine, University of Southern California, Los Angeles, CA, USA

David P Osborn BA, MA, MSc, PhD, MRCPsych, FHEA
Reader and Consultant Psychiatrist, UCL Mental Health Sciences Unit, UCL, London, UK

Richard S Panush MD, MACP, MACR
Professor of Medicine, Division of Rheumatology, Department of Medicine, Keck School of Medicine, University of Southern California, Los Angeles, CA, USA

Henry P Parkman MD
Professor of Medicine, Gastrointestinal Section, Temple University School of Medicine, Philadelphia, PA, USA

Philip M Preshaw BDS, PhD, FDS RCS(Edin), FDS(Rest Dent) RCS(Edin)
Professor of Periodontology and Consultant in Restorative Dentistry, School of Dental Sciences and Institute of Cellular Medicine, Newcastle University, Newcastle upon Tyne, UK

Zeeshan Ramzan MD
Gastroenterology Fellow, Gastrointestinal Section, Temple University School of Medicine, Philadelphia, PA, USA

Kenneth M Shaw MD, FRCP
Honorary Consultant Physician, Queen Alexandra Hospital, Portsmouth Hospitals NHS Trust; Emeritus Professor of Medicine, University of Portsmouth, Portsmouth, UK

Kevin Shotliff MD, FRCP, DCH
Consultant Physician and Honorary Senior Lecturer (Imperial College), Chelsea and Westminster Hospital, London, UK

Sharon Tuck BSc(Hons), PG Cert
Podiatry Pathway Lead – At Risk Foot, Podiatry Service, Solent NHS, St James Hospital, Portsmouth, UK

Gerald F Watts DSc, DM, PhD, FRACP, FRCP
Winthrop Professor of Medicine, Head of Metabolic Research Centre and Lipid and Hypertension Services, Royal Perth Hospital, School of Medicine and Pharmacology, University of Western Australia, Perth, Western Australia, Australia

Preface to Third Edition

For the individual person diagnosed with diabetes today, we believe that the prospects of future good health are substantially better than they were a generation ago. Greater scientific understanding of underlying molecular and metabolic mechanisms, innovative technologies and new therapies, along with expanding evidence-based clinical management, have all contributed to a major risk reduction to the individual in terms of developing long-term complications of diabetes. However, for the population as a whole with escalating numbers of people developing diabetes within the current global pandemic of 'diabesity', the overall prevalence of diabetic complications has not diminished. Indeed, the consequences of diabetes now so predominate present-day health-care services and costs that changing concepts in the way prevention and clinical care of such need to be addressed. It is also evident that complication risk differs from one individual to another for a variety of reasons. How much differences are due to genetic susceptibility or to metabolic variation is unclear, but recognizing that some people with diabetes are more at risk than others does lead to the principle of risk stratification and personalized individual clinical management.

A large number of substantive clinical trials in recent years have consolidated a firm evidence base for the treatment of diabetes aimed at reducing long-term complications, not forgetting the parallel need to ensure the present day-to-day quality of life as well. Treatment guidelines derived from expert bodies and consensus opinion have defined important surrogate markers of risk, particularly hypertension, dyslipidaemia and hyperglycaemia (in that order), and the defining of 'quality' target-based standards has been associated with significant progress in risk factor management. Research studies indicate that good blood pressure control, optimal lipid status and improved glycaemia will all contribute to a substantial reduction in long-term microangiopathic diabetic complications, and the positive expectation is that this will be replicated in the real world of the diabetes population as a whole. With the current pattern of diabetes complications changing towards a greater emphasis on macroangiopathy, particularly coronary heart disease, the importance of early metabolic control and its potential, beneficial, long-term 'legacy' effect have highlighted the significance of early detection of diabetes through screening and ensuring optimal control in the early years after diagnosis.

Providing clinical support for people with diabetes has become almost as complex as the nature of diabetes itself. Most diabetes care these days is well provided within a primary care community setting, but, for those identified with higher risk or when developing complications are detected, involvement of a multidisciplinary team and liaison with specialist services will be needed. Integrated models of diabetes care are evolving to meet overall clinical needs according to local circumstances, with the configuration of clinical care pathways enabling those at highest risk to be individually managed. The epidemiology of long-term diabetes complications is changing, with greater understanding of underlying causative mechanisms and improved metabolic control arising from better therapeutic regimens and more structured models of care. The development of diabetic complications should not be seen as inevitable, but sadly the consequences of diabetes are still prevalent and it is evident that some are more at risk than others. Significant strides have been made towards mitigating the more classic complications of retinopathy and nephropathy, whereas other diabetes-related issues, such as mental health and certain cancers, are becoming increasingly clinically significant. In our preface to the previous edition of this book, we conceded that there was still much more to be done to reduce the considerable burden of diabetes both to the individual and to society, but we also recognized that many advances had been made. Much progress has indeed been made in the understanding of how complications arise and how they can be prevented, while ensuring that in today's world such knowledge is shared between professionals and people with diabetes alike.

With this new edition of *Diabetes: Chronic Complications*, we have extensively revised earlier chapters on traditional complications, providing the latest science and current therapeutic guidance. In addition, as other long-term problems related to diabetes continue to emerge, we have introduced a number of new chapters, including mental health, disorders of the mouth, cancer and problems of the liver. Illustrative case histories and a selection of multiple choice questions have also been included. We are most grateful to all of the authors who have contributed their expertise and experience. Although, for the purpose of this book, these complications of diabetes are considered separately, the reality is that development of one complication will signal increased susceptibility to other problems. Most of the complications discussed have issues specific to the particular organ or tissue concerned, but equally all have shared generic components and common management considerations.

Even today the discussion of diabetic complications can still be emotive and subject to misunderstanding, but with the substantial knowledge and evidence base that are now available to everyone involved in diabetes care, much wisdom is in place to secure a life with diabetes but very positive moves towards a life without complications. In this book we have endeavoured to provide a practical analysis and reflection on current issues related to the prevention and management of long-term diabetic complications, knowledge that we trust will be found useful by all involved in the clinical practice of diabetes care, and importantly knowledge that can be shared to advantage with the many individuals now living with diabetes who wish to enjoy long-term good health free of complications.

Kenneth M. Shaw
Michael H. Cummings

CHAPTER 1

Diabetes and the Eye

Kevin Shotliff and Nigel Davies
Chelsea and Westminster Hospital, London, UK

 Key points

- Of people with diabetes in the UK 2 per cent are thought to be registered blind.
- Of patients with type 1 diabetes 87–98 per cent have retinopathy seen after 30 years of the disease.
- Eighty-five per cent of those with type 2 diabetes on insulin and 60 per cent on diet or oral agents have retinopathy after 15 years of the disease.
- Optical coherence tomography (OCT) is a technique allowing visualization of retinal layers and assessment of maculopathy.
- New treatments such as intravitreal therapy and vitrectomy are emerging as treatments that maintain or improve vision but laser remains the primary treatment of choice.

 Therapeutic key points

- Poor glycaemic control is associated with worsening of diabetic retinopathy and improving glycaemic control improves outcome.
- Systolic hypertension is associated with retinopathy in type 1 and type 2 diabetes; reducing this improves retinopathy.
- Reducing lipid levels with fibrates and statins has been shown to improve retinopathy.
- Intraretinal injections of vascular endothelial growth factor (VEGF) receptor blockers may improve maculopathy.
- Laser therapy remains the primary treatment of choice for sight-threatening diabetic retinopathy, both proliferative disease and maculopathy.

Diabetes: Chronic Complications, Third Edition. Edited by Kenneth M. Shaw, Michael H. Cummings.
© 2012 John Wiley & Sons, Ltd. Published 2012 by John Wiley & Sons, Ltd.

1.1 Introduction

Since the invention of the direct ophthalmoscope by Helmholtz in 1851 and von Yaeger's first description of changes in the fundus of a person with diabetes 4 years later, there has been increasing interest in the retina because it contains the only part of the vasculature affected by diabetes that is easily visible. Interestingly, these first retinal changes described in 1855 were actually hypertensive, not diabetic.

Despite the target outlined in the St Vincent Declaration in 1989 to reduce blindness caused by diabetes by one-third within 5 years, and the advances made in laser therapy and vitreoretinal surgical techniques, diabetic retinopathy remains the most common cause of blindness in the working-age population of the western world. Furthermore, with predictions of a dramatic increase in the number of people diagnosed with diabetes, the detection and treatment of diabetic retinopathy continues to be a focal point for healthcare professionals. Indeed the recent National Service Framework (NSF) for Diabetes has prioritized diabetic retinopathy by setting specific targets associated with retinal screening and implementing the development of a National Screening Programme.

Visual loss from diabetic retinopathy has two main causes: maculopathy, described as disruption of the macular region of the retina, leading to impairment of central vision; and retinal ischaemia, resulting in proliferative diabetic retinopathy.

As well as the retina, other parts of the eye can also be affected in people with diabetes. Cataracts are more prevalent and are actually the most common eye abnormality seen in people with diabetes, occurring in up to 60 per cent of 30–54 year olds. The link between diabetes and primary open-angle glaucoma, however, continues to be disputed. Vitreous changes do occur in people with diabetes, such as asteroid hyalosis, seen in about 2 per cent of patients. These small spheres or star-shaped opacities in the vitreous appear to sparkle when illuminated and do not normally affect vision. Branch retinal vein occlusions and central retinal vein occlusions are associated with hypertension, hyperlipidaemia and obesity, and are often found in people with diabetes. Hypertensive retinopathy features several lesions in common with diabetic retinopathy, and care must be taken not to confuse the two conditions.

1.2 Epidemiology of diabetic retinopathy

Currently 2 per cent of the UK diabetic population is thought to be registered blind,[1] which means that a person with diabetes has a 10- to 20-fold increased risk of blindness. The prevalence of diabetic retinopathy depends on multiple factors and, as for many microvascular complications, is more common in the ethnic minorities compared with white people.

A prevalence of 25–30 per cent for a general diabetic population is often quoted. Every year about 1 in 90 North Americans with diabetes develops proliferative retinopathy and 1 in 80 develops macular oedema.

In patients with type 1 diabetes:[2,3]

- <2 per cent have any lesions of diabetic retinopathy at diagnosis
- 8 per cent have it by 5 years (2 per cent proliferative)
- 87–98 per cent have abnormalities 30 years later (30 per cent of these having had proliferative retinopathy).

In patients with type 2 diabetes:[4,5]

- 20–37 per cent can be expected to have retinopathy at diagnosis
- 15 years later, 85 per cent of those on insulin and 60 per cent of those on diet or oral agents will have abnormalities.

The 4-year incidence of proliferative retinopathy in a large North American epidemiological study was 10.5 per cent in patients with type 1 diabetes, 7.4 per cent in patients with older-onset/type 2 diabetes taking insulin and 2.3 per cent in patients with type 2 diabetes not on insulin.[2,3,5]

Currently in the UK, maculopathy is a more common and therefore more significant sight-threatening complication of diabetes. This is due to the much greater number of people with type 2 diabetes compared with type 1, and the fact that maculopathy tends to occur in older people. About 75 per cent of those with maculopathy have type 2 diabetes and there is a 4-year incidence of 10.4 per cent in this group.[5] Although patients with type 2 diabetes are 10 times more likely to have maculopathy than those with type 1, 14 per cent of patients with type 1 diabetes who become blind do so because of maculopathy.[1]

The risk factors for development/worsening of diabetic retinopathy are:

- duration of diabetes
- type of diabetes (proliferative disease in type 1 and maculopathy in type 2)
- poor diabetic/glycaemic control
- hypertension
- diabetic nephropathy
- recent cataract surgery
- pregnancy
- alcohol (variable results which may be related to the type of alcohol involved, e.g. effects are worse in Scotland than in Italy)
- smoking (variable results, but appears worse in young people with exudates and older women with proliferative disease)
- ethnic origin.

1.3 Retinal anatomy

To understand how diabetic retinopathy is classified and treated, a basic grasp of retinal anatomy is essential. The retina is the innermost of three successive layers of the globe of the eye, the others being:

- the sclera – the rigid outer covering of the eye, which includes the cornea
- the choroid – the highly vascularized middle layer of the eye, which has the largest blood flow in the entire body.

The retina comprises two parts: the neurosensory retina, the photoreceptive part composed of nine layers and the retinal pigment epithelium (Figure 1.1).

The normal retina is completely transparent to visible wavelengths of light, its bright red/orange reflex the result of the underlying vasculature of the choroid. The retina has a number of distinct features. The optic nerve (often described as the optic disc) is a circular structure varying in

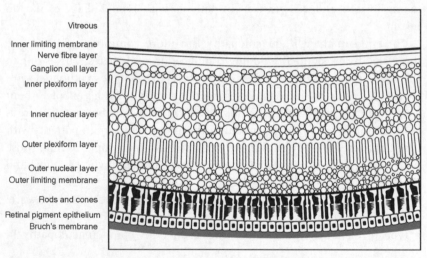

Vitreous
Inner limiting membrane
Nerve fibre layer
Ganglion cell layer
Inner plexiform layer
Inner nuclear layer
Outer plexiform layer
Outer nuclear layer
Outer limiting membrane
Rods and cones
Retinal pigment epithelium
Bruch's membrane

Figure 1.1 Cross-section of the retina illustrating the 10 layers of the retina: inner limiting membrane (glial cell fibres forming the barrier between the retina and the vitreous body), optic nerve fibres (axons of the third neuron), ganglion cells (cell nuclei of multipolar ganglion cells of the third neuron), inner plexiform layer (synapses between axons of the second neuron and dendrites of the third neuron), inner nuclear layer (cell nuclei of the amacrine cells, bipolar cells and horizontal cells), outer plexiform layer (synapses between axons of the first neuron and dendrites of the second neuron), outer nuclear layer (cell nuclei of rods and cones, the first neuron), outer limiting membrane (porous plate of processes of glial cells, which rods and cones project through), rods and cones (true photoreceptors), retinal pigment epithelium (single layer of pigmented epithelial cells) and Bruch's membrane.

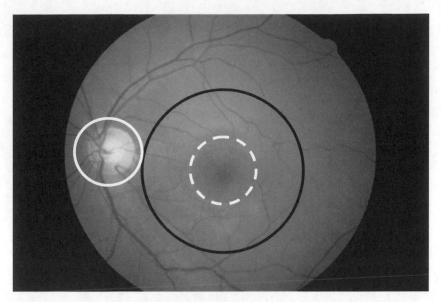

Figure 1.2 Fundus photograph illustrating the normal retina with optic nerve head (optic disc) circled in white, macula circled in black and fovea circled with a broken white line.

colour from pale pink in the young to yellow/orange in older people. It is located approximately 15° nasally from the visual axis and slightly superior (Figure 1.2). The optic nerve is essentially a 'cable' connecting the eye to the brain, which carries information from the retina to the visual cortex via the optic chiasma. The optic nerve may exhibit a central depression known as the optic or physiological cup. Both the central retinal vein and artery leave and enter the eye through the optic nerve. The 'blind spot' on visual field testing occurs because the optic disc contains no photoreceptor rod and cone cells.

The macula is the round area at the posterior pole within the temporal vessel arcades 3–4 mm temporal to and slightly lower than the optic disc (Figure 1.2). It is approximately 5 mm in diameter. At the centre of the macula and roughly the same size as the optic disc is the fovea, a depression in the retinal surface. The fovea is the point at which vision is sharpest; the foveola, the thinnest part of the retina and forming the base of the fovea, contains only cone cells, giving this area anatomical specialization for high-resolution vision in relatively bright levels of light. The fovea is 0.3 mm in diameter. At the very centre of the foveola lies the umbo, a tiny depression corresponding to the foveolar reflex.

The fovea features an avascular zone of variable diameter extending beyond the foveola, which is usually about 0.5 mm in diameter (Figure 1.3).

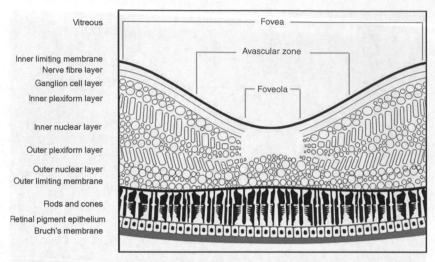

Figure 1.3 Cross-section of the retina at the fovea illustrating the fovea, foveola and foveal avascular zone.

The five innermost layers of the retina, from the inner limiting membrane to the inner nuclear layer, receive their blood supply from the central artery of the retina.

This enters the retina at the optic disc and forms four branches. There are three retinal capillary plexus which supply the inner and middle retina: the radial peripapillary plexus around the optic disc, which is at the level of the nerve fibre layer, a superficial capillary plexus at the junction of the ganglion cells and inner plexiform layers, and a deep capillary plexus, at the junction of the inner nuclear layer with the outer plexiform layer. The five outer layers of the retina, from the outer plexiform layer to the pigment epithelium, receive their blood supply from the capillaries of the choroid by means of diffusion.

The retinal veins exit the retina at the optic disc and with the arteries form the four vessel arcades of the retina – superior and inferior temporal arcades and superior and inferior nasal arcades (Figure 1.4). Retinal arteries appear bright red, with a sharp reflex strip that becomes lighter with age, and retinal veins are a darker red with little or no reflex strip.

The retinal pigment epithelium (RPE) is the base layer of the retina. The level of adhesion between the RPE and the sensory retina is weaker than that between the RPE and Bruch's membrane, resulting in a potential space. A retinal detachment is the separation of the sensory retina from the RPE as a result of subretinal fluid infiltrating this potential space.

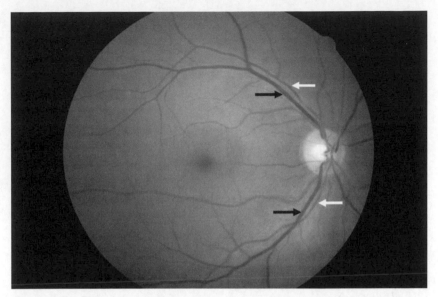

Figure 1.4 Retinal veins (black arrows) and retinal arteries (white arrows) of the superior and inferior temporal arcades.

1.4 Pathophysiology and anatomical changes of diabetic retinopathy

The pathophysiology of diabetic retinopathy is still being unravelled. Hyperglycaemia and the other metabolic effects of diabetes all play a part in triggering a series of biochemical and anatomical changes that manifest as the systemic complications of the disease.

Biochemical changes
The pathways that are affected by high blood glucose and lack of insulin and contribute to the damage include accumulation of advanced glycosylated end-products, oxidative stress, inflammation, the accumulation of sorbitol via the aldose reductase pathway, activation of protein kinase C, the release of VEGFs, fibroblastic growth factors and platelet-derived growth factors. There is also involvement of the renin–angiotensin system and recently there has been the finding that erythropoietin is a promoter of neovascularization in ischaemic tissues.

Anatomical changes
The initial microscopic anatomical change is thickening of basement membranes around the body. Basement membranes can act as passive

regulators of growth factors, by binding them to their components and thus providing an altered biochemical environment.

Glycated haemoglobin has a greater affinity for oxygen than haemo-globin, which may reduce oxygen delivery to tissues, and red blood cell membranes become more rigid, which can impede their flow along the small retinal capillaries. Increased platelet adhesiveness can accelerate plaque formation in vessels.

As the basement membrane thickens, it loses its negative charge and becomes 'leakier'. In normal retinal capillaries there is a one-to-one rela-tionship between endothelial cells and pericytes, which is the highest ratio for any capillary network in the body. Pericytes may control endothe-lial cell proliferation, maintain the structural integrity of capillaries and regulate blood flow. In diabetes there is a significant loss of pericytes in the retinal capillaries, which, along with increased blood viscosity, abnormal fibrinolytic activity and reduced red cell deformity may lead to capillary occlusion, tissue hypoxia and the stimulus for new vessel formation.

Classification of diabetic retinopathy

The classification of diabetic retinopathy, as shown in Figure 1.5, is based on visible/ophthalmoscopic features, but the unseen changes described above occurring before these help explain the clinical findings.

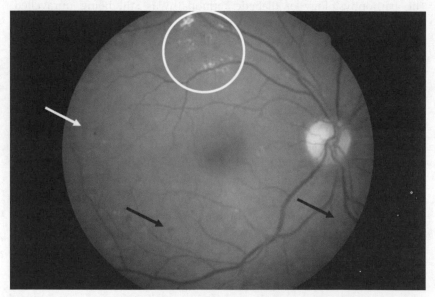

Figure 1.5 Background diabetic retinopathy with microaneurysm (white arrow), haemorrhages (black arrows) and hard exudates (white circles).

The natural progression is from background to pre-proliferative/pre-maculopathy then to proliferative retinopathy/maculopathy and ultimately sight-threatening disease.

Non-proliferative diabetic retinopathy (Figure 1.5)

Capillary microaneurysms are the earliest feature seen clinically, as red 'dots'.

- Small intraretinal haemorrhages or 'blots' also occur, as can haemorrhage into the nerve fibre layer, often flame shaped.
- With increased capillary leakage intraretinal oedema occurs. The RPE acts as a pump to remove water from the retina, but serum proteins that leak into the deeper retinal layers can not pass through the outer limiting membrane. Retinal oedema therefore persists as the protein accumulation holds water molecules osmotically. At the border of the areas of capillary leakage, serum lipids deposit in the retina, forming exudates.

Pre-proliferative retinopathy (Figure 1.6)

- Cotton-wool spots or soft exudates are infarcts in the nerve fibre layer occurring at areas of non-perfusion. Axoplasmic transport is disrupted

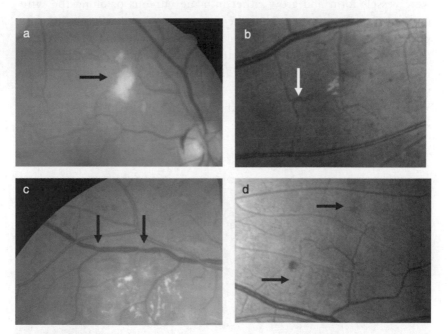

Figure 1.6 Pre-proliferative diabetic retinopathy with (a) cotton-wool spots, (b) venous loop, (c) venous beading and (d) IRMAs (intraretinal microvascular abnormalities).

in the nerve fibres of ganglion cells, giving oedematous infarcts that are seen as pale/grey fuzzy-edged lesions.

- Intraretinal microvascular abnormalities (IRMAs) are tortuous dilated hypercellular capillaries in the retina, which enlarge enough to be visible and occur in response to retinal ischaemia.
- Further changes include alternating dilatation and constriction of veins (venous beading), and other venous alterations such as duplication and loop formation.
- There are also large areas of capillary non-perfusion occurring in the absence of new vessels. These ischaemic areas may not be visible with an ophthalmoscope but can be seen on fluorescein angiography.

The Early Treatment of Diabetic Retinopathy Study (ETDRS) suggested that certain of these features matter and suggested a '4–2–1' rule:[6]

- four quadrants of severe haemorrhages or microaneurysms
- two quadrants of IRMAs
- one quadrant with venous beading.

If a patient has one of these features, there is a 15 per cent risk of developing sight-threatening retinopathy within the next year. If two are present this rises to a 45 per cent risk.

Proliferative retinopathy (Figure 1.7)
New vessels form and grow either into the vitreous or along the vitre-oretinal interface (this tends to occur in younger patients in whom the posterior vitreous face is well formed). The vitreous forms a reservoir for the angiogenic agents released by the ischaemic retina and acts as scaffolding for neovascularization and fibrosis. There are two forms of new vessels:

- those on the disc or within one disc diameter of the disc (NVDs)
- new vessels elsewhere (NVEs).

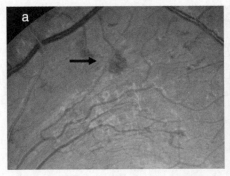 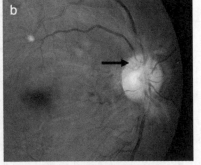

Figure 1.7 Proliferative diabetic retinopathy with (a) neovascularization on the surface of the retina (NVE) and (b) neovascularization at the optic disc (NVD).

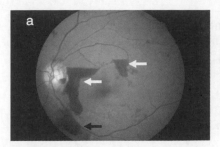
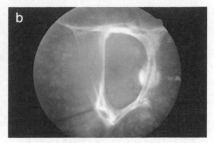

Figure 1.8 Advanced diabetic retinopathy with (a) pre-retinal haemorrhages (white arrows) and vitreous haemorrhage (black arrow), and (b) fibrous proliferation.

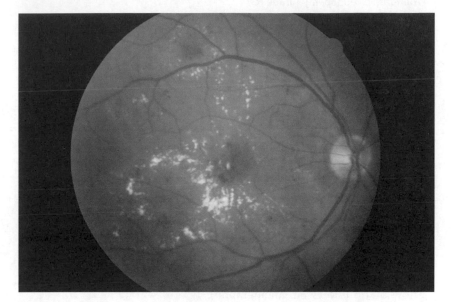

Figure 1.9 Diabetic maculopathy with retinal haemorrhages and hard exudates.

Both give no symptoms but cause the problems of advanced retinopathy (Figure 1.8) such as haemorrhage, scar tissue formation, traction on the retina and retinal detachment, which actually result in loss of vision.

Diabetic maculopathy

Oedema in the macula area can distort central vision and reduce visual acuity. Any of the above changes can coexist with maculopathy. The changes seen can be:

- oedematous (clinically it may just be difficult to focus on the macula with a hand-held ophthalmoscope, or visual acuity may have altered or may worsen when a pinhole is used)
- exudative (with haemorrhages, hard exudates and circinate exudates – Figure 1.9)

Box 1.1 Classification, features and grading scheme for diabetic retinopathy

Mild-to-moderate non-proliferative retinopathy (grade R1)
Microaneurysms
Haemorrhages
Hard exudates

Severe non-proliferative retinopathy (grade R2)
Soft exudates/cotton-wool spots
Intraretinal microvascular abnormalities (IRMAs)
Venous abnormalities (e.g. venous beading, looping and reduplication)

Proliferative retinopathy (grade R3)
New vessels on the disc or within one disc diameter of it (NVD)
New vessels elsewhere (NVE)
Rubeosis iridis (± neovascular glaucoma)

Maculopathy (grade Mo – absent M1 – present)
Haemorrhages and hard exudates in the macula area
Reduced visual acuity with no abnormality seen

Other grades
R0: normal fundus appearance
A: advanced eye disease including vitreous haemorrhage, fibrosis and retinal detachments
P: evidence of previous laser therapy
U: un-gradable image
OL: other non-diabetic changes/lesion seen

- ischaemic (capillary loss occurs but clinically the macula may look normal on direct ophthalmoscopy, although poorly perfused areas will show up on fluorescein angiography)
- any combination of these (Box 1.1).

1.5 Diagnosis and clinical investigation

Slit-lamp biomicroscopy
Indirect ophthalmoscopy with a slit-lamp biomicroscope performed by an Ophthalmologist is considered to be the gold standard for diagnosing diabetic retinopathy. The use of high magnification biomicroscope lenses such as a 78-, 66- or 60-D lens allows the detection of retinal oedema and neovascularization because of the level of stereoscopic vision achieved.

Fundus photographs
Colour fundus photographs are used extensively in screening (see below) and are also an important part of documenting the changes when the

patient is under the care of an Ophthalmologist. The current generation of retinal cameras now produce very-high-resolution digital images.

Optical coherence tomography

Optical coherence tomography (OCT) is a relatively new method of tissue imaging that has rapidly become an important part of assessment of patients with maculopathies of any cause.

OCT is based on the optics of a Michelson interferometer and produces a set of images that show changes in refractive index through tissues. This allows visualization of layers that correspond to the anatomical layers in the retina. The most recent devices use a Fourier transform method to produce high-resolution images with a short acquisition time.

The field of view is small, but covers the macula and fovea, which are arguably the most important areas of retina required for our day-to-day vision. OCT can also be used to image the optic nerve head.

Figure 1.10 shows a Fourier domain OCT of the normal macula, with the different retinal layers labelled.

There are several advantages of OCT, which include delineation of sites of anatomical change, storage of images and comparison of images taken at a later time. Many OCT devices contain image registration software that allows a direct assessment of change occurring during the process of disease evolution or as a result of intervention.

Some examples of OCT scan in patients with diabetes are shown in Figures 1.11 and 1.12.

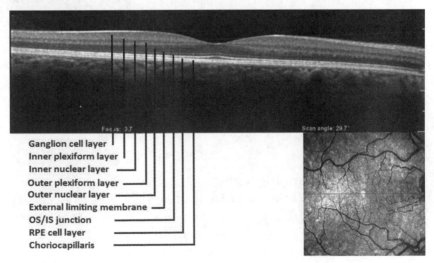

Ganglion cell layer
Inner plexiform layer
Inner nuclear layer
Outer plexiform layer
Outer nuclear layer
External limiting membrane
OS/IS junction
RPE cell layer
Choriocapillaris

Figure 1.10 A Fourier domain optical coherence tomography (OCT) of the normal macula.

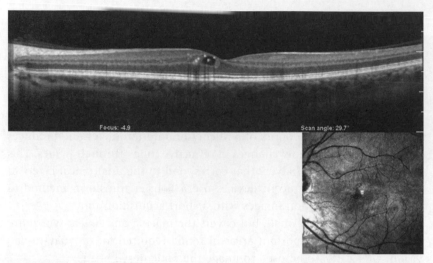

Figure 1.11 Optical coherence tomography (OCT) scan of patient with diabetic macular oedema.

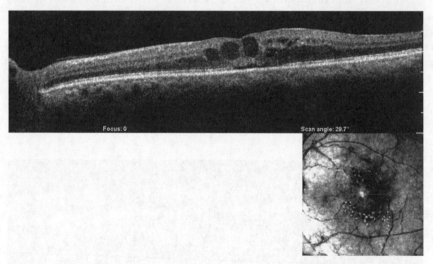

Figure 1.12 Optical coherence tomography (OCT) scan of patient with cystic diabetic macular oedema.

Free fluorescein angiography

Retinal angiography was introduced in the 1960s and remains a mainstay investigation of retinal disease. Free fluorescein angiography (FFA) systems are now digital and a series of images is acquired that tracks the passage of fluorescein through the posterior segment vasculature.

In diabetes, FFA is crucial to the assessment of the presence of ischaemia (hypofluorescence), vascular leakage (late hyperfluorescence) and neo-

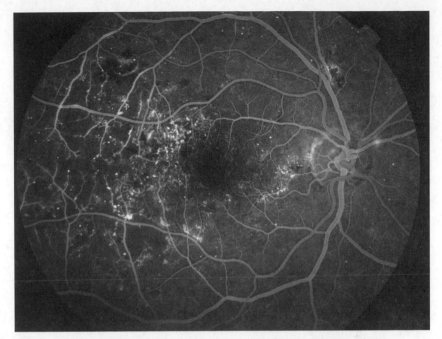

Figure 1.13 Early phase image showing loss of perifoveal capillaries and temporal capillaries in a patient with type 1 diabetes.

vascularization at the optic disc and elsewhere. The presence of leakage from vessels around the macular area guides the application of laser treatment. Examples of angiographic images are shown in Figures 1.13–1.16.

OCT scanning and fluorescein angiography are used together to investigate and monitor anatomical and vascular changes in retinal disease.

1.6 Screening for diabetic retinopathy

Diabetic retinopathy meets the World Health Organization's four cardinal principles that determine whether a health problem is suitable for screening:

1. The condition should be an important health problem with a recognizable pre-symptomatic state – as the most common cause of blindness in the working population of the western world with a well-recognized pattern of changes visible in the eye, diabetic retinopathy fulfils this.
2. An appropriate screening procedure, which is acceptable both to the public and healthcare professionals, should be available – retinal photography is accepted by patients and the medical profession.

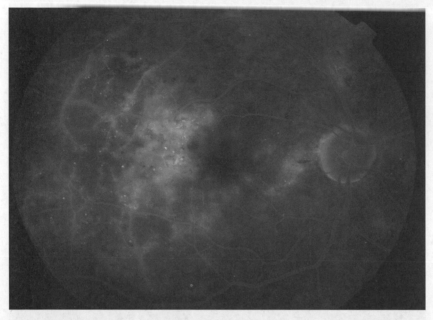

Figure 1.14 Late phase angiogram showing leakage of fluorescein in the temporal area of the macula.

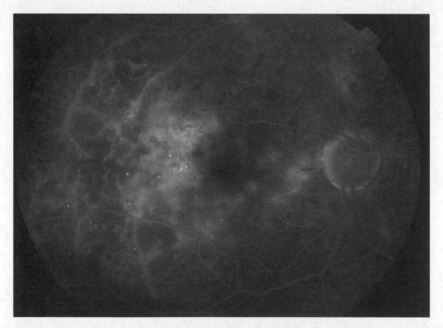

Figure 1.15 Early phase angiogram showing severe capillary shutdown, microaneurysms, and vessel dilatation and tortuosity in a patient with type 2 diabetes.

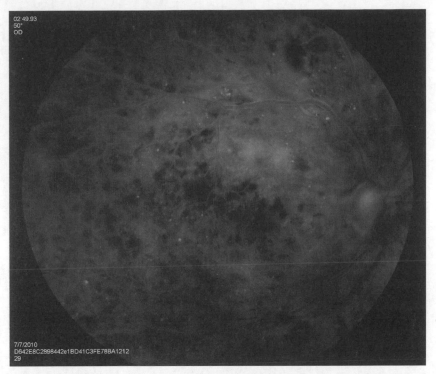

Figure 1.16 Late phase showing diffuse fluorescein leakage.

3. Treatment for patients with recognizable disease should be safe, effective
   and universally agreed – laser therapy for advanced disease, although
   not without risk, is accepted as a good evidence-based therapy to prevent
   blindness, and newer medical therapies are in development.
4. The economic cost of early diagnosis and treatment should be considered in relation to total expenditure on healthcare, including the consequences of leaving the disease untreated.

To detect diabetic retinopathy the retina must first be visualized. Several
methods of retinal examination can be used:

• Indirect ophthalmoscopy with the slit-lamp.
• The direct method, using a hand-held ophthalmoscope, is performed as
  part of everyday practice by many doctors. The practicalities of ophthalmoscopy, including the high costs in terms of the level of specialist
  training and experience required (indirect method), varying results
  depending on the person carrying out the examination (direct method)
  and the fact that no permanent visual record is retained (both methods),
  mean that ophthalmoscopy has been deemed unsuitable as the basis for
  a comprehensive national screening programme.[7]
• Digital retinal photography (Figure 1.17) with mydriasis provides a
  permanent record, which can be interpreted with a high degree of

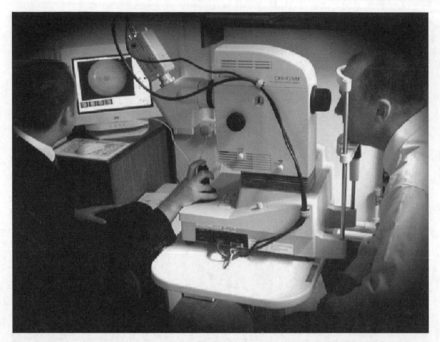

Figure 1.17 Screening for diabetic retinopathy using a digital fundus camera.

accuracy and is relatively inexpensive. Photography and grading of resulting images by trained technicians have demonstrated a higher level of sensitivity and specificity than any other screening method and provide a permanent record for quality assurance and audit.

In light of this, the National Screening Committee has recommended digital retinal photography as the screening method of choice (see www.diabetic-retinopathy.screening.nhs.uk). A comprehensive National Screening Programme is currently being implemented to meet targets set out in the National Service Framework (NSF) for Diabetes. Although NSF targets are based on annual screening, results from a study by the Royal Liverpool University Hospital concluded that a 3-year screening interval may be appropriate for patients with no retinopathy and well-controlled diabetes.[8] During pregnancy, women with diabetes should be screened each trimester, regardless of their level of control or the absence of any existing retinopathy.

A full retinal screening examination should include the following:
- Visual acuity (VA) – using a standard Snellen chart; if the VA is worse than 6/9 it should be rechecked with a pinhole to correct for refractive errors. If it does not then correct to 6/9 or better, or if it has worsened by more than two lines on a Snellen chart in the last year, an ophthalmology review may be needed because some maculopathy cannot be seen easily with a hand-held ophthalmoscope. Cataracts are, however,

a more likely cause. If vision gets worse with a pinhole, it should be assumed that maculopathy is present until proven otherwise. It should be remembered that high blood glucose readings can give myopia (difficulty in distance vision) and low blood glucose hypermetropia (difficulty in reading), although this is not universal.

- Examination of the eye through a dilated pupil: although retinal photography has overtaken this, the ability to examine an eye, including the anterior chamber, lens and fundus, should not be lost as a skill, because significant disease is often picked up using this method in opportunistic screening and in those who cannot get to a site where photography is possible, such as bed-bound and infirm patients in nursing homes.
- Retinal photographs: over 90 per cent of people can have good quality photographs take. Digital images are used because they require a less intense flash and can be repeated immediately if the view is inadequate. The photographs/images obtained should then be graded/assessed by a trained observer using a standardized grading scheme, as demonstrated in Box 1.1. In the future, scanning laser ophthalmoscopes and computer grading software may also be used.

Reasons for immediate referral to an ophthalmologist are:

- proliferative retinopathy – untreated NVD carries a 40 per cent risk of blindness in under 2 years and laser treatment reduces this
- rubeosis iridis/neovascular glaucoma
- vitreous haemorrhage
- advanced retinopathy with fibrous tissue or retinal detachments.

Reasons for early referral to an ophthalmologist (within 6 weeks) are:

- pre-proliferative changes
- maculopathy
- A fall of more than two lines on a Snellen chart.

Reasons for routine referral are:

- cataracts
- non-proliferative retinopathy with large circinate exudates not threatening the macula/fovea.

1.7 Management: Risk factor reduction, medical and surgical management

Medical treatment

Glycaemic control

There is good epidemiological evidence for an association between poor glycaemic control and worsening of retinopathy, and that improving glycaemic control improves outcome:

- The Diabetes Control and Complications Trial (DCCT)[9] looked at intensive glycaemic control in patients with type 1 diabetes over 6.5 years and showed a 76 per cent reduction in the risk of initially developing retinopathy in the tight glycaemic control group, compared with the control group. The rate of progression of existing retinopathy was slowed by 54 per cent and the risk of developing severe non-proliferative or proliferative retinopathy was reduced by 47 per cent.
- The United Kingdom Prospective Diabetes Study (UK PDS)[4,10] looked at patients with type 2 diabetes over 9 years and showed a 21 per cent reduction in progression of retinopathy and a 29 per cent reduction in the need for laser therapy in those with better glycaemic control.

The DCCT, UK PDS and several previous studies also showed an initial worsening of retinopathy in the first 2 years in the tight/improved glycaemic control groups, so all patients therefore need careful monitoring over this period. This is particularly important in high-risk groups such as pregnant women. The long-term benefits, however, outweigh this initial risk.

Blood pressure

There is good evidence for an association between both systolic and diastolic hypertension and retinopathy in type 1 patients although the link may only be with systolic hypertension in patients with type 2 diabetes. The UK PDS looked at blood pressure control in these patients and showed that the treatment group, with a mean blood pressure (BP) of 144/82 mmHg, when compared with a control group with a mean of 154/87 mmHg, had a 35 per cent reduction in the need for laser therapy.[11]

Adequate BP control, e.g. <140/80 in patients with type 2 diabetes, is therefore advocated. Using angiotensin-converting enzyme (ACE) inhibitors as first-line therapy for this is also suggested, with experimental evidence showing that these agents may have anti-angiogenic effects by altering local growth factor levels as well as any benefit from reducing blood pressure. Studies using enalapril and lisinopril have both shown a reduction in the progression of retinopathy in patients with type 1 diabetes.

The EURODIAB controlled study of lisinopril in type 1 diabetes (EUCLID)[12] showed a 50 per cent risk reduction in retinopathy progression and a 80 per cent risk reduction in development of proliferative retinopathy, although the follow-up was relatively short (2 years). There are data from the use of candesartan (DIRECT study[13]) and enalapril and losartan (RASS study[14]) that also show reduction in progression of retinopathy. These studies suggest that drugs acting on the renin–angiotensin system may have significant benefit in the management of hypertension in the context of diabetes.

Lipid control and therapy

Experimental evidence suggests that oxidized low-density lipoprotein (LDL)-cholesterol may be cytotoxic for endothelial cells. Epidemiological data also suggest an association between higher LDL-cholesterol and worse diabetic retinopathy, especially maculopathy with exudates. A total cholesterol >7.0 mmol/l gives a fourfold greater risk of proliferative retinopathy than a total cholesterol <5.3 mmol/l. A worse outcome from laser therapy in those treated for maculopathy has also been seen if hyperlipidaemia is present. Aggressive lipid lowering is therefore advocated, especially in maculopathy.

The Fenofibrate Intervention and Event Lowering in Diabetes (FIELD) study assessed the effect of fenofibrate on cardiovascular events in patients with type 2 diabetes.[15] A tertiary end-point showed a 30 per cent reduction in the need for retinal laser in the treatment group (3.4% vs 4.9%, $p = 0.0002$).

The ACCORD study[16] compared tight glycaemic control with standard control and also lipid control with fenofibrate and simvastatin with placebo and simvastatin, and for systolic blood pressure control. The progression of retinopathy was clearly reduced in the tight control groups, 7.3 per cent versus 10.4 per cent for glycaemic control and intensive lipid control (6.5% combination vs 10.2% placebo and statin). There was no significant difference in progression in the blood pressure groups.

The Joint British Diabetes Societies and the American Diabetes Association recommend that the total cholesterol level be <4 mmol/l and the LDL level <2.0 mmol/l.

The control of lipid levels with statin medications has also become very important in the management of diabetes. The therapeutic effects of statins are related not only to their lipid-lowering effects[17] but also to additional pleotropic effects, related to the action on isoprenoid levels in the HMG (hydroxymethylglutaryl) pathway. As a result, statins are anti-inflammatory, anti-platelet, anti-thrombotic and profibrinolytic. The function of vascular endothelial cells is improved, nitric oxide availability is enhanced, adhesion of leukocytes to intracellular adhesion molecules (ICAM-1) on endothelial cells is reduced and expression of VEGF can be reduced.

All of these effects can be seen to offset the pathogenic mechanisms caused by diabetes, dyslipidaemia and hypertension.

There are some data to show that statin therapy is of benefit in diabetic retinopathy and maculopathy. The Collaborative Atorvastatin Diabetes Study (CARD[18]) showed a trend in reduction in laser treatment in the treatment group compared with placebo, but there was no impact on progression of retinopathy. Studies also show a reduction in exudate in patients taking statins, but these involved small numbers and duration of treatment.

At present no large randomized controlled trial data are available and this may be difficult to perform because statins are already becoming accepted medications as part of the management of patients with diabetes.

Antiplatelet therapy

In view of the altered rheological properties of patients with diabetes, these agents have been tried but the results are variable. Some studies suggest that aspirin and ticlopidine may slow the progression of retinopathy, but the benefit is small. The other benefits of aspirin should, however, make it advisable in most patients with no contraindications.

Protein kinase C inhibition

Ruboxistaurin is an oral PKC-β inhibitor. A large randomized controlled trial did not show significant effect on progression of maculopathy but there was a reduction in the incidence of moderate vision loss.[19]

Lifestyle advice

Although stopping smoking reduces macrovascular risk, its effect on retinopathy is less clear. Alcohol consumption and physical activity also show no consistent effect.

Surgical management

Maculopathy – laser and intravitreal therapy

Laser treatment

The rationale for laser treatment in the macula is to cause closure of retinal microaneurysms and also mild thermal damage to the RPE cells, which has an effect on the outer blood–retinal barrier and allows increased egress of fluid from the retina; it also stimulates RPE cells into increased pumping activity.

The ETDRS studied the effect of focal or grid laser treatment to the macula. Clinically significant macula oedema was defined as:

- Retinal thickening within 500 μm of the foveal centre
- Exudate associated with thickening within 500 μm of foveal centre
- An area of thickening >1500 μm diameter, any part of which is closer than 1500 μm to the foveal centre.

The ETDRS showed that argon laser therapy (given to one eye, with the other eye in the same patient used as a non-treated control) reduced the rate of moderate vision loss (three lines on the ETDRS chart) at 3 years from 24 per cent in the non-treated eyes compared with 12 per cent in the treated group.[6]

Although the laser energy used is set to produce a very mild burn, continuous wave laser pulses of 0.1 s duration also cause thermal damage to photoreceptors and choriocapillaris, and thus damage retinal sensitivity.

To reduce this collateral damage, micropulse lasers have been developed. These produce a train of very short pulses for each laser shot, each pulse lasting just a few microseconds. This allows for energy absorption by the melanin in RPE cells with local thermal effect. The interpulse interval allows the melanosomes to cool without causing a significant temperature rise in the nearby photoreceptors or choriocapillaris. The arrival of the next pulse causes another local RPE temperature rise and overall there is a cumulative effect.

Typically, laser shots delivered with these systems do not produce visible burns. There are emerging data in the literature that demonstrate an effect in terms of oedema reduction equivalent to the conventional laser, but a clear preservation of visual sensitivity as assessed by microperimetry.[17]

Intravitreal therapy

There are some patients who have oedema that is greatest in the centre of the fovea and those whose oedema does not respond to repeated laser treatment. In these patients, intravitreal administration of therapeutic agents has been studied.

Intravitreal steroids, such as triamcinolone and dexamethasone, have been assessed. Although initially promising, the reduction in oedema is short-lived and the treatment complicated by progression of cataract and raised intraocular pressure in a relatively high proportion of patients. A DRCR.net study comparing laser alone with intravitreal triamcinolone alone showed that at 2- and 3-year time points the visual outcome was significantly better with laser.[20]

More recently intravitreal administration of VEGF receptor blockers has been assessed. These agents are either selective aptamers (pegaptanib sodium, Macugen) of the VEGF 165 isoform receptor or monoclonal antibodies to all VEGF-A receptors (ranibizumab, Lucentis and bevacizumab, Avastin). Initial studies were case series indicating that these agents were useful in many conditions of retinal oedema and ischaemia resistant to other treatments. Randomized controlled trial data are emerging in diabetes that show a beneficial effect on both degree of oedema and improvement in VA with the use of these agents.[21,22]

The intravitreal therapies need to be administered frequently (at 4-weekly intervals initially, with monthly monitoring and re-treatment) to be effective and each treatment carries the low risk of surgical complication. There is also the potential for systemic side effects from the blockage of VEGF receptors elsewhere in the body, which needs to be evaluated in the long term.

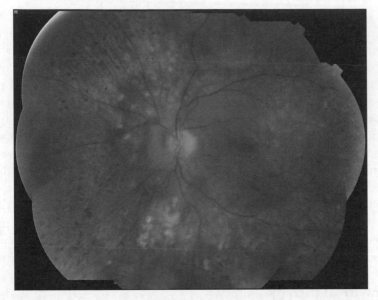

Figure 1.18 Panretinal photocoagulation laser therapy.

Laser therapy for maculopathy therefore currently remains the primary treatment of choice in diabetic maculopathy. It is likely that the new treatments will have a significant part to play in the management of patients who do not respond to laser therapy, but their exact role has yet to be clarified.

Proliferative diabetic retinopathy

Panretinal laser photocoagulation (Figure 1.18) was introduced in the early 1970s after the clinical observation that patients with retinal degenerations and coexistent diabetes did not develop proliferative retinopathy. The Diabetic Retinopathy Study showed a 50 per cent reduction in the risk of severe vision loss (five lines or more) in patients treated with panretinal photocoagulation (PRP).

Treatment is with a continuous wave laser in 0.05- to 0.2-second pulses, and overall 1200–1600 burns of diameter 500 μm or 3000–6000 burns of diameter 200 μm are applied to the peripheral fundus. The treatment is performed in two or three sessions and a remarkable reduction in neovascularization is achieved.

Complications of the laser treatment include loss of visual field (including the field required for driving), reduction of night-time vision, increased glare and a mild reduction in visual acuity. Overall the benefits of the treatment far outweigh the side effects.

Scanning laser systems are now available that deliver the treatment in preset patterns, making administration faster and more uniform.

Vitrectomy

Pars plana vitrectomy has become a safe and commonly performed technique in ophthalmology and is used with very good effect in some patients with advanced diabetic eye disease.

Indications for vitrectomy include persistent vitreous haemorrhage precluding retinal laser treatment, traction retinal detachment and macular oedema associated with a thickened posterior vitreous face (vitreomacular traction or epiretinal membrane).

Vitrectomy is often accompanied by endolaser after the vitreous has been cleared, using a small laser probe held just over the surface of the retina.

The procedure has the advantage of removing the reservoir for angiogenic agents and also the scaffolding structure for neovascularization. Complications, however, include retinal detachment and cataract formation, both of which need further surgery.

Cataract surgery

Cataract extraction

Cataracts can cause a significant reduction in vision and the metabolic disturbances of diabetes are a known cause. Approximately 15 per cent of patients undergoing a cataract extraction can be expected to have diabetes. Small-incision, sutureless cataract surgery is now the accepted practice and the surgical risks are very low.

Cataract surgery can, however, have an impact on the whole eye. In diabetes, patients with no or minimal retinopathy do not appear to have an increased risk of progression after surgery. Patients who have previously had retinal laser for maculopathy have a significant risk of recurrence of oedema after surgery, and those with pre-existing macular oedema may worsen considerably and should therefore receive early postoperative management of their retinal condition.

Patients with active proliferative retinopathy should be treated with laser and be in a quiescent state before cataract surgery. If the cataract prevents laser treatment, they should receive PRP at the time of surgery or immediately afterwards (next day).

1.8 Conclusion

The management of diabetes and diabetic eye disease has changed considerably in recent years and will continue to do so.

Tight control of glucose, blood pressure and serum lipid levels is becoming paramount in the reduction of diabetic complications.

Screening for diabetic retinopathy is performed and has a good chance of detecting those with pre-symptomatic sight-threatening disease.

The mainstay of treatment for both maculopathy and proliferative retinopathy remains laser treatment and the modalities for laser delivery are improving. New adjunctive treatments such as intravitreal therapy and vitrectomy are emerging as treatments that maintain or improve vision.

Case study

A 47-year-old man had had type 2 diabetes for 11 years. He also had hypertension and dyslipidaemia. His medication was metformin, gliclazide, ramipril and simvastatin. He had developed peripheral neuropathy in his hands and feet and also retinopathy. He was referred to the eye clinic from a retinal screening programme with retinopathy grade R2 in both eyes.

He was followed at regular intervals and, despite good medical control, the retinopathy progressed. Figure 1.19 shows new vessels on the left optic nerve head and in Figure 1.20 there is a small area in the superotemporal vascular arcade of the right eye. Fluorescein angiography confirmed bilateral proliferative retinopathy (Figures 1.21 and 1.22). There was a significant degree of fluorescein leakage around both maculas and a small area of macular oedema in the left eye.

Laser treatment with panretinal photocoagulation was performed in both eyes, the laser scars being visible in Figures 1.23 and 1.24. After the panretinal laser treatment the degree of macular oedema in the left eye worsened. Figure 1.25 shows a comparative spectral domain optical coherence tomography scan. This area was treated with focal laser treatment. One month later the degree of oedema was lessening significantly, as shown in Figure 1.26. The patient remains under regular review in the clinic.

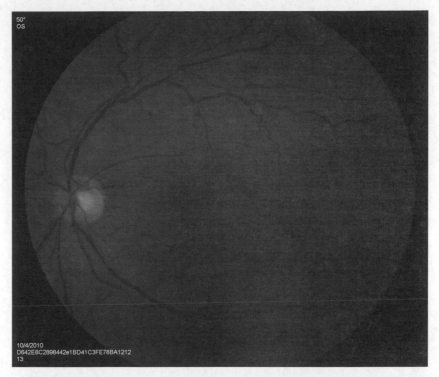

Figure 1.19 A retinal macula view photograph of the left eye showing new vessels on the optic nerve head.

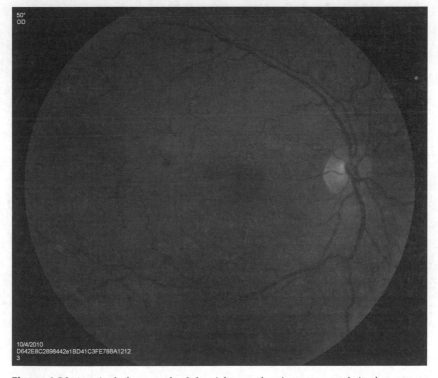

Figure 1.20 A retinal photograph of the right eye showing new vessels in the superotemporal vascular arcade.

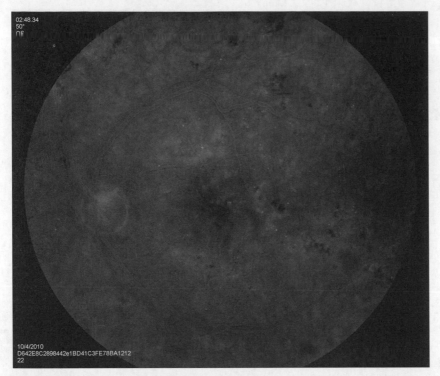

Figure 1.21 Fluorescein angiogram of Figure 1.19.

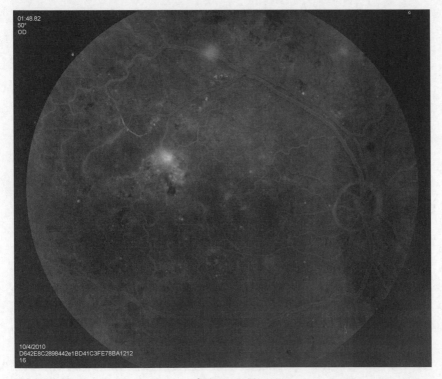

Figure 1.22 Fluorescein angiogram of Figure 1.20.

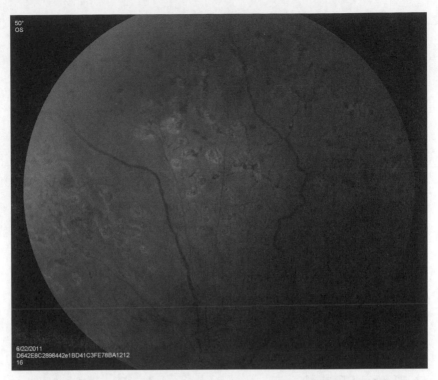

Figure 1.23 Retinal photograph showing scars from panretinal photocoagulation.

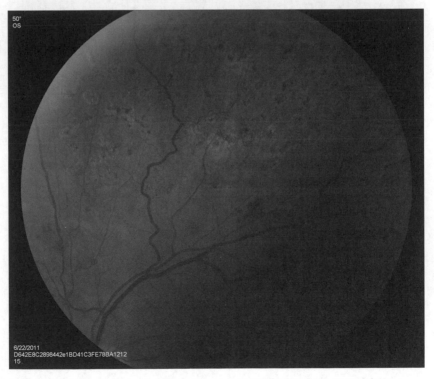

Figure 1.24 Retinal photograph showing scars from panretinal photocoagulation.

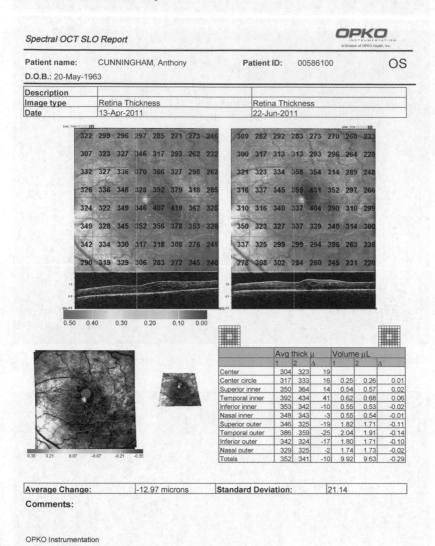

Spectral OCT SLO Report

OPKO
INSTRUMENTATION
A Division of OPKO Health, Inc.

Patient name:	CUNNINGHAM, Anthony	Patient ID:	00586100	OS

D.O.B.: 20-May-1963

Description		
Image type	Retina Thickness	Retina Thickness
Date	13-Apr-2011	22-Jun-2011

		Avg thick μ			Volume μL		
		1	2	Δ	1	2	Δ
Center		304	323	19			
Center circle		317	333	16	0.25	0.26	0.01
Superior inner		350	364	14	0.54	0.57	0.02
Temporal inner		392	434	41	0.62	0.68	0.06
Inferior inner		353	342	-10	0.55	0.53	-0.02
Nasal inner		348	343	-3	0.55	0.54	-0.01
Superior outer		346	325	-19	1.82	1.71	-0.11
Temporal outer		386	359	-25	2.04	1.91	-0.14
Inferior outer		342	324	-17	1.80	1.71	-0.10
Nasal outer		329	325	-2	1.74	1.73	-0.02
Totals		352	341	-10	9.92	9.63	-0.29

Average Change:	-12.97 microns	Standard Deviation:	21.14

Comments:

OPKO Instrumentation

Figure 1.25 A Spectral domain optical coherence tomography scan pre-laser therapy.

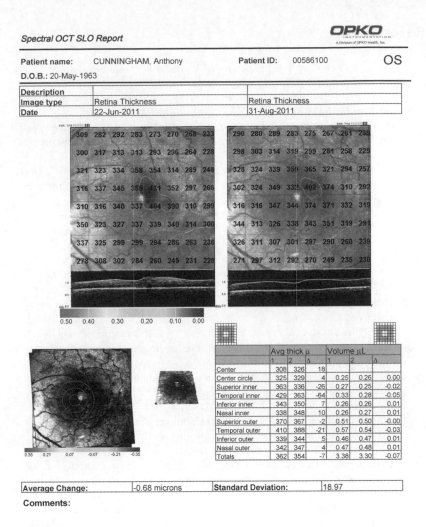

Figure 1.26 A comparative Spectral domain optical coherence tomography scan post-laser therapy.

References

1. Evans J, Rooney C, Aswood F, Dattani N, Wormald R. Blindness and partial sight in England and Wales. *Health Trends* 1996;**38**:5–12.
2. Klein R, Klein BEK, Moss SE. Epidemiology of proliferative diabetic retinopathy. *Diabet Care* 1992;**15**:1875–1891.
3. Klein R, Klein BEK, Moss SE, Davis MD, DeMets DL. The Wisconsin Epidemiological Study of Diabetic Retinopathy: II. Prevalence and risk of diabetic retinopathy when age at diagnosis is less than 30 years. *Arch Ophthal* 1984;**102**:520–526.
4. Kohner EM, Aldington SJ, Stratton IM, et al., United Kingdom Prospective Diabetes Study 30. Diabetic retinopathy at diagnosis of non- insulin dependent diabetes mellitus and associated risk factors. *Arch Ophthal* 1998;**116**:297–303.
5. Klein R, Klein BEK, Moss SE, Davis MD, DeMets DL. The Wisconsin Epidemiological study of Diabetic Retinopathy. III. Prevalence and risk of diabetic retinopathy when age at diagnosis is 30 or more years. *Arch Ophthal* 1984;**102**:527–532.
6. Early Treatment Diabetic Retinopathy Study Group. Early photocoagulation for diabetic retinopathy. ETDRS Report number 9. *Ophthalmology* 1991;**98**(suppl): 767–785.
7. Freudenstein U, Verne J. A national screening programme for diabetic retinopathy. *BMJ* 2001;**323**:4–5.
8. Younis N, Broadbent DM, James M, Harding SP, Vora JP. Incidence of sight threatening retinopathy in patients with type 2 diabetes in the Liverpool diabetic eye study: a cohort study. *Lancet* 2003;**361**:195–200.
9. DCCT Research Group. The effect of intensive treatment of diabetes on the development and treatment and progression of long-term complications in insulin dependent diabetes mellitus. *N Engl J Med* 1993;**329**:977–1034.
10. Stratton IM, Kohner EM, Aldington SJ, et al. Progression of diabetic retinopathy at diagnosis of non-insulin dependent diabetes in the United Kingdom Prospective Diabetes Study. *Diabetologia* 2001;**44**:156–163.
11. UK Prospective Diabetes Study Group. Tight blood pressure control and risk of macro-vascular and microvascular complications in type 2 diabetes (UKPDS 38). *BMJ* 1998;**317**:703–712.
12. Chaturvedi N, Sjolie AK, Stephenson JM, et al. Effect of lisinopril on progression of retinopathy in normotensive people with type 1 diabetes. The EUCLID Study Group. EURODIAB Controlled Trial of Lisinopril in Insulin-Dependent Diabetes Mellitus. *Lancet* 1998;**351**:28–31.
13. Sjølie AK, Klein R, Porta M, et al., DIRECT Programme Study Group. Effect of candesartan on progression and regression of retinopathy in type 2 diabetes (DIRECT-Protect 2): a randomised placebo-controlled trial. *Lancet* 2008;**372**: 1385–1393.
14. Klein R, Moss SE, Sinaiko AR, et al. The relation of ambulatory blood pressure and pulse rate to retinopathy in type 1 diabetes mellitus: the renin-angiotensin system study. *Ophthalmology* 2006;**113**:2231–2236.
15. Keech AC, Mitchell P, Summanen PA, et al., FIELD study investigators. Effect of fenofibrate on the need for laser treatment for diabetic retinopathy (FIELD study): a randomised controlled trial. *Lancet* 2007;**370**:1687–1697.
16. Chew EY, Ambrosius WT, Davis MD, et al., ACCORD Eye Study Group. Effects of medical therapies on retinopathy progression in type 2 diabetes. *N Engl J Med* 2010;**363**:233–244.

17. Bonetti PO, Lerman LO, Napoli C, Lerman A. Statin effects beyond lipid lowering – are they clinically relevant? *Eur Heart J* 2003;**24**:225–248.
18. Colhoun HM, Betteridge DJ, Durrington PN, et al., CARDS investigators. Primary prevention of cardiovascular disease with atorvastatin in type 2 diabetes in the Collaborative Atorvastatin Diabetes Study (CARDS): multicentre randomised placebo-controlled trial. *Lancet* 2004;**364**:685–696.
19. Schwartz SG, Flynn HW Jr, Aiello LP. Ruboxistaurin mesilate hydrate for diabetic retinopathy. *Drugs Today (Barc)* 2009;**45**:269–274 (Review).
20. Beck RW, Edwards AR, Aiello LP, et al. Diabetic Retinopathy Clinical Research Network (DRCR.net). Three-year follow-up of a randomized trial comparing focal/grid photocoagulation and intravitreal triamcinolone for diabetic macular edema. *Arch Ophthalmol* 2009;**127**:245–251.
21. Nicholson BP, Schachat AP. A review of clinical trials of anti-VEGF agents for diabetic retinopathy. *Graefes Arch Clin Exp Ophthalmol* 2010;**248**:915–930.
22. Parravano M, Menchini F, Virgili G. Antiangiogenic therapy with anti-vascular endothelial growth factor modalities for diabetic macular oedema. *Cochrane Database Syst Rev* 2009;(**4**):CD007419.

Useful websites

www.nice.org.uk: diabetic retinopathy: early management and screening
www.diabetic-retinopathy.screening.nhs.uk/overview-of-screening-models.html: preservation of sight in diabetes: a risk reduction program
www.rcophth.ac.uk: Royal College of Ophthalmologists

Useful addresses

The Partially Sighted Society
Queen's Road, Doncaster DN1 2NX, UK
Tel: 01302 323132

Royal National Institute for the Blind
224 Great Portland Street, London W1, UK
Tel: 0207 3881266

Action for Blind People
14–16 Verney Road, London SE16 3DZ, UK
Tel: 0207 7328771

CHAPTER 2

Diabetic Chronic Kidney Disease

Richard J MacIsaac,[1] George Jerums[2] and Gerald F Watts[3]

[1]Department of Endocrinology and Diabetes, St Vincent's Hospital and University of Melbourne, Fitzroy, Victoria, Australia
[2]Endocrine Centre Austin Health and University of Melbourne, Heidelberg Repatriation Hospital, Heidelberg West, Victoria, Australia
[3]School of Medicine and Pharmacology, University of Western Australia, Royal Perth Hospital, Perth, Western Australia, Australia

---

⭐ Key points

- Diabetic chronic kidney disease (CKD) is the leading cause of end-stage kidney disease in the western world.

- Screening people with diabetes for markers of CKD and initiation of measures to retard the progression of kidney disease are therefore now considered part of routine clinical practice

- Diabetic CKD is staged on the basis of both glomerular filtration rate (GFR) and level of urinary albumin excretion.

- Urinary albumin can be quantified by measuring the urinary albumin:creatinine ratio (ACR) or albumin excretion rate (AER).

- The estimated GFR (GFR) is derived from the Modification of Diet in Renal Disease (MDRD) formula or the newer Chronic Kidney Disease Epidemiology Collaboration (CKD-EPI) equation.

- The MDRD formula underestimates true GFR values >60 ml/min per $1.73\,m^2$ and the CKD-EDI formula possibly improves this underestimation.

- People with diabetes, especially those with CKD, have increased cardiovascular (CV) morbidity and mortality.

Diabetes: Chronic Complications, Third Edition. Edited by Kenneth M. Shaw, Michael H. Cummings.
© 2012 John Wiley & Sons, Ltd. Published 2012 by John Wiley & Sons, Ltd.

Therapeutic key points

- The finding of persistently elevated levels of urinary albumin or a GFR <60 ml/min per 1.73 m^2 should mandate for correcting hyperglycaemia, hypertension, dyslipidaemia and smoking.
- Interrupting the renin–angiotensin system (RAS) with an angiotensin-converting enzyme (ACE) inhibitor or an angiotensin receptor blocker (ARB) results in renal and CV protection beyond the effects of blood pressure lowering alone.
- All people with microalbuminuria should be considered for treatment with an RAS blocker and a statin.
- A HbA1c <6.5 per cent should be the general target for the prevention of diabetic CKD, whereas, in advanced CKD, a higher target could be accepted according to the clinical context.
- The general target blood pressure for people with diabetic CKD is 130/80 mmHg. If persistent proteinuria is present aim for <125/75 mmHg.

2.1 Introduction

It has been recognized for some time that the incidence of diabetes is increasing worldwide mainly because of a dramatic increase in type 2 diabetes. This increase prevalence is the result of the combination of obesity, urbanization and an ageing population. The public health impact of this phenomenon is enormous, because diabetes is now the leading cause of end-stage renal disease (ESRD) in western countries. Chronic kidney disease (CKD) in people with diabetes has traditionally been referred to as 'diabetic nephropathy'. Diabetic nephropathy has been defined as persistent clinically detectable proteinuria that is associated with an elevation in blood pressure (BP) and a decline in glomerular filtration rate (GFR), and has been reported to occur in 25–40 per cent of people with either type 1 or type 2 diabetes. People with diabetes, especially those with CKD, have an increased cardiovascular (CV) morbidity and mortality. Therefore, the early identification of people at greatest risk and the subsequent initiation of renal and CV protective treatments are of the utmost importance.

Microalbuminuria is an early component in a continuum of progressive increase in albumin excretion rates (AERs) that usually characterises diabetic CKD. The term refers to a subclinical increase in urinary albumin excretion. By definition, it corresponds to an AER of 20–200 µg/min (30–300 mg/day) or an albumin:creatinine ratio (ACR) of 2.5–35 in males and 3.5–35 in females (Table 2.1). The development of microalbuminuria has been equated with incipient nephropathy, but it is also a risk factor for macrovascular disease in people with diabetes.[1] Although recent work has

Table 2.1 Classification of albuminuria for people with diabetes

	AER		ACR (mg/mmol)	
	µg/min	mg/day	Females	Males
Normoalbuminuria	<20	<30	<3.5	<2.5
Microalbuminuria	20–200	30–300	3.5–35	2.5–25
Macroalbuminuria	>200	>300	>35	>25

ACR, albumin:creatinine ratio; AER, albumin excretion rate.

Table 2.2 Stages of chronic renal disease according to the National Kidney Foundation

Stage	Description	GFR (ml/min per 1.73 m^2)
1	Kidney damage with normal or increased GFR	≥90
2	Kidney damage with a mild decrease in GFR	60–89
3	Kidney damage with a moderate decrease in GFR	30–59
4	Kidney damage with a severe decrease in GFR	15–29
5	Kidney failure	<15 (or dialysis)

GFR, glomerular filtration rate.

suggested that some individuals with diabetes and impaired renal function may not have an elevated level of urinary albumin excretion, measuring albumin excretion is still the best non-invasive means of predicting and following diabetic kidney disease.[2] The staging of diabetic CKD is also based on the estimated glomerular filtration rate (eGFR) and classification according to the National Kidney Foundation (NKF) guidelines (Table 2.2).

This chapter summarizes the aetiology and structural and functional changes of diabetic CKD. Clinical interventions aimed at preventing or ameliorating the progression of this devastating complication of diabetes are also outlined.

2.2 Epidemiology and natural history

Prevalence and incidence of diabetic CKD

Although diabetes remains the leading cause of ESRD in the western world, a recent analysis has shown that the age-adjusted rate of adults with diabetes who start treatment for ESRD in the USA is declining. During 1996–2007, the number of ESRD cases attributable to diabetes increased, as did the number of people with diagnosed diabetes. However, as the rate of increase in the number of people diagnosed with diabetes was greater than the rate of increase in cases of ESRD, the age-adjusted rate for people with diabetes entering renal replacement programmes decreased by 35 per cent between 1996 and 2007.

Microalbuminuria is an early component in a continuum of progressive increased urinary albumin excretion that usually characterizes diabetic CKD. Microalbuminuria is a relatively common finding in the general population, with a prevalence rate of around 7 per cent. The level of urinary albumin excretion is a powerful predictor of both all-cause and CV mortality in the general population, even in the absence of diabetes. Community-based surveys have shown that the prevalence of microalbuminuria for people with diabetes ranges between 16 and 28 per cent. It appears that both the absolute level and the rate of progression of urinary albumin excretion are independent predictors of all-cause mortality and renal and CV events in individuals with diabetes.[3]

For individuals with type 1 diabetes, approximately 10–20 per cent develop microalbuminuria after 5–10 years of diagnosis. In another study of normoalbuminuric individuals, 18 per cent progressed to microalbuminuria after 9 years of follow-up. New insights into the epidemiology of diabetic CKD have been highlighted in recent follow-up studies of large interventional trials in people with type 1 diabetes – the Diabetes Control and Complications Trial (DCCT)/Epidemiology of Diabetes Interventions and Complications (EDIC) study – and type 2 diabetes – the UK Prospective Diabetes Study (UKPDS). In contrast to type 1 diabetes, the finding of microalbuminuria is not uncommon at the time of diagnosis for individuals with type 2 diabetes, with one study suggesting that the prevalence could be around 18 per cent. In that study the severity of hyperglycaemia at diagnosis was an important risk factor for an elevated urinary albumin level. In a 19-year follow-up study of participants with type 1 diabetes in DCCT/EDIC, a total of 89 of 1439 participants developed stage 3 CKD (eGFR <60 ml/min per $1.73 \, m^2$), resulting in a cumulative incidence of 11.4 per cent. For these patients, 24 per cent remained normoalbuminuric, 16 per cent developed microalbuminuria and 61 per cent developed macroalbuminuria before reaching stage 3 CKD. The finding of macroalbuminuria was associated with a markedly increased rate of fall in eGFR of 5.7%/year versus 1.2%/year for participants with normoalbuminuria.[4]

During the intervention phase of the UKPDS an observational study showed that 24.9 per cent of patients with type 2 diabetes developed microalbuminuria within 10 years of the diagnosis of diabetes, but only 0.8 per cent developed ESRD. Annual rates of transition between normo-, micro-, macroalbuminuria, and end-stage CKD ranged between 2 and 3 per cent per year. Furthermore, a recent 15-year follow-up study of patients enrolled in the UKPDS has shown that 38 per cent of patients developed albuminuria (microalbuminuria or macroalbuminuria) and 29 per cent developed renal impairment (Cockcroft–Gault estimated a creatinine clearance <60 ml/min or doubling of plasma creatinine). Interestingly, in approximately half of the patients who developed renal impairment (51 per cent) there was no preceding increase in urinary albumin excretion.[5]

Natural history of diabetic CKD

The natural history of the albuminuric pathway that is associated with a decline in GFR, especially in type 1 diabetes, has several well-characterized stages as summarized in Table 2.3.[6] The main features of the first stage are hyperfiltration and renal hypertrophy. The second stage consists of a 'silent phase' associated with normal urinary albumin excretion or intermittent episodes of microalbuminuria. This silent phase may last for many years and most patients with diabetes will remain in this phase for their lifetime. The next phase (stage 3) is characterized by persistent micro-albuminuria. Usually GFR will be preserved in individuals with type 1 or type 2 diabetes during this stage, as long as they remain normotensive and their AER does not rise progressively. However, in type 2 diabetes, the onset of hypertension and macrovascular disease commonly precedes or accompanies this stage and subsequently promotes a rise in AER and a decline in GFR. A schematic representation of the traditional evolution of diabetic CKD for individuals with type 1 or type 2 diabetes based on progression from normo- to micro- to macroalbuminuria is shown in Figure 2.1.

The fourth stage, 'diabetic nephropathy', is characterized by clinically detectable proteinuria, hypertension and a subsequent decline in GFR. In the absence of antihypertensive therapy, GFR has been estimated to decrease by up to 10–15 ml/min per year during this stage. In comparison the normal age-related decline in GFR for healthy individuals after the age of 40 years is estimated to be approximately 1 ml/min per year. The final stage (stage 5) occurs when individuals progress to ESRD. At this stage GFR has usually decreased to below 15 ml/min, necessitating the commencement of kidney replacement therapy.

In the last 15 years the concept of progressive increases in AER during the microalbuminuric phase being a reliable predictor of diabetic CKD has been challenged. This original paradigm was based on studies published in the early 1980s showing that the finding of microalbuminuria was

Table 2.3 Stages in the albuminuric pathway to end-stage renal disease (ESRD)

Stage	Characteristics	Diabetes	Duration [year]	AER (µg/min)	BP (mmHg)	GFR (ml/min)	Treatment effects
1	Hyperfiltration and nephromegaly	Type 1	0–5	↑ then <20	N	↑	
		Type 2	Not clearly defined		↑	↑ or N	
2	Normoalbuminuria and ↑ GBMT and mesangial expansion	Type 1	5–15	<20	N	↑	Reversed by strict glycaemic control
		Type 2	Not clearly defined	↑ 10–20%/year	↑	N	Effects of BP control not documented
3	Microalbuminuria (incipient DN)	Type 1	10–20	20–200	N then ↑	N	Attenuated by strict glycaemic control.
		Type 2	0–15	↑ 20–40%/year	↑ (↑Δ 3 mmHg/year)	↓ 3–5/year	Attenuated, arrested or reversed by strict BP control based on RAS inhibition
4	Overt DN (macroalbuminuria)	Type 1	15–25	>200	↑ (↑ Δ 5 mmHg/year)	↓ Δ 8–12/year[a]	Faster progression with poor glycaemic control (observational studies only)
		Type 2	5–20[b]			↓ Δ 4–12/year[a]	
5	ESRD	Type 1	20–30	>200	↑	↓ (<20)	Attenuated by strict BP control based on RAS inhibition
		Type 2	10–20[b]				

BP, blood pressure, including isolated systolic BP in elderly people with type 2 diabetes; DN, diabetic nephropathy – in type 2 diabetes, this may include hypertensive, ischaemic, atherosclerotic and non-diabetic glomerular disease as well as DN; ESRD, end-stage renal disease; GBMT, glomerular basement membrane thickening; N, normal; ras, renin–angiotensin system.

[a]Rise in serum creatinine is a late and insensitive index of progression of overt DN and indicates loss of 50 per cent or more of renal function.

[b]Many people with type 2 diabetes do not reach stage 4 or 5 because of increased cardiovascular mortality associated with stages 3 and 4.

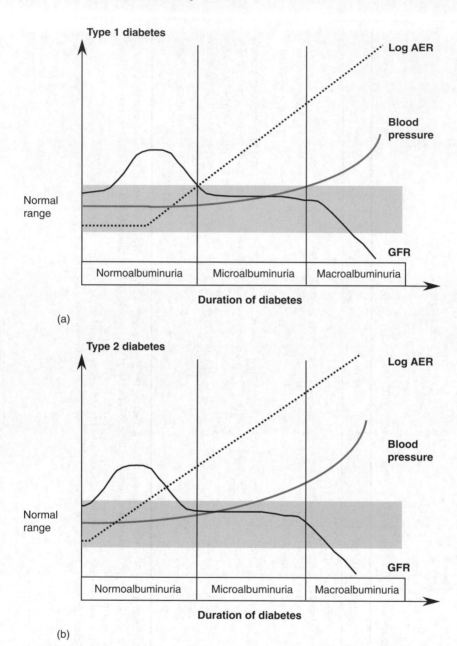

Figure 2.1 Natural history of 'albuminuric chronic kidney disease' in (a) type 1 and (b) type 2 diabetes in the absence of interventions that modify albumin excretion rate (AER).

associated with a risk of progression to overt proteinuria of 60–80 per cent over 6–14 years in people with type 1 diabetes. More recently, spontaneous remission of microalbuminuria has been reported to occur in approximately 50 per cent of patients with diabetes whereas rates of progression of microalbuminuria to macroalbuminuria only range between 11 and 35 per cent. Furthermore, detection of onset of an early GFR decline has been possible at the stage of new-onset microalbuminuria, well before the onset of overt nephropathy. This finding has been facilitated by the use of markers such as cystatin C which accurately detect a decline in GFR before reaching 60 ml/min per 1.73 m^2. In addition, two studies published in the early 1990s demonstrated that some patients with diabetes could develop a low creatinine clearance (CrCl) while remaining normoalbuminuric.[7,8]

The prevalence of normoalbuminuric CKD in people with diabetes has been reported in recent studies to be approximately 25 per cent after accounting for the use of renin–angiotensin system (RAS)-blocking agents. Although the demographic and laboratory profile of people with diabetes and normoalbuminuric low GFR remains to be fully defined, it appears to be more common in elderly women. Furthermore, distinct sets of risk factors for the development of low GFR or increased AER have been described in recent studies, which again promotes the concept of a rise in AER and a decrease in GFR as complementary rather than obligatory manifestations of diabetic CKD.[8]

2.3 Pathophysiology

Initiators and promoters of diabetic CKD

Genetic factors clearly influence the development of diabetic CKD.[9] Possible candidate genes are those regulating the renin-angiotensin system (RAS), hypertension, dyslipidaemia, hyperglycaemia and immune responses. However, the role of genotyping in assessment of microalbuminuria and guiding the management of diabetic renal disease remains undefined. Family history of CV disease, hypertension, renal disease and dyslipidaemia should nevertheless be routinely elicited in all diabetic patients. The following are candidates implicated in the susceptibility to develop diabetic nephropathy:

- Angiotensin-converting enzyme (ACE)
- Angiotensinogen
- Angiotensin II receptor (type 1)
- Aldose reductase
- Apolipoprotein E
- Atrial natriuretic peptide

- Heparin sulphate
- Intercellular adhesion molecule-1 (ICAM-1)
- Matrix metalloproteinase
- Methylene metalloprotease-9 (MM-9)
- Na^+/H^+ exchanger
- Nitric oxide synthase
- Plasminogen activator inhibitor-1 (PAI-1)
- Peroxisome proliferator-activated receptor (PPAR)
- Type 4 collagen
- β-Adrenergic receptor
- Vascular endothelial growth factor (VEGF).

The stage of microalbuminuria usually evolves over 10–15 years with defined initiators and promoters such as levels of glycaemia, blood pressure control and smoking. Exercise-induced microalbuminuria has also been demonstrated to be predictive of later persistent microalbuminuria. Given that microalbuminuria is an indicator that the kidney is being damaged, especially in type 1 diabetes, undue exercise could be detrimental to early diabetic CKD; however, more work is required to clarify the clinical impact of exercise on the progression of microalbuminuria.[1]

After the transition to the macroalbuminuric or overt nephropathy stage, the rate of progression of renal disease is influenced by a number of factors, including the level of blood pressure, hyperglycaemia, the level of proteinuria or albuminuria, the presence of retinopathy, smoking and possibly anaemia. Non-modifiable risk factors include male gender and ethnicity (Box 2.1). In particular, higher rates of ESRD due to diabetes

---

Box 2.1 Initiators and promoters of diabetic chronic kidney disease

Initiators of diabetic neuropathy (DN)

- Hyperglycaemia
- Predisposing genes

Promoters of DN

- Hyperglycaemia
- Hypertension
- Dyslipidaemia
- Insulin resistance
- Smoking
- Procoagulant state
- Long duration of diabetes
- Anaemia
- Ethnicity/westernization

have been reported for Pima Indians, Mexican Americans, Asians, South Pacific Islanders, New Zealand Maoris and Australian Aborigines than people of white European origin. However, it is not clear if these inter-population differences are due to genetic changes in the predisposition to diabetic nephropathy or to environmental, social or cultural factors.

The pathophysiology of diabetic CKD involves the activation of metabolic, inflammatory and haemodynamic pathways. Metabolic pathways are mainly driven by chronic hyperglycaemia that results in increased protein kinase C (PKC) activity, abnormalities in polyol metabolism, increased secretion of profibrotic cytokines such as transforming growth factor-β (TGF-β) and connective tissue growth factor (CTGF), and non-enzymatic glycosylation leading to the glycation of glomerular and tubular proteins and the production of advanced glycation end-products (AGEs). The resultant generation of reactive oxygen species (ROS) and an inflammatory process play a pivotal role in the development of diabetic CKD.

Haemodynamic pathways that result in systemic and intraglomerular hypertension are driven by the activation of vasoactive systems such as the renin–angiotensin–aldosterone and endothelin systems. It should be appreciated that each of the above pathways can influence the other. For example, activation of the renin–angiotensin–aldosterone system promotes endothelial dysfunction, inflammation and the expression of TGF-β and CTGF. The final common manifestation of the above pathways is usually the accumulation of excess connective tissue which leads to fibrosis or scarring of the kidney.[7]

The role of abnormal indicators of protein glycation in the pathogenesis of experimental diabetic CKD has been highlighted recently. It has been proposed that activation of the receptor for advanced glycation endproducts (RAGE), via a decrease in angiotensin II type 2 receptors, plays a key role in promoting the development and progression of diabetic kidney disease. Other postulated promoters of diabetic CKD that are currently being extensively investigated are hyperfiltration and abnormal uric acid metabolism. The role of these two factors in the pathogenesis of diabetic CKD remains to be fully elucidated. The efficacy of treating modifiable initiators and promoters of diabetic CKD is discussed in later.

Structural changes observed in diabetic CKD

The structure of a nephron, the functional unit of the kidney, is shown in Figure 2.2. Diabetic CKD primarily affects the glomerulus in type 1 diabetes (Figure 2.3). In patients with type 1 diabetes, morphological changes occur in the renal arterioles, interstitium and tubules, but the development of a glomerulopathy is considered the hallmark of diabetic

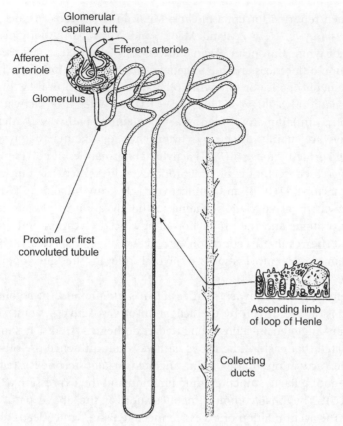

Glomerular
capillary tuft

Efferent arteriole

Afferent
arteriole

Glomerulus

Proximal or first
convoluted tubule

Ascending limb
of loop of Henle

Collecting
ducts

Figure 2.2 Structure of a nephron, the functional unit of the kidney. Diabetic renal disease primarily affects the glomerulus.

nephropathy. This glomerulopathy is characterized by thickening of the glomerular basement membrane (GBM) and mesangial expansion. These changes have even been observed in normoalbuminuric patients and, although there is a fair degree of overlap with microalbuminuric patients, the overall severity of these changes increases with the onset of microalbuminuria.

Compared with type 1 diabetic nephropathy, there is a wider heterogeneity of renal ultrastructural morphology in type 2 diabetes. Three patterns of renal ultrastructural changes have been described for microalbuminuric patients with type 2 diabetes and normal GFR:

1. Normal or near normal renal structure
2. Typical diabetic glomerulopathy
3. An atypical pattern of renal injury comprising: tubulointerstitial lesions, advanced glomerular arteriolar hyalinosis and global glomerulosclero-

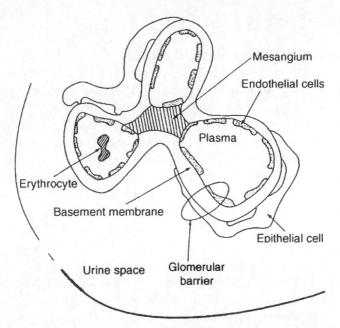

Figure 2.3 Diagrammatic, high-powered, cross-sectional representation of the glomerular capillary lobule of kidney. To get into the urine space, albumin has to pass from the plasma across the endothelial cells, basement membrane and epithelial cells. In diabetic renal disease the basement membrane increases in thickness and the mesangium expands to invade the glomerular barrier. Increase in albumin in the urine reflects damage to the glomerular barrier filtration rate (GFR); normal GFR ranges between 70 and 120 ml/min per 1.73 m^2.

sis. Furthermore, renal morphological changes that could be ascribed to other well-recognized forms of non-diabetic renal disease were uncommon.[10] At present there have been no detailed studies of renal structure in normoalbuminuric individuals with type 2 diabetes regardless of GFR.

For individuals with type 2 diabetes and macroalbuminuria, three patterns of renal morphology are generally described with most of these people expected to have a low GFR:

1. Non-diabetic renal disease
2. Typical diabetic glomerulopathy
3. Atypical diabetic nephropathy with interstitial and vascular changes.

It is estimated that approximately 10–30 per cent of people with type 2 diabetes and proteinuria may have recognized forms of non-diabetic renal ultrastructural changes.

2.4 Management

Diagnosis and clinical investigation

The diagnosis of diabetic CKD is based on the measurement of elevated levels of urinary albumin excretion and decreased GFR. Patients with diabetic CKD do not usually need to progress to a renal biopsy. Indications for considering a biopsy could include heavy proteinuria in the absence of diabetic retinopathy, an abnormal urinary sediment, the rapid progression of proteinuria or systemic features that suggest the presence of another disease process associated with the development of proteinuria.

A person with diabetic CKD is at substantially increased risk for the development and progression of CV disease (CVD). Therefore, clinical assessment should aim to address reducing the risk of CVD as well as progression to ESRD. Diabetic CKD is associated with multiple comorbidities apart from CVD, including hypertension, dyslipidaemia, anaemia, and bone and mineral metabolism disorders. Awareness of these comorbidities and the adoption of a multifactorial management approach can reduce the risk of the development and progression of the micro- and macrovascular complications of diabetes which frequently occur in people with diabetes and concurrent CKD.

Management of diabetic CKD

The factors and goals that have been shown to delay the progression of diabetic CKD are outlined in Table 2.4. The remainder of this section focuses on the following management issues in patients with diabetic CKD: selecting the right glucose-lowering therapies, RAS blockade, novel therapies, low-protein diets, the correction of anaemia, the use of aspirin, lifestyle modification and preparation for renal replacement therapy. The management of the individual risk factors for diabetic CKD, namely hyperglycaemia, hypertension and dyslipidaemia, is discussed in the next section.

Multifactorial interventions

The management of people with diabetic CKD involves strict attention to the common risk factors for kidney and CVD, namely hyperglycaemia, hypertension, dyslipidaemia and smoking. However, it is worth noting that multi-interventional, target-driven strategies, as shown in the Steno-2 study, aim for a HbA1c <6.5 per cent, systolic BP <130 mmHg, diastolic BP <80 mmHg, fasting cholesterol <4.5 mmol/l and fasting triglycerides <1.7 mmol/l, which includes the universal use of RAS blockers, aspirin, the aggressive use of statins and attention to lifestyle factors, a decrease in the risk for developing proteinuria of 60 per cent, and for CV events of

Table 2.4 Important factors and targets for delaying the progression of diabetic CKD

Factor	Target
Glycaemic control	HbA1c <6.5% for prevention, but a higher target could be accepted according to the clinical context
Blood pressure	<130/80 mmHg – general target <125/75 mmHg – if there is proteinuria or eGFR <60 ml/min per 1.73 m^2
Lipid control	Statins for all people with micro- or macroalbuminuria. Consider statin use if eGFR <60 ml/min per 1.73 m^2 Aim for LDL <2.5 mmol/l for primary prevention Consider a fibrate if TG >2.5 mmol/l and HDL <1.0 mmol/l
RAS inhibition	ACE inhibitor or ARB for all people with micro- or macroalbuminuria
Albuminuria	Aim to reduce to the lowest level possible, especially for people with macroalbuminuria
Aspirin	Approximately 100 mg daily If there is micro- or macroalbuminuria or if eGFR <60 ml/min per 1.73 m^2
Smoking	Stop
Weight	Aim for a BMI <25 kg/m^2

It should be noted that these are general targets and need to be individualized according to a patient's age and comorbidities.
ACE, angiotensin-converting enzyme; ARB, angiotensin receptor blocker; BMI, body mass index; CKD, chronic kidney disease; (e)GFR, (estimated) glomerular filtration rate; HbA1c, glycated haemoglobin; HDL, high-density lipoprotein; RAS, renin–angiotensin system; TG, triglyceride.

approximately 50 per cent in people with type 2 diabetes and microalbuminuria followed for 8 years.[11] This result was achieved despite the fact that only a minority of individuals reached the study's glycaemic goal. Furthermore, a 5-year observational study, which monitored the development of complications after completion of the interventional phase of the Steno-2 study, has shown that the risk of developing ESRD was significantly reduced in people originally assigned to the above multifactorial, target-driven management strategy compared with those who originally received conventional treatment.[12]

Glucose-lowering therapies

Metformin is excreted by the kidneys and when GFR declines the blood level of metformin rises; this inhibits the oxidation of lactate which can result in the potentially fatal complication of lactic acidosis. We recommend limiting the use of metformin to a maximum of 500 mg twice daily in people with an eGFR <60 ml/min per 1.73 m^2, and ceasing the medication completely when the eGFR falls to <30 ml/min per 1.73 m^2. Most of the sulfonylureas are renally excreted and dosages may need to be reduced as CKD progresses. Glibenclamide should not be used in elderly people and in those with an eGFR <60 ml/min per $1.73\,m^2$. Possibly glipizide is the safest sulfonylurea to use in the setting of reduced GFR.

The thiazolidinediones are not renally excreted and most likely are beneficial in terms of reducing AER. They need to be used with caution in people with CKD because they also promote fluid retention. The dipeptidyl peptidase (DPP)-4 inhibitor, linagliptin is the only currently available member of this drug class that does not undergo significant renal excretion. Current evidence suggests that it can safely be used in people with diabetes and a severe decrease in GFR or even in those with ESRD. The use of acarbose is not endorsed for people with reduced renal function. The handling of insulin by the kidneys is also altered because, as renal function declines, a reduction in insulin doses is sometimes required to avoid hypoglycaemia. One of the new glucagon-like peptide (GLP)-1 analogues, exenatide, is renally excreted and is not approved for use in people with GFR <30 ml/min per $1.73\,m^2$. However, another medication of this class, liraglutide, is not renally excreted and is most probably safe to use in patients with low GFR.

RAS blockade

In patients with diabetes, activation of intrarenal RAS produces haemodynamic and non-haemodynamic effects that contribute to the development and progression of diabetic CKD. There is now good evidence to suggest that interrupting the renin–angiotensin system with an angiotensin-converting enzyme (ACE) inhibitor or an angiotensin receptor blocker (ARB) results in renal and CV protective effects, over and above those observed by BP lowering alone. In a landmark trial, Lewis et al. demonstrated that the ACE inhibitor captopril reduced the risk of achieving the combined endpoint of death, dialysis and transplantation, compared with BP control alone achieved with non-RAS-blocking agents in individuals with type 1 diabetes and advanced nephropathy (macroalbuminuria).[13] In another important study, captopril significantly reduced the progression from micro- to macroalbuminuria and prevented an increase in AER in patients with type 1 diabetes.[14] A subsequent systematic review of the effects of ACE inhibition in patients traditionally classified as normotensive, who also had microalbuminuria, has been performed.[15] It concluded that use of ACE inhibitors significantly reduced the progression to macroalbuminuria and increased the chances of remission to normoalbuminuria. The beneficial effects of ACE inhibitors were observed to be weakest at the lowest levels of microalbuminuria, but did not differ according to other baseline risk factors.

For individuals with type 2 diabetes both ACE inhibitors and the use of an ARB have been shown to reduce urinary albumin excretion and CV events for individuals with microalbuminuria. Slowing of the progression to ESRD in individuals with type 2 diabetes, hypertension and macroalbuminuria has been shown in clinical trials comparing the use of an ARB with placebo, superimposed on background antihypertensive therapy.

Dual blockade of the RAS with an ACE inhibitor and ARB in individuals with type 2 diabetes and microalbuminuria has been demonstrated to be more effective in reducing BP and decreasing albuminuria than either agent as monotherapy.[16] However, the recent ONgoing Telmisartan Alone and in combination with Ramipril Global Endpoint Trial (ONTARGET), involving patients at high risk of vascular disease, with most not having diabetes or renal dysfunction, showed that combination therapy was not superior to ACE inhibition alone with regard to CV and renal outcomes.[17] Indeed, combination therapy was associated with an increased risk of adverse renal outcomes, mainly acute dialysis. Regardless of these findings, the effectiveness of combining an ACE inhibitor and an ARB remains unclear in the setting of established diabetic CKD with proteinuria, and this is currently being evaluated in clinical trials. The combination of an ACE inhibitor and ARB is generally not advised, but can still be considered a therapeutic option in patients with progressive albuminuria in the macroalbuminuric range or in patients with refractory hypertension (>160/100 mmHg).

Combining an ACE inhibitor with a diuretic or a calcium-channel blocker may also produce greater reductions in AER than monotherapy with an ACE inhibitor. The renal and CV outcomes seen with these combinations are discussed below. In addition, salt restriction potentiates the effects of interruption of the RAS in reducing albuminuria in hypertensive individuals with type 2 diabetes.[18]

The use of ACE inhibitors or ARBs in patients with diabetic CKD is associated with an initial fall in GFR due to a reduction in glomerular capillary pressure. This results in an elevation in serum creatinine up to 35 per cent above baseline, which then stabilizes in the first 2–4 months of therapy. This early limited acute rise in serum creatinine after the initiation of RAS blockers is reversible and associated with long-term preservation of kidney function. Hyperkalaemia can also occur after the initiation of RAS-blocking agents. It is recommended that both serum creatinine and potassium levels be measured approximately 1 week after the initiation of RAS-blocking agents. This recommendation needs to be tailored according to a patient's baseline GFR.

Novel therapies

Despite the availability of current therapies that target the renin–angiotensin system, people with diabetic CKD still progress to ESRD.

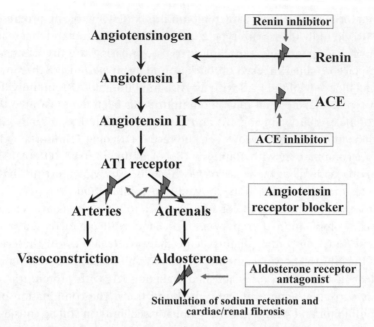

Figure 2.4 Potential sites for blocking the renin–angiotensin system.

Commonly used strategies that are based on RAS blockage are only partially effective because the use of ACE inhibitors or ARBs interferes with negative feedback mechanisms, resulting in a reactive increase in renin activity. One potentially novel renoprotective approach involving RAS blockade is to directly inhibit the action of renin and hence the conversion of angiotensinogen to angiotensin I (Figure 2.4). In the Aliskiren in the Evaluation of Proteinuria in Diabetes (AVOID) clinical trial, the oral direct renin inhibitor, aliskiren, reduced ACR in overtly proteinuric individuals with type 2 diabetes who were already receiving maximal recommended doses of an ACE inhibitor.[19] There was a small reduction in BP with aliskiren (2/1 mmHg), but the authors of the study concluded that the beneficial effects on albuminuria were independent of BP changes. Furthermore, adverse events, including hyperkalaemia, were similar in patients taking an ACE inhibitor who were then randomized to aliskiren or placebo therapy. However, it should be noted that participants in that study, although having overt proteinuria, still had relatively well-preserved renal function with a mean eGFR of 67 ml/min per 1.73 m². This promising intervention has yet to be shown to improve clinical outcomes.

Recently, paricalcitol, a vitamin D receptor activator, has been shown to reduce albuminuria in individuals with type 2 diabetes and ACR levels in the macroalbuminuric range without an increased incidence of hypercalcaemia or other serious adverse events.[20] Whether vitamin D activation treatment results in a preservation of GFR has yet to be tested in clinical trials. The potential benefits of vitamin D are most probably the result of an interaction with multiple pathways that promote the development and progression of renal dysfunction, including the renin–angiotensin system. In contrast, other vitamins, such as vitamin B complexes (containing folic acid, vitamin B_6 and vitamin B_{12}), have been shown to have no effect on proteinuria and to cause a significant decline in GFR compared with placebo-treated individuals. Benfotiamine also does not appear to have any effect on reducing urinary albumin excretion in patients with type 2 diabetes. Other agents such as endothelin antagonists reduce albuminuria but appear to have an unacceptable side-effect profile to allow their use in clinical practice.

Protein restriction

Although the American Diabetes Association guidelines for the management of diabetic CKD recommends a protein intake of 0.8 g/kg per day in individuals with overt nephropathy, it should be remembered that it is extremely difficult to get patients to follow a long-term low-protein diet.

Anaemia correction

Anaemia is common in patients with diabetes and is emerging as a potential risk factor for the progression of diabetic CKD. However, evidence has emerged from randomized controlled trials that correcting anaemia with an erythropoiesis-stimulating agent (ESA) in patients with diabetes and CKD before dialysis and targeting a haemoglobin level of 130 g/l is associated with an increased risk of serious adverse outcomes with no evidence of any beneficial effect. Therefore, treatment of anaemia in individuals with diabetes, and predialysis CKD, with ESAs is generally not recommended. However, it still may be reasonable to consider treatment with an ESA if Hb <100 g/l, and targeting levels of 100–120 g/l. It is important that patients are screened for other reversible causes of anaemia, such as iron deficiency, and treated appropriately.

Aspirin

Currently there is uncertainty about the universal use of aspirin for the prevention of CV events among patients with diabetes. An ongoing trial should help to clarify this situation. However, given the increased CV risk that CKD confers on individuals with diabetes it is reasonable to consider aspirin for the primary prevention of CVD in people with diabetes and CKD. Clopidogrel does not appear to be a suitable alternative antiplatelet drug for these individuals.

Lifestyle factors

Obesity in itself is associated with the development of a specific form of focal segmental glomerulosclerosis that is characterized by massive proteinuria and glomerular lesions. The pathophysiology of this condition includes insulin resistance, hypertension, adiponectin deficiency and hyperaldosteronism. It is possible that this condition could contribute to the development of proteinuria in obese people with diabetes. There is some evidence that weight loss reduces proteinuria and stabilizes progression of CKD in people with and without diabetes. Weight loss in all people with diabetic CKD should be encouraged and promoted through the use of diets low in calories, fat and salt. As shown in the case report weight loss achieved with bariatric surgery can be associated with a significant reduction in albuminuria and blood pressure.

Several observational studies have documented an association between smoking and diabetic CKD. However, no studies have assessed the renal effects of smoking cessation. In particular, smoking appears to promote the initiation of microalbuminuria and the subsequent transition to macroalbuminuria. There is some evidence to suggest that cessation of smoking retards the progression of diabetic CKD in type 1 diabetes. A similar effect is likely for individuals with type 2 diabetes. Smoking is already an established risk factor for CVD and may possibly also play a role in the onset and progression of diabetic CKD. Even though there is a lack of definitive interventional studies for smoking, the above evidence provides a strong rationale for the inclusion of smoking cessation in the management of individuals with type 2 diabetes and CKD.

When to refer to a nephrologist

In general, individuals with a GFR <30 ml/min per $1.73\,m^2$ should be referred to a nephrologist in preparation for the start of renal replacement therapy. Other situations when it may be appropriate to refer include the finding of nephritic range proteinuria, an unexplained decline in eGFR of >20 ml/min per $1.73\,m^2$ from one review to the next, haemoglobin levels <10 g/dl when other causes of anaemia are excluded, and the detection of abnormalities of bone metabolism, when there are difficulties in achieving BP targets or when the diagnosis of the underlying cause for CKD is unclear.

Prevention, screening and monitoring

Prevention

Diabetic CKD does not occur in the absence of hyperglycaemia, so preventing the transition from normal glucose tolerance to diabetes is the ultimate means of preventing the development of this complication. Studies investigating the prevention of diabetic CKD have mainly focused on the development of microalbuminuria. However, attention is also being placed on the concept of trying to prevent an early decline in GFR (before reaching 60 ml/min per 1.73 m^2). Very good BP control appears to be an important factor in preventing the development of microalbuminuria in type 2 diabetes. Recent studies have also investigated the role of RAS-blocking agents in preventing the development of microalbuminuria.

ACE inhibitors attenuate the progression from normoalbuminuria to microalbuminuria in individuals with type 2 diabetes and hypertension. However, the ARB, losartan, or the ACE inhibitor, enalapril, did not reduce the 5-year cumulative incidence of microalbuminuria compared with placebo treatment in normotensive individuals with type 1 diabetes. Furthermore, the use of RAS-blocking agents did not slow the development of early renal ultrastructural characteristic of diabetic nephropathy.[21] Possibly, there has to be sufficient intrarenal RAS activation, in hypertensive patients or those with late nephropathy, before the benefits of blocking the renin–angiotensin system become apparent.

Screening and monitoring

Screening patients at risk for diabetic CKD usually involves testing for the presence of persistent microalbuminuria and estimating the GFR. Laboratory-based screening for microalbuminuria can be achieved in a number of ways:

- A 24-hour urine collection for the estimation of AER, accepted as the gold standard with the added advantage of allowing for the estimation of creatinine clearance
- A spot urine collection for the estimation of the ACR
- A timed 4-hour or overnight collection for the estimation of AER.

Alternatively, screening for microalbuminuria can be performed on spot or early morning urine samples using point-of-care testing or special reagent strips. However, these approaches can usually measure only urinary albumin concentration and sometimes the result is only semi-quantitative. There is therefore also no adjustment for urinary creatinine levels to account for variations in urinary concentration. If a positive result for microalbuminuria is found using the above methods, it is recommended that a confirmation test measuring ACR or AER be ordered.

The reference ranges of albuminuria for AER and ACR 24-h urine collections and spot urine samples for ACR are shown in Table 2.1. At least two out of three consecutive estimations of albuminuria should fall into the microalbuminuric range before a diagnosis of persistent microalbuminuria is made. Increases in albuminuria into the microalbuminuric range may occur transiently with exercise, urinary tract infection, uncontrolled hyperglycaemia and cardiac failure.[22] Potential sources of 'false positives' when measuring microalbuminuria are as follows:

- Exercise
- Acute fluid intake
- Haematuria
- Menstrual flow
- Urinary infection
- Renal papillary necrosis
- Semen.

In individuals with type 1 diabetes, it is recommended that screening for microalbuminuria start approximately 5 years after diagnosis, because the development of diabetic complications is rare before this time. In contrast, given that approximately 20 per cent of people newly diagnosed with type 2 diabetes have microalbuminuria, it is recommended that all those with type 2 diabetes be screened at the time of diagnosis. An algorithm for screening for microalbuminuria is shown in Figure 2.5.

Current gold standard methods for determining GFR, employing the clearance of radioisotopes or non-radiolabelled markers, are time-consuming and expensive, and thus not easily adaptable to routine clinical practice. Therefore, creatinine has been used as an endogenous marker of GFR for many decades. Unfortunately, the influence of non-renal factors on serum creatinine levels, including age, gender, ethnicity, muscle mass

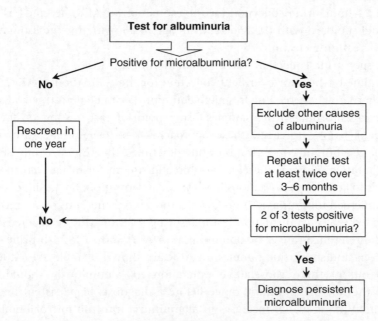

Figure 2.5 Screening strategy for microalbuminuria.

and dietary protein intake, limit its usefulness as a marker of GFR. To overcome the limitations of using creatinine alone, equations to estimate GFR based on serum creatinine have been developed that include variables such as age, sex, race and measurements of body size, i.e. the modification of diet in renal disease (MDRD) equation.[23]

Recently, studies have highlighted the limitations of existing creatinine-based methods for estimating renal function in diabetes. In summary, for patients with a GFR in the normal or hyperfiltering range, GFR is grossly underestimated by the MDRD formula by approximately 10–40 ml/min per 1.73 m^2. To overcome the limitations of the MDRD equation, a new creatinine-based formula, based on the original variables used in the MDRD formula, has been devised to improve estimation of GFR in individuals with a GFR >60 ml/min per 1.73 m^2, i.e. the Chronic Kidney Disease Epidemiology Collaboration (CKD-EPI) equation.[24] However, it should be noted that the CKD-EPI equation has yet to be rigorously tested in individuals with diabetes with high–normal GFR levels. In contrast, recent studies have suggested that estimates of GFR based on serum cystatin C levels provide a simple and accurate method for detecting and monitoring an early decline in renal function. Although cystatin C is well established as a research tool, it has yet to make the transition to use in routine clinical practice.

Once the urinary albumin threshold for microalbuminuria has been reached, AER or ACR should be measured every 3–6 months. A measurement of serum creatine to allow for automatic reporting of an eGFR should also be made very 3–6 months. However, as discussed above, existing methods for eGFR measurement are robust only below a threshold of 60 ml/min per 1.73 m^2. The implication is that approximately half of total kidney filtration rate can be lost before it is possible to detect a decline in renal function using current clinical paramenters.

Risk factor management

This section focuses on the management of the modifiable risk factors associated with the development and progression of diabetic CKD: hyperglycaemia, hypertension and dyslipidaemia.

Hyperglycaemia

Diabetic CKD does not occur in the absence of hyperglycaemia and glycaemic control is the main determinant of the onset of nephropathy. The DCCT in type 1 diabetes and the UKPDS in type 2 diabetes have demonstrated the strong relationship between glycaemic control and the risk of the development of diabetic microvascular complications without a clear-cut HbA1c threshold. In the DCCT, development of microalbuminuria was reduced by 34 per cent and macroalbuminuria by 56 per cent via achieving tight glycaemic control (HbA1c <7.0%).[25] An interventional analysis of the UKPDS[26] demonstrated that reducing mean HbA1c levels from 7.9 per cent to 7.0 per cent was associated with an absolute risk reduction of developing overt nephropathy of 11 per cent over 12 years and a risk reduction of 30 per cent for the transition from normo- to microalbuminuria in type 2 diabetes.

Recently, the Action in Diabetes and Vascular Disease: Preterax and Diamicron-MR-controlled evaluation (ADVANCE) study examined the effects of tight glycaemic control on renal events in 5571 patients with type 2 diabetes.[27] Patients were randomized to intensive glycaemic control, achieving a HbA1c of 6.5 per cent, or standard glycaemic control, achieving a HbA1c of 7.3 per cent. After a mean follow-up of 5 years the total number of renal events was reduced by 11 per cent (26.9% vs 30%) in patients randomized to intensive versus standard glycaemic control. The incidence of new microalbuminuria was reduced by 9 per cent with intensive therapy, occurring in 23.7 per cent of patients in that group compared with 25.7 per cent in the standard treatment arm. New-onset macroalbuminuria was reduced by 30 per cent (2.9% in the intensive glycaemic vs 4.1% in the standard glycaemic arm). New or worsening nephropathy, defined as progression of albuminuria by at least one stage (from normoalbuminuria to either micro- or macroalbuminuria) was 21 per cent lower with intensive therapy. Progression to ESRD was also reduced with intensive glycaemic control versus standard glycaemic control (0.4% vs 0.6%). However, the difference in this end-point failed to reach statistical significance. For patients who had micro- or macroalbuminuria at baseline, remission to normoalbuminuria occurred in 57 per cent of patients treated with intensive glycaemic control compared with 15 per cent of patients in the standard control group.

Similarly, in the Action to Control Cardiovascular Risk Diabetes (ACCORD) trial, intensive glycaemic control resulted in a 21 per cent reduction in the development of microalbuminuria and a 32 per cent reduction in the development of macroalbuminuria.[28] In the ACCORD study, tight glycaemic control achieved a median HbA1c of 6.3 versus 7.6 per cent in the standard glucose control group. The randomized trial was discontinued after 3.7 years due to excess mortality in the intensive glycaemic arm, but all participants continued to be followed for a total of 5 years. At the end of 5 years HbA1c levels were 7.2 per cent in patients originally randomized to intensive glycaemic control versus 7.6 per cent in patients originally randomized to conventional glycaemic control. At the end of 5 years, the results were similar to those seen at the end of randomization, with incident microalbuminuria being reduced by 15 per cent and incident macroalbuminuria by 29 per cent. At the end of the interventional phase of the ACCORD trial, an increase was noted in the composite outcome of doubling of serum creatinine or a 20 ml/min per 1.73 m^2 decrease was noted in eGFR with intensive glycaemic control. The authors attributed this finding to a resolution of hyperfiltration with intensive glycaemic control. However, it is unlikely that resolution of hyperfiltration as such explains a doubling of creatinine, because this would require a drop in GFR from >130 ml/min per 1.73 m^2 (the threshold for hyperfiltration) to a final GFR of <65 ml/min per 1.73 m^2.

Once the stage of overt proteinuria or ESRD has been reached, it is controversial whether improving glycaemic control further retards the progression of renal failure in diabetes. Possibly a HbA1c of 6.5 per cent should be the general target for the prevention of diabetic CKD, whereas in advanced CKD a higher target could be accepted according to the clinical context. Regardless of the above, it is also important to individualize HbA1c targets, taking into account a patients age, comorbidities, risk for hypoglycaemia and the type of glucose-lowering agents prescribed.

Hypertension

In individuals with type 1 diabetes, high BP is usually due to underlying diabetic renal disease and typically BP only starts to increase around the time of transition from micro- to macroalbuminuria. In contrast, hypertension may be detected in approximately a third of patients with type 2 diabetes at the time of diagnosis. In this setting the aetiology of hypertension is most probably multifactorial and possibly represents a component of the metabolic syndrome. Regardless of the sequence or underlying causes of hypertension in type 1 and type 2 diabetes, many studies have demonstrated that high BP accelerates the progression of diabetic CKD and that aggressive BP lowering slows the deterioration in renal function.

In general, the BP target for people with diabetes should be <130/80 mmHg. If persistent proteinuria is present, a more stringent target of <120/75 mmHg is recommended. Some experts, such as Parving, have suggested that the optimal BP for patients with diabetes, especially those with proteinuria, is a presyncopal BP. As discussed below, antihypertensive medications that interrupt the RAS appear to have renal protective effects over and above those expected from BP-lowering effects alone. However, achieving BP goals commonly requires the combination of three to four different antihypertensive medications, especially in patients with type 2 diabetes. People with diabetes, especially those with renal disease, are also at higher risk of CVD, so achieving BP targets offers both renal and CVD protection. It is recommended that initial antihypertensive therapy be commenced with an agent that inhibits the RAS. As discussed below diuretics and calcium-channel blockers are useful second agents in patients with diabetic CKD. The choice of antihypertensive agents will depend to some extent on the patient's clinical circumstances, because these may preclude certain drug combinations (e.g. the combination of β blockers and non-dihydropyridine calcium-channel blockers), or dictate the early introduction of specific antihypertensive agents.

In the Avoiding Cardiovascular Events in Combination Therapy in Patients Living with Systolic Hypertension (ACCOMPLISH) study, 11506 patients (60% with diabetes) received treatment with the ACE inhibitor benazepril combined with either the thiazide diuretic hydrochlorothiazide (HCT) or amlodipine.[29] The differences in systolic BP between the two combinations was <1 mmHg over the trial period and the use of both BP-lowering combinations achieved excellent BP control, 132/73 mmHg for the benazepril and amlodipine group and 133/74 mmHg in the benazepril and HCT group.

The trial was terminated early at 36 months, because the benazepril and amlodipine combination was found to be superior to the benazepril and HCT combination in reducing the primary composite end-point of CV events and death. Furthermore, the benazepril and amlodipine combination resulted in significantly fewer patients achieving the renal end-point of doubling of serum creatinine concentration or the development of ESRD. However, it is worth noting that for participants with diabetes and CKD in the ACCOMPLISH study, the renal outcomes and death from CV causes was similar in both treatment arms of the study.[30]

The effects of BP lowering on renal outcomes have been studied in detail by the ADVANCE investigators.[31] In that study approximately 5000 participants were randomized to receive perindopril and indapamide or placebo, in addition to other antihypertensive agents. Participants treated with perindopril and indapamide achieved BP levels of 135/75 mmHg, whereas those receiving placebo achieved BP levels of 140/77 mmHg. The composite primary renal microvascular outcomes in that study included the development of macroalbuminuria, the doubling of serum creatinine to a level of >200 μmol/l, requirement for renal replacement therapy or death from renal disease over 5 years. Secondary renal outcomes included the separate components of the combined renal primary end-point, the development of new microalbuminuria, and progression or regression of micro- (30–300 μg/mg) or macroalbuminuria (>300 μg/mg).

Treatment with perindopril and indapamide resulted in a relative reduction in total renal events by 21 per cent ($p < 0.0001$) when compared with placebo over the 4.3 years of the trial. The event rate of the individual components of the primary renal outcome was not separately reduced, but there was an 18 per cent reduction in new or worsening macroalbuminuria that just failed to reach significance ($p = 0.055$). In contrast, there was a highly significant 21 per cent reduction in the development of new-onset microalbuminuria with active treatment ($p < 0.0001$).

The ACCORD–BP study is one of the few randomized clinical trials to achieve BP levels below the recommended thresholds of 130/80 mmHg for people with diabetes.[32] In that study, 4733 participants with type 2 diabetes were randomly assigned to intensive BP-lowering therapy, targeting a systolic BP of <120 mmHg, or standard therapy, targeting a systolic BP of <140 mmHg. The primary composite outcome was non-fatal myocardial infarction, non-fatal stroke or death from CV causes. The mean follow-up was 4.7 years. After 1 year of the trial, the mean systolic BP was 119 mmHg in the intensive therapy group and 134 mmHg in the standard therapy group. The annual rate of the primary outcome was 1.87 per cent in the intensive therapy group and 2.09 per cent in the standard therapy group, a non-significant difference. The mean eGFR rates were significantly lower in the intensive therapy group at the last study visit. There were also significantly more instances of an eGFR <30 ml/min per 1.73 m^2 in the intensive therapy group (99 vs 52 events, $p < 0.001$). The frequency of macro- but not microalbuminuria at the end of the study was significantly lower in the intensive therapy group, and there was no between-group difference in the frequency of ESRD.

Although observation studies suggest a continuous relationship between BP levels and renal and CV events in people with diabetes, very few interventional studies have achieved BP levels below the recommended thresholds of 130/80 mmHg. The results of both the ACCORD-BP trial and INternational VErapamil SR Trandolapril Study (INVEST), which have attained BP levels of <130/80 mmHg, suggest that lowering BP levels below these levels has little impact on reducing clinical events below those seen with moderate BP control equivalent to approximately 135/85 mmHg.[33]

Ambulatory blood pressure monitoring (ABPM) provides measurements of several variables that are of potential value in estimating the risk of clinical outcomes in diabetes. These include an estimate of 'true' BP levels and the identification of the 'white-coat' effect, measurement of the diurnal rhythm of BP that allows patients to be classified into nocturnal 'dippers' and 'non-dippers' (reduction in BP <10%), and the recording of BP random variability and ambulatory heart rate. However, it should be noted that the clinical trial information presented above has been based on clinical BP recordings.

Dyslipidaemia

Several cross-sectional and prospective studies have shown associations between dyslipoproteinaemia, specifically elevation in apolipoprotein B (apoB)-100 containing lipoproteins and low high-density lipoprotein (HDL), and albuminuria in individuals with diabetes.[34,35] A sub-study from the Collaborative Atorvastatin Diabetes Study (CARDS) showed that, over approximately 4 years, atorvastatin ameliorated the expected decline in eGFR in patients with elevated levels of urinary albumin (net improvement of 0.38 ml/min per 1.73 m^2 per year, $p = 0.03$) compared with placebo treatment.[36] Similar effects have not been observed in interventional studies involving participants with type 1 diabetes. It is important to emphasize that intensive treatment of dyslipidaemia in people with diabetes should be considered not only to ameliorate renal injury but also to avoid CV complications.[37] To date there is no evidence to suggest that statins reduce CV events in people who have already developed ESRD. However, the Study of Heart And Renal Protection (SHARP) showed that the combination of simvastatin and ezetimibe decreased total CV events in patients with CKD, some of whom had diabetes (approximately 25% of the study population). Statin doses do not generally need to be altered as GFR starts to decline, although there may be increased risk of myopathy with all statins with more advanced CKD; lowering the dose of the statin and adding ezetimibe may allow low-density lipoprotein (LDL)-cholesterol and apo B targets to be achieved with reduced risk of musculoskeletal side effects.

In the Fenofibrate Intervention and Event Lowering in Diabetes (FIELD) and ACCORD studies, the use of fenofibrate was shown to reduce albuminuria.[38,39] A further analysis of the FIELD study has shown that fenofibrate causes an acute but sustained plasma creatinine increase which does not reflect changes in true GFR.[40] At the end of the interventional phase of the FIELD study, plasma creatinine levels were re-measured 8 weeks after treatment cessation. After this washout period, eGFR had fallen less from baseline for patients treated with fenofibrate (1.9 ml/min per 1.73 m^2) than for those on placebo treatment (6.9 ml/min per 1.73 m^2), sparing 5.0 ml/mim/1.73 m^2 of GFR ($p < 0.001$). Greater preservation of eGFR with fenofibrate was observed in patients with baseline hypertriglyceridaemia alone or when combined with a low HDL-cholesterol level. Furthermore, fenofibrate reduced urinary ACR by 24 per cent versus 11 per cent with placebo treatment ($p < 0.001$). There was 14 per cent less progression and 18 per cent more regression of albuminuria in fenofibrate-compared with placebo-treated patients ($p < 0.001$). However, ESRD event frequency was similar for fenofibrate- and placebo-treated patients ($n = 21$ vs 26, $p = 0.48$). The FIELD investigators interpreted these findings to mean that use of fenofibrate is associated with a reduction in albuminuria and a slowing in eGFR decline despite initial and reversible increases in plasma creatinine.

Both the FIELD and the ACCORD lipid studies show that fenofibrate slows the progression of diabetic retinopathy.[41] The mechanisms by which fenofibrate exerts this beneficial effect on albuminuria, eGFR and the diabetic eye are still unknown. Fibrates are renally excreted and, in patients with CKD, the dose of fibrate should be decreased to reduce the risk of severe myopathy and rhabdomyolysis, especially when used in combination with statins. However, it should be noted that the risk of myositis is higher with gemfibrozil compared with fenofibrate use.

2.5 Conclusion

In summary, screening people with diabetes for early markers of diabetic CKD and initiation of measures to retard the progression of renal dysfunction are now considered part of routine clinical practice. In addition it is necessary to measure, assess and manage CV risk factors aggressively. We recommend that annual screening for microalbuminuria and the measurement of eGFR be performed in people who have had type 1 diabetes for at least 5 years and in those with type 2 diabetes starting at the time of diagnosis. In particular, the finding of microalbuminuria and/or a reduced eGFR should be a mandate for intensifying treatment of the common risk factors for renal disease and CVD, i.e. hyperglycaemia, hypertension, dyslipidaemia and smoking.

Case study

A 47-year-old white woman has had diabetes and microalbuminuria but a normal eGFR since 1998, when she was 155 cm tall and weighed 93 kg (body mass index [BMI] 39 kg/m²). She was given lifestyle and dietary advice and then treated with a combination of sulfonylurea and metformin from 1998 to 1999. Thereafter, twice daily premixed insulin and metformin were used because of poor glycaemic control. Her blood pressure (BP).which had risen to 150/90 mmHg, was treated with a dihydropyridine calcium channel blocker from 2000 and in combination with an ACE inhibitor from 2001 onwards. After starting an ACE inhibitor her eGFR decreased transiently from 90 ml/min per 1.73 m² to 75 ml/min per 1.73 m², but then stabilized and increased 3 months later to 80 ml/min per 1.73 m². Her lipid profile consisted of an elevated low-density lipoprotein (LDL)-cholesterol level of 3.5 mmol/l (<2.5 mmol/l), a low HDL-cholesterol level of 0.9 mmol/l (>1.0 mmol/l) and an elevated triglyceride level of 2.7 mmol/l (<1.5 mmol/l). She was commenced on a statin. Because of inadequate glycaemic control and weight gain, gastric stapling was performed in August 2002.

Serial measurements of albumin excretion rate (AER), eGFR, systolic, body weight and glycated haemoglobin (HbA1c) are shown in Figure 2.6. The horizontal interrupted lines represent the

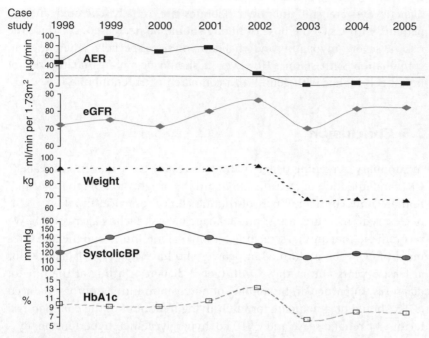

Figure 2.6 Case study: serial measurements of albumin excretion rate (AER), estimated glomerular filtration rate (eGFR), systolic, body weight and glycated haemoglobin (HbA1c). The horizontal interrupted lines represent the targets or thresholds for normoalbuminuria (AER <20 μg/min), normal range GFR (70–120 ml/ min per 1.73 m², shown as a shaded area), systolic BP (BP <130 mmHg) and good glycaemic control (HbA1c <7.0%).

targets for normoalbuminuria (AER <20 μg/min), normal range GFR (70–120 ml/min per 1.73 m², shown as a shaded area), systolic BP (<130 mmHg) and good glycaemic control (HbA1c <7.0%). The following changes were documented for 12 months after August 2002:

Weight loss of 25 kg

HbA1c decline from 13.5% to <7.0%

BP decline of 10/5 mmHg, to <130/80 mmHg

AER decline from >70 μg/min to <20 μg/min (from micro- to normoalbuminuria)

The eGFR remained within the normal range.

Triglyceride/HDL-cholesterol abnormalities should correct with sustained weight loss.

Questions

1. Which two interventions reduced the level of albuminuria?

Answer: transient decrease after starting ACE inhibitors in late 2001 and long-term reduction after gastric stapling in late 2002.

2. What is the most likely explanation for the overall improvement in Rosemary's therapeutic indices?
Answer: weight loss after gastric stapling.

3. What is the likely pathogenetic explanation for Rosemary's response to gastric stapling?
Answer: weight loss leading to improved insulin sensitivity which promoted improved glycaemic and blood pressure control.

3. In retrospect, what were the least effective interventions in this patient?
Answer: Dietary advice for weight loss and exercise. Dihydropyridine calcium channel blockade to reduce her levels of microalbuminuria.

4. Why did her eGFR decrease after starting an ACE inhibitor and what is the significance of this decrease?
Answer: the initiation of an ACE inhibitor or an angiotensin receptor blocker decreases intraglomerular pressure and hence GFR. This decrease in GFR is associated with a good long-term prognosis in terms of preservation of renal function.

5. Why was she started on a statin when she has a normal lipid profile?
Answer: patients with diabetes and microalbuminuria are at an exaggerated risk for cardiovascular disease. It is recommended that all patients with microalbuminuria be treated with a statin, if tolerated.

References

1. Watts GF, Jasik M, Cooper ME. The implications of the detection of proteinuria and microalbuminuria in insulin and non-insulin dependent diabetes. *Aust N Z J Med* 1995;**25**:157–161.
2. Caramori ML, Fioretto P, Mauer M. The need for early predictors of diabetic nephropathy risk: is albumin excretion rate sufficient? *Diabetes* 2000;**49**:1399–1408.
3. MacIsaac RJ, Jerums G, Cooper ME. New insights into the significance of microalbuminuria. *Curr Opin Nephrol Hypertens* 2004;**13**:83–91.
4. Molitch ME, Steffes M, Sun W, et al. Development and progression of renal insufficiency with and without albuminuria in adults with type 1 diabetes in the diabetes control and complications trial and the epidemiology of diabetes interventions and complications study. *Diabetes Care* 2010;**33**:1536–1543.
5. Retnakaran R, Cull CA, Thorne KI, et al. Risk factors for renal dysfunction in type 2 diabetes: U.K. Prospective Diabetes Study 74. *Diabetes* 2006;**55**:1832–1839.

6. Mogensen CE. Microalbuminuria, blood pressure and diabetic renal disease: origin and development of ideas. *Diabetologia* 1999;**42**:263–285.

7. Jerums G, Premaratne E, Panagiotopoulos S, et al. New and old markers of progression of diabetic nephropathy. *Diabetes Res Clin Pract* 2008;**82**:S30–S37.

8. Jerums G, Panagiotopoulos S, Premaratne E, et al. Integrating albuminuria and GFR in the assessment of diabetic nephropathy. *Nat Rev Nephrol* 2009;**5**:397–406.

9. Seaquist ER, Goetz FC, Rich S, et al. Familial clustering of diabetic kidney disease. Evidence for genetic susceptibility to diabetic nephropathy. *N Engl J Med* 1989;**320**:1161–1165.

10. Fioretto P, Mauer M, Brocco E, et al. Patterns of renal injury in NIDDM patients with microalbuminuria. *Diabetologia* 1996;**39**:1569–1576.

11. Gaede P, Vedel P, Larsen N, et al. Multifactorial intervention and cardiovascular disease in patients with type 2 diabetes. *N Engl J Med* 2003;**348**:383–393.

12. Gaede P, Lund-Andersen H, Parving HH, et al. Effect of a multifactorial intervention on mortality in type 2 diabetes. *N Engl J Med* 2008;**358**:580–591.

13. Lewis EJ, Hunsicker LG, Bain RP, et al. The effect of angiotensin-converting-enzyme inhibition on diabetic nephropathy. The Collaborative Study Group. *N Engl J Med* 1993;**329**:1456–1462.

14. Viberti G, Mogensen CE, Groop LC, et al. Effect of captopril on progression to clinical proteinuria in patients with insulin-dependent diabetes mellitus and microalbuminuria. European Microalbuminuria Captopril Study Group. *JAMA* 1994;**271**:275–279.

15. ACE Inhibitors in Diabetic Nephropathy Trialist Group. Should all patients with type 1 diabetes mellitus and microalbuminuria receive angiotensin-converting enzyme inhibitors? A meta-analysis of individual patient data. *Ann Intern Med* 2001;**134**:370–379.

16. Mogensen CE, Neldam S, Tikkanen I, et al. Randomised controlled trial of dual blockade of renin-angiotensin system in patients with hypertension, microalbuminuria, and non-insulin dependent diabetes: the candesartan and lisinopril microalbuminuria (CALM) study. *BMJ* 2000;**321**:1440–144.

17. ONTARGET Investigators, Yusuf S, Teo KK, et al. Telmisartan, ramipril, or both in patients at high risk for vascular events. *N Engl J Med* 2008;**358**:1547–1559.

18. Ekinci EI, Thomas G, Thomas D, et al. Effects of salt supplementation on the albuminuric response to telmisartan with or without hydrochlorothiazide therapy in hypertensive patients with type 2 diabetes are modulated by habitual dietary salt intake. *Diabet Care* 2009;**32**:1398–1403.

19. Parving HH, Persson F, Lewis JB, et al. Aliskiren combined with losartan in type 2 diabetes and nephropathy. *N Engl J Med* 2008;**358**:2433–2446.

20. de Zeeuw D, Agarwal R, Amdahl M, et al. Selective vitamin D receptor activation with paricalcitol for reduction of albuminuria in patients with type 2 diabetes (VITAL study): a randomised controlled trial. *Lancet* 2010;**376**:1543–1551.

21. Mauer M, Zinman B, Gardiner R, et al. Renal and retinal effects of enalapril and losartan in type 1 diabetes. *N Engl J Med* 2009;**361**:40–51.

22. Watts GF, Kubal C, Chinn S. Long-term variation of urinary albumin excretion in insulin-dependent diabetes mellitus: some practical recommendations for monitoring microalbuminuria. *Diabetes Res Clin Pract* 1990;**9**:169–177.

23. Stevens LA, Coresh J, Greene T, et al. Assessing kidney function – measured and estimated glomerular filtration rate. *N Engl J Med* 2006;**354**:2473–2483.

24. Stevens LA, Schmid CH, Greene T, et al. Comparative performance of the CKD Epidemiology Collaboration (CKD-EPI) and the Modification of Diet in Renal Disease (MDRD) Study equations for estimating GFR levels above 60 mL/min per 1.73 m². *Am J Kidney Dis* 2010;**56**:486–495.

25. The effect of intensive treatment of diabetes on the development and progression of long-term complications in insulin-dependent diabetes mellitus. The Diabetes Control and Complications Trial Research Group. *N Engl J Med* 1993;**329**:977–986.

26. UKPDS 33. Intensive blood-glucose control with sulphonylureas or insulin compared with conventional treatment and risk of complications in patients with type 2 diabetes (UKPDS 33). UK Prospective Diabetes Study (UKPDS) Group. *Lancet* 1998;**352**:837–353.

27. ADVANCE Collaborative Group, Patel A, MacMahon S, et al. Intensive blood glucose control and vascular outcomes in patients with type 2 diabetes. *N Engl J Med* 2008;**358**:2560–2572.

28. Ismail-Beigi F, Craven T, Banerji MA, et al. Effect of intensive treatment of hyperglycaemia on microvascular outcomes in type 2 diabetes: an analysis of the ACCORD randomised trial. *Lancet* 2010;**376**:419–330.

29. Jamerson K, Weber MA, Bakris GL, et al. Benazepril plus amlodipine or hydrochlorothiazide for hypertension in high-risk patients. *N Engl J Med* 2008;**359**: 2417–2428.

30. Bakris GL, Sarafidis PA, Weir MR, et al. Renal outcomes with different fixed-dose combination therapies in patients with hypertension at high risk for cardiovascular events (ACCOMPLISH): a prespecified secondary analysis of a randomised controlled trial. *Lancet* 2010;**375**:1173–1181.

31. Patel A, ADVANCE Collaborative Group, MacMahon S, et al. Effects of a fixed combination of perindopril and indapamide on macrovascular and microvascular outcomes in patients with type 2 diabetes mellitus (the ADVANCE trial): a randomised controlled trial. *Lancet* 2007;**370**:829–840.

32. ACCORD Study Group, Cushman WC, Evans GW, et al. Effects of intensive blood-pressure control in type 2 diabetes mellitus. *N Engl J Med* 2010;**362**:1575–1585.

33. Cooper-DeHoff RM, Gong Y, Handberg EM, et al. Tight blood pressure control and cardiovascular outcomes among hypertensive patients with diabetes and coronary artery disease. *JAMA* 2010;**304**:61–68.

34. Watts GF, Naumova R, Slavin BM, et al. Serum lipids and lipoproteins in insulin-dependent diabetic patients with persistent microalbuminuria. *Diabet Med* 1989;**6**: 25–30.

35. Watts GF, Powrie JK, O'Brien SF, et al. Apolipoprotein B independently predicts progression of very-low-level albuminuria in insulin-dependent diabetes mellitus. *Metabolism* 1996;**45**:1101–1107.

36. Colhoun HM, Betteridge DJ, Durrington PN, et al. Effects of atorvastatin on kidney outcomes and cardiovascular disease in patients with diabetes: an analysis from the Collaborative Atorvastatin Diabetes Study (CARDS). *Am J Kidney Dis* 2009;**54**: 810–819.

37. Jandeleit-Dahm K, Bonnet F. Treatment of diabetic nephropathy: control of serum lipids. In: Boner G, Cooper M (eds), *Management of Diabetic Nephropathy*. London: Martin Dunitz, 2003:135–41.

38. Keech A, Simes RJ, Barter P, et al. Effects of long-term fenofibrate therapy on cardiovascular events in 9795 people with type 2 diabetes mellitus (the FIELD study): randomised controlled trial. *Lancet* 2005;**366**:1849–1861.

39. ACCORD Study Group, Ginsberg HN, Elam MB, et al. Effects of combination lipid therapy in type 2 diabetes mellitus. *N Engl J Med* 2010;**362**:1563–1574.
40. Davis TM, Ting R, Best JD, et al. Effects of fenofibrate on renal function in patients with type 2 diabetes mellitus: the Fenofibrate Intervention and Event Lowering in Diabetes (FIELD) Study. *Diabetologia* 2010;**54**:280–290.
41. ACCORD Study Group, Chew EY, Ambrosius WT, et al. Effects of medical therapies on retinopathy progression in type 2 diabetes. *N Engl J Med* 2010;**363**:233–244.

CHAPTER 3

Diabetes and the Liver

Lisa Jones and Anna Mae Diehl

Division of Gastroenterology and Hepatology, Duke University, Durham, North Carolina, USA

 Key points

- Non-alcoholic fatty liver disease (NAFLD) is a spectrum of liver damage that ranges from simple steatosis to steatohepatitis (non-alcoholic steatohepatitis or NASH) to cirrhosis.
- NAFLD is frequently associated with type 2 diabetes, leading to significant malignancy and cardiovascular-related morbidity and mortality.
- Complex interactions of insulin resistance, inflammatory cytokines and fibrogenic factors contribute to disease progression.
- Liver biopsy remains the gold standard for the diagnosis of fatty liver disease.
- There is no single effective therapy for the treatment of NAFLD; however, lifestyle modifications aimed at weight reduction and tight glycaemic control should be implemented in an effort to mitigate disease progression.

 Therapeutic key points

- Available treatment strategies attempt to alter the various pathways that lead to pathogenesis of NAFLD.
- Pharmacological interventions such as insulin-sensitizing agents have been studied in a wide variety of patient populations but yield inconsistent results.
- Although optimal treatment strategies have yet to be established, a reasonable management plan should include weight reduction in obese individuals and tight glycaemic control.
- Periodic laboratory surveillance and regular physician visits are warranted to detect progression of liver disease. Advanced liver disease management focuses on reducing complications.
- Patients without significant contraindications with further hepatic decompensation should be evaluated for liver transplantation.

Diabetes: Chronic Complications, Third Edition. Edited by Kenneth M. Shaw, Michael H. Cummings.

3.1 Introduction

Non-alcoholic fatty liver disease (NAFLD) is the most common cause of chronic liver disease in the western world. The syndrome encompasses a spectrum of histopathological changes in the liver, ranging from benign fatty infiltration (steatosis) to steatosis with inflammation with or without necrosis (steatohepatitis) to cirrhosis.

Fatty liver disease was considered to be a manifestation of alcoholic liver disease until 30 years ago when the first cases of fatty liver in patients without a history of significant alcoholic consumption were described.[1] The study also noted that these histological changes were most prevalent in individuals with morbid obesity and type 2 diabetes. Today, we recognize that metabolic syndrome (dyslipidaemia, hypertension, truncal obesity and insulin resistance) is a risk factor for the development of fatty liver disease. The prevalence of type 2 diabetes is estimated to be 6.4 per cent.[2] Likewise, the prevalence of obesity worldwide in both developed and developing countries is approaching epidemic numbers. Fatty liver disease is closely associated with type 2 diabetes and obesity. Those with the more severe form of the disease are at higher risk for cirrhosis, hepatocellular cancer and ultimately death. Given the large, and increasing, number of individuals with type 2 diabetes and/or obesity, NAFLD will probably also reach epidemic proportions.

In this chapter, we review the natural history, pathogenesis and management of fatty liver disease in patients with diabetes.

3.2 Epidemiology

NAFLD is rapidly becoming the most common cause of end-stage liver disease in the western world. A large US-based study estimated the prevalence of fatty liver to be almost 33 per cent in the general population.[3] The worldwide prevalence of NAFLD is largely unknown, because prevalence estimates vary depending on the studied population and diagnostic criteria (i.e. imaging, liver biopsy, postmortem examination, biochemical assays) used to determine these rates. The highest prevalence of NAFLD is reported in the bariatric surgery population, with rates nearing 90 per cent, emphasizing the association between obesity and fat deposition in the liver.[4] The high prevalence of NAFLD directly impacts health-care resources. A 2008 analysis of health-care utilization indicated that individuals with fatty liver disease have 26 per cent higher health-care costs over a 5-year period compared with the general population.[5]

As mentioned above, 30 years ago a strong association between type 2 diabetes and NAFLD was discovered. In 2007, Targher and colleagues utilized ultrasonography and serological assays to determine the prevalence of NAFLD among patients with type 2 diabetes in an Italian-based primary care clinic. This cross-sectional study reported a 70 per cent prevalence. Diabetic patients with NAFLD were more likely to be male, older and have had diabetes for a longer duration than those without NAFLD.[6]

Although reported prevalence estimates of NAFLD in patients with diabetes have varied across studies, they continue to highlight the significant association between these two conditions.

3.3 Natural history

The severity of the various histological forms of NAFLD predict clinical prognosis. Simple steatosis is associated with a more indolent course than non-alcoholic steatohepatitis (NASH). Patients with steatosis have similar mortality rates to the general population. In addition, only 1 per cent of such patients are thought to progress to cirrhotic liver disease.[7] Conversely, NASH is associated with liver-related mortality and has a higher fibrosis progression rate, with at least 8 per cent of patients developing cirrhosis within 5 years.[8] Matteoni and colleagues' retrospective analysis of a small cohort of patients with biopsy-proven NAFLD identified the link between liver histology and clinical outcomes by demonstrating significantly higher liver-related morbidity and mortality in patients with NASH, both with and without evidence of fibrosis, than patients with simple steatosis.[9] Mortality rates from cardiovascular disease and malignancy were also noted to be increased in NASH. Indeed, death was more likely to result from these conditions than from the underlying liver disease itself.

The presence of NAFLD clearly has an impact on the prognosis in patients with diabetes. This was first suggested by a number of small, observational studies that demonstrated that NAFLD was an independent risk factor for mortality in patients with diabetes. This suspicion was validated by a 2010 retrospective analysis of almost 300 patients with diabetes, who were followed over an average period of 10 years after the presence of NAFLD was confirmed using either abdominal ultrasonography or liver biopsy. Those with diabetes and NAFLD had a 2.4-fold higher risk of mortality than patients with diabetes alone. Malignancy was the most common cause of death (33%) in patients with diabetes and NAFLD, although hepatic- and cardiovascular-related complications also contributed significantly to mortality.[10]

The high proportion of malignancy- and cardiovascular-related deaths among individuals with NAFLD suggests that the metabolic derangements associated with fatty liver disease may contribute to the pathogenesis of diseases outside the liver. The types of cancers that decrease survival in patients with NAFLD have yet to be fully established in large cohort studies. Newer investigations suggest a rise in hepatocellular carcinoma (HCC) in these patients. A large case–control study conducted in the USA attempted to examine the potential link between HCC and diabetes: 2061 patients with HCC were compared with 6100 patients without cancer as case controls. Forty-three per cent of the patients with HCC were diagnosed with diabetes in the 3 years before the discovery of their HCC. After adjusting for HCC-related risk factors such as viral hepatitis, haemochromatosis and alcoholic liver disease, diabetes was associated with a two to threefold increase in the risk of HCC. The prevalence of NAFLD was not known in this population, however.[11] Thus, although diabetes appears to be an independent risk factor for HCC, it is difficult to ascertain whether the HCC typically develops in the context of NAFLD-related cirrhosis. Therefore, whether or not insulin resistance promotes hepatocarcinogenesis in the absence of underlying liver fibrosis remains unknown.

3.4 Pathogenesis

The exact pathogenic mechanisms that cause NAFLD remain the focus of extensive investigation through studies of multiple animal models and patients enrolled in clinical trials. It appears that complex interactions among insulin resistance, inflammatory cytokines and fibrogenic factors lead to development and progression of NALFD. A 'two-hit' theory has been widely adopted to explain the pathogenesis of NAFLD. The first 'hit' is attributed to alterations in fatty acid metabolism that perpetuate triglyceride (TG) deposition in the liver (i.e. steatosis). The 'second hit' occurs when inflammatory cytokines respond briskly, inciting oxidative stress which, in its most severe form, leads to hepatocellular injury and death (i.e. NASH). In a subgroup of individuals with NASH, regenerative responses cannot keep pace with ongoing hepatocyte death, and a fibrous matrix is deposited instead of replacing dead hepatocytes. Progressive fibrosis distorts the normal hepatic architecture, ultimately resulting in cirrhosis. The tissue remodelling process that occurs during fibrogenic repair of NASH-related liver damage also promotes the outgrowth of malignant hepatocytes, and this enhances hepatocarcinogenesis.

Steatosis

Lipid metabolism is normally a tightly regulated process. Dietary ingestion and subsequent intestinal absorption of fat supplies free fatty acids (FFAs) for lipid metabolism. In addition, FFAs are released from adipocytes during lipolysis. In NAFLD, hepatic uptake and synthesis of FFAs are increased. This expands the hepatic pool of FFAs and stimulates TG synthesis. FFAs

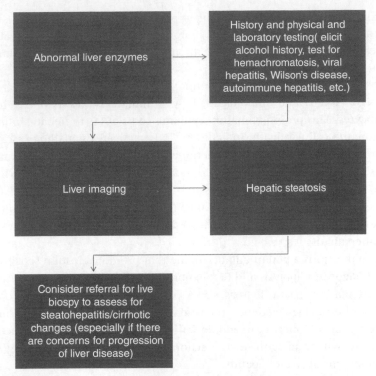

Figure 3.1 Diagnostic evaluation in non-alcoholic fatty liver disease.

that are not incorporated into TG, and that are released from existing TG droplets within hepatocytes, normally undergo oxidation within hepatic mitochondria – microsomes and peroxisomes. However, chronically increased exposure of hepatocytes to FFAs sometimes overwhelms the liver's ability to oxidize FFAs, expanding the hepatocyte FFA pool and driving further TG production. TG is normally packaged into very-low-density lipoproteins and secreted from the liver. However, when the rate of TG synthesis exceeds the rate of TG export, pathological accumulation of TGs occurs within hepatocytes (i.e. hepatic steatosis).[12]

From steatosis to steatohepatitis

It is important to emphasize that esterification of FFAs to generate TGs is an effective mechanism for detoxifying FFAs. Thus, TGs themselves are not hepatotoxic. Rather, the risk of lipotoxicity increases when TG synthesis cannot increase sufficiently to prevent FFAs from accumulating. FFAs may injure hepatocytes via several mechanisms. First, their accumulation may deregulate hepatocyte gene expression, because FFAs modulate the activity of certain types of transcription factors. Second, FFAs may directly interact with and damage other vital cellular macromolecules.

Third, the oxidation of FFAs results in potentially toxic by-products, such as reactive oxygen species (ROS). Lipotoxicity related to FFA accumulation increases the rate of hepatocyte death and incites progression from simple steatosis to steatohepatitis.

Two adipocytokines central to this process include tumour necrosis factor α (TNFα) and adiponectin. FFAs stimulate synthesis of TNFα in adipocytes. This proinflammatory cytokine contributes to hepatic inflammation and cellular death. In addition, TNFα activates signalling cascades responsible for the promotion of peripheral insulin resistance by activating translocation of the nuclear transcription factor NF-κB. Nuclear NF-κB, in turn, induces expression of genes that encode interleukins IL8 and IL6, and other proinflammatory cytokines that incite recruitment of inflammatory cells and exacerbate insulin resistance, within both the liver and extrahepatic tissues.

Adiponectin is a potent adipocytokine that promotes insulin sensitivity and antagonizes lipolysis and FFA export from adipocytes into the peripheral circulation. It also increases FFA oxidation and decreases new fatty acid synthesis. Obese patients and patients with diabetes have low circulating levels of adiponectin. In addition, their adiposity promotes production of TNFα, which antagonizes the action of adiponectin, potentiating the development of steatohepatitis.

Insulin regulation

Insulin is a key regulatory hormone in glucose and lipid metabolism. Resistance to insulin in peripheral tissues promotes hyperglycaemia and lipolysis. The latter increases the supply of FFAs to the liver, increasing the risk for hepatic lipotoxicity. Insulin resistance also triggers compensatory production of the hormone in the pancreas, thereby perpetuating hyperinsulinaemia. Excess insulin exacerbates cellular resistance to insulin. In hepatocytes, this inhibits normal downregulation of gluconeogenesis in the postprandial state, and potentiates development of postprandial hyperglycaemia (i.e. glucose intolerance). Postprandial hyperglycaemia, in turn, provides an additional stimulus for pancreatic insulin production, thereby exacerbating hyperinsulinaemia and further desensitizing insulin signalling in target cells (i.e. causing insulin resistance).

Progression to fibrosis

Free fatty acids also serve as ligands for peroxisome proliferator-activated receptor (PPAR) α. PPARα promotes the synthesis of the enzymes that catalyse FFA oxidation, and this upregulates β oxidation of FFAs. The derivatives of this process are ROSs. Increased ROS production increases the risk for oxidative stress, which, in turn, further disrupts mitochondrial function and generates more ROSs. Patients with NAFLD do not produce adequate levels of antioxidants and pre-existing antioxidants are over-

whelmed by excess ROSs, leading to the generation of toxic lipid interme-
diates. Hepatocellular death results from overwhelming oxidative stress,
which triggers regenerative responses to replace dead hepatocytes. The
resultant wound-healing process activates quiescent hepatic stellate cells
to become myofibroblastic.

Liver fibrosis occurs when myofibroblastic hepatic stellate cells prolifer-
ate and secrete excessive collagen-based extracellular matrix. Injured
hepatocytes perpetuate this process by releasing growth factors and mor-
phogens that promote proliferation of myofibroblastic stellate cells. An
insulin-resistant state also stimulates production and connective tissue
growth factor and other profibrogenic factors which exacerbate this fibrogenic response. Fortunately, however, few patients with NASH develop
sufficient fibrosis to cause cirrhosis. Hence, it is likely that more complex
interactions of genetic, metabolic and environmental factors determine the
body's ability to repair liver damage without excessive fibrogenesis.

Intestinal contribution to NAFLD

Small bowel bacterial overgrowth and intestinal permeability are associated with increased microbial production of ethanol and acetaldehyde.
Hepatic uptake of acetaldehyde incites hepatic steatosis, whereas intesti-
nally derived endotoxins perpetuate hepatic $TNF\alpha$ production, further
contributing to hepatocellular injury. Gut-derived bacterial products and
diet-derived FFAs also activate toll-like receptors on hepatic stellate cells,
stimulating those cells to become myofibroblastic and produce collagen.

Summary

The spectrum of NAFLD results from excessive exposure of hepatocytes
to FFAs. This stimulates hepatocyte TG synthesis, which buffers hepatocytes from FFA-mediated lipotoxicity. However, when the ability of hepatocytes to detoxify FFAs (via esterification to form TGs or elimination via
oxidation) is overwhelmed, FFAs accumulate, leading to hepatocellular
oxidative stress, inflammation and, sometimes, fibrogenesis. More research
is needed to further elucidate the interaction of biochemical, genetic susceptibility and environmental factors which leads to the progression of the
disease in order to clarify why some, but not other, individuals with steatosis develop NASH, and why only a subset of those with NASH become
cirrhotic or develop HCC.

3.5 Diagnosis of NAFLD

History and physical examination

The evaluation for the presence of NAFLD is generally triggered by elevated liver enzymes and the presence of excessive liver fat on imaging

during routine evaluation. If abnormal liver tests are identified, a thorough physical examination and in-depth review of medical, personal and family history is warranted. It is especially important to utilize historical and serological data to exclude other potential aetiological precipitants of liver disease (i.e. viral or autoimmune hepatitis, Wilson's disease, haemochromatosis). A detailed assessment of alcohol intake is also necessary to confidently exclude the presence of alcoholic liver disease. This is especially important given that there are no serological or radiographic studies that can distinguish alcoholic liver disease from non-alcoholic liver disease. Acceptable limits of alcohol intake are 2 drinks (or 20 g of ethanol) per day in men and 1 drink (or 10 g) in women. Alcoholic liver disease should be considered if intake is in significant excess of these limits. In general, patients with NAFLD without cirrhosis are often asymptomatic, although patients may report vague right upper quadrant abdominal pain and general malaise. A history of significant right upper quadrant abdominal pain should trigger further evaluation of the gallbladder and biliary tree. In addition, the history may reveal signs of advancing liver disease, such as weight gain or weight loss, increasing abdominal girth consistent with oedema and/or ascites, jaundice and gastrointestinal bleeding.

Hepatomegaly is a common physical examination finding, although the examination typically uncovers consequences of long-standing obesity and insulin resistance such as arthritis, acanthosis nigrans and central adiposity. Examination findings suggestive of advanced liver disease include splenomegaly, muscle wasting, ascites and/or lower extremity oedema.

Serological evaluation

Liver enzymes, such as ALT and AST, can be elevated in NAFLD, although normal laboratory values do not exclude the possibility of fatty liver disease. Generally, abnormal liver tests demonstrate a predominance of ALT levels over AST. Hence the ratio AST:ALT is typically less than 1. Aminotransferase elevation is also generally less than two to four times the upper limit of the normal values, and rarely exceeds a tenfold elevation. Until very recently, there were no biochemical tests that distinguished steatosis from steatohepatitis. However, emerging data suggest that circulating levels of keratin 8/18, an apoptotic cleavage product, are higher in NASH than in steatosis.[13] There are also serological clues to suggest the presence of advanced liver disease, including a low platelet count, decreased albumin and a prolonged prothrombin time.

Serological biomarkers of fibrosis have been investigated to identify patients with fibrosis, replacing liver biopsies as the gold standard in differentiating between pathological changes in the liver. Although several non-invasive markers are under development, very few have consistently been validated against liver biopsy in all stages of fibrosis. Existing data suggest that such tests are most useful in predicting patients who are at the extreme ends of the fibrosis spectrum (i.e. either no fibrosis or cirrhosis), but not reliable in distinguishing among various intermediate stages of fibrosis. The latter question is, unfortunately, the most clinically relevant because fibrosis stage predicts which patients are most likely to become cirrhotic eventually.

A thorough battery of tests should include testing for viral hepatitis, haemochromatosis, Wilson's disease, autoimmune hepatitis and α_1-antitrypsin deficiency, given that there is no one blood test that is diagnostic of NAFLD. If the above studies are, in fact, unrevealing in a patient with the metabolic syndrome, the diagnosis of NAFLD can be made. Further testing is then required to determine the severity of liver injury (i.e. to distinguish NASH from steatosis) and fibrosis (i.e. to detect subclinical cirrhosis)

Radiographic studies

Abdominal ultrasonography and computed tomography (CT) are frequently utilized imaging modalities for the detection of hepatic steatosis. Characteristic findings on ultrasonography are increased echogenicity of the liver parenchyma. Although relatively inexpensive, the sensitivity and specificity significantly decrease in the presence of visceral adiposity. A liver with significant steatosis appears to be hypodense compared with surrounding organs on CT. Magnetic resonance imaging (MRI) provides a more detailed assessment, given its ability to quantify the amount of fatty infiltration using differences in signal intensity between fat and water. Despite its ability to quantify steatosis, MRI is an expensive test limited to patients without severe obesity and implantable devices. Unfortunately, no radiological study can reliably distinguish steatosis from NASH, or advancing fibrosis. The most promising emerging technology is the Fibroscan, which uses transient elastography (ultrasound-based technology) to determine liver stiffness. The device can distinguish those without fibrosis from those with advanced fibrosis, although the sensitivity is altered in the presence of acute liver injury or significant cholestasis. Its efficacy is also severely limited by obesity.[14] In addition, transient elastography is not useful for distinguishing steatosis from steatohepatitis, or separating patients without fibrosis from those with minimal fibrosis. Thus, establishing severity of tissue damage in NAFLD can be done by only histological evaluation of liver tissue. Although seemingly invasive, the histological features have been demonstrated to correlate with clinical prognosis.

Liver biopsy

Liver biopsy remains the most reliable tool to diagnosis NAFLD and to assess the severity of related liver injury and extent of fibrosis. It is performed using either a percutaneous or a transjugular approach. The advantage of percutaneous liver biopsy is that it does not require fluoroscopic guidance or sedation and can be performed at the bedside. A transjugular approach is performed by interventional radiologists. The procedure is typically done under minimal sedation, but generally reserved for patients with severe coagulopathy or ascites.[15]

The severity of fibrotic changes is important in assessing the risk of progression to end-stage liver disease. Liver biopsy can also be used to confirm the suspicion for NASH, given the unavailability of serological means to diagnose the disorder definitively.

Benign fatty liver appears predominately as macrovesicular steatosis, although some accumulation of microvesicular fat may also occur. Steatohepatitis (NASH) is characterized by the occurrence of liver cell death and lobular infiltration with lymphocytes, neutrophils and other inflammatory cells in fatty livers. Extreme hepatocyte injury in NASH causes ballooning degeneration of hepatocytes, a hallmark of this condition. Ballooning results when massive oxidative damage to cytoskeletal proteins overwhelms normal mechanisms that ubiquitinate damaged cytokeratins in order to target them for proteosomal degradation. The progressive retention of damaged structural proteins results in hepatocyte endoplasmic reticulum (ER) stress. Compensatory mechanisms repress further synthesis of cytoskeletal proteins, depriving hepatocytes of structural elements that prevent them from swelling. Meanwhile, the ER stress confounds efforts to clear the ubiquitinated keratins, causing clumps of ubiquitinated cytokeratins (so called Mallory–Denk bodies) to form in the swollen (ballooned) cells.

Recently, it has been demonstrated that ER stress stimulates ballooned hepatocytes to produce profibrogenic factors that incite neighbouring stromal cells to elaborate fibrous matrix. This finding helps to explain evidence that hepatocyte ballooning enhances the likelihood of developing cirrhosis, and why initial deposition of fibrous matrix in NASH typically occurs around injured hepatocytes (dubbed 'pericellular fibrosis'). As oxidative stress is typically greatest in perivenular (zone 3) hepatocytes, this promotes deposition of fibrous matrix around terminal hepatic venules. Some patients with NASH also develop periportal fibrosis, and it has been suggested that the latter process accompanies the expansion of progenitor populations that are attempting to regenerate the injured parenchyma. In any case, the intensity of both perivenular and periportal fibrosis parallels the severity of hepatocellular injury and death. When hepatocyte injury is severe and protracted, fibrous septa bridge adjacent portal tracts and perivenular areas, eventually generating islands (nodules) of parenchyma that are surrounded by fibrosis. This extreme state of architectural distortion is dubbed cirrhosis (Plate 3.1).

Established criteria for the diagnosis of NASH have been proposed.[16] Although this scoring system has been universally accepted in clinical practice, it has become widely used to quantify the effects of therapeutic interventions on hepatic histology during NAFLD treatment trials.

Management

There is no single established treatment for NAFLD. Available treatment strategies attempt to alter the various pathways that lead to pathogenesis of NAFLD. Targeted therapy antagonizes the mechanisms central to the development of obesity, insulin resistance, intrahepatic oxidative stress and inflammation. Therapies also aim to halt the progression of fibrosis. Newer interventions, both on the market and in development, aim to slow progression of and potentially reverse advanced disease. The diversity of potential treatment modalities (lifestyle modification, medication, surgical intervention) reflects the complex pathogenesis of the disease.

Lifestyle interventions

Weight reduction via dietary modification is central to management of the metabolic syndrome. Insulin resistance contributes to the development of both type 2 diabetes and NAFLD, so similar lifestyle modifications are recommended for both conditions. There are no formal guidelines to aid practitioners in providing recommendations to their patients because the degree of calorie restriction and the ideal macronutrient composition necessary to alter the pathogenesis of the metabolic syndrome and its sequelae are unknown. The Look Ahead diabetes prevention trial recently published findings demonstrating that intensive lifestyle medication with calorie restriction and exercise reversed radiographic evidence of steatosis. In addition, patients with the greatest weight loss (>10%) had significantly reduced the extent of steatosis.[17] Thus, it seems reasonable to recommend interventions aimed at modest weight reduction. Another more recently published prospective trial of lifestyle intervention confirmed the benefits of this approach by documenting improved liver histology in NAFLD patients who lost weight during the study.[18]

The ideal distribution of fats, protein and carbohydrates for the dietary treatment of NASH is undefined. Patients with NASH tend to consume excess of carbohydrates and fat, suggesting that dietary habits influence pathogenesis of the disease. More specifically, patients with NAFLD are more likely to consume diets high in fructose. High fructose consumption leads to increased inflammation, lipogenesis, hypertriglyceridaemia and insulin resistance. The histological progression of fatty liver disease is also influenced by fructose intake. Among a group of obese individuals, fructose-enriched diets increased the chance of having NAFLD.[19] Moreover, among individuals with established NAFLD, those who consumed large amounts of fructose were more likely to have advanced fibrosis.[20] Previous studies have suggested a benefit to both low-carbohydrate and low-fat diets. Review of the major dietary recommendations suggest that a diet with a low glycaemic index and fewer calories (as recommended to patients with diabetes) may be an appropriate strategy for patients with NAFLD, although the impact of these recommendations on histological improvement is largely unknown. Unfortunately, the success rate of weight loss maintenance in patients with obesity is low. Although there is no clear evidence to recommend specific dietary changes, it is reasonable that an individualized approach to lifestyle modifications should be adopted in patients with diabetes to promote adherence increasing the chance for sustained weight loss over time. Given this history, it is tempting to recommend bariatric surgery as a strategy to achieve sustained weight reduction. However, a recent Cochran meta-analysis demonstrated inconsistent effects of bariatric surgery on hepatic necroinflammation and noted some reports of fibrosis progression. Hence, the authors advised against recommending bariatric surgery simply to treat NAFLD.[21]

Pharmacotherapy

Insulin-sensitising agents

Pharmacological agents aim to increase insulin sensitivity, inhibit the chaotic inflammatory response and halt the progression to fibrosis. Insulin-sensitizing agents are the most extensively studied pharmacological treatment for NAFLD.

Thiazolidinediones (TZDs) attenuate insulin resistance in peripheral tissues via activation of the PPARγ. This activation leads to increased intracellular adiponectin availability. Adiponectin ameliorates new fatty acid and TG synthesis, increases fatty acid oxidation, and promotes antifibrotic and anti-inflammatory factors. Despite favourable evidence demonstrating the beneficial effects of this class of drugs, uniformity in histological improvement across the spectrum of NAFLD has not been demonstrated.[22] In addition, the sustainability of the response has been questioned. Twenty-one patients with NASH were treated with pioglitazone and followed prospectively for 48 weeks. Nine of these subjects were followed for a minimum of 48 weeks after treatment. Over time, insulin sensitivity decreased, as did serum levels of adiponectin. Histology also revealed progression of hepatic steatosis and inflammation, although fibrotic changes remained stable.[23] It appears that long-term follow-up exposes the harmful effects of weight gain associated with TZDs, and its ability to reverse the initial beneficial effects of insulin sensitivity.

Metformin has also been evaluated, but only in small, uncontrolled, clinical trials. There are some promising outcomes in mice models;

however, these have yet to be validated consistently in patients with NAFLD.[24]

A large, randomized, placebo-controlled trial that compared the relative efficacies of treatment with either pioglitazone or vitamin E with placebo in non-diabetic, non-cirrhotic adult patients with biopsy-proven NASH has just been published. Both agents improved liver histology. However, not all treated patients benefited: many in the pioglitazone-treatment arm gained weight and some in the vitamin E group developed diabetes.[25] Hence, insulin sensitizers are clearly not the panacea for NASH, and further research is needed to identify better therapies.

Antioxidant therapy

Oxidative stress contributes to the brisk inflammatory response in NASH pathogenesis. α-Tocopherol (vitamin E) prevents lipid peroxidation, subsequently suppressing free radical formation and inhibiting the action of TNFα. Vitamin E may also have antifibrotic effects via inhibition of the gene expression of fibrogenic factors, such as transforming growth factor (TGF) β1. Various clinical trials demonstrate modest improvement in serum aminotransferase levels and steatosis, but fail to consistently show histological improvement.[26] As mentioned above, the most promising evaluation of the beneficial effects of vitamin E comes from a recent, randomized, placebo-controlled trial in people who do not have diabetes but have NASH. Improvement in the histological appearance of the liver was greater in patients in the vitamin E arm of the trial compared with placebo.

Further exploration into the pathogenic mechanisms promoting the progression of fatty liver disease will prompt new investigation into possible therapeutic interventions.

End-stage liver disease

Monitoring for progression of liver disease should occur periodically through blood tests, as described above, and outpatient visits. If serological tests suggest advanced liver disease, a repeat liver biopsy to confirm the clinical suspicion may be warranted.

Once advanced liver disease develops, management focuses on early detection and management of known complications. Common complications of advanced liver disease include development of ascites, gastrointestinal bleeding secondary to oesophageal varices, hepatic encephalopathy and renal dysfunction. Surveillance for oesophageal varices with upper endoscopy is performed if no history of prior endoscopy exists. Patients are also screened biannually for HCC using cirrhosis protocol MRI or CT. Ultrasonography is an acceptable alternative in patients who have contraindications to these tests. However, ultrasound examinations are not as sensitive in detecting smaller lesions. Suitable candidates with further decompensation of end-stage liver disease secondary to NAFLD should undergo evaluation for liver transplantation.

3.6 Conclusions

Non-alcoholic fatty liver disease is common in patients with type 2 diabetes. Complex metabolic pathways contribute to the histological features of the disease. The foundation of management should aim to achieve modest and sustainable weight reduction and improvement in glycaemic control. The clinical significance of advancing liver disease is clear, so future investigation is needed to exploit systemic repair pathways that halt and reverse the progression to cirrhotic liver disease.

Case study

A 55-year-old woman with a history of insulin-dependent type 2 diabetes, hypertension and morbid obesity presents to a gastroenterologist for a new patient visit. Routine outpatient labs revealed significant elevations in her liver enzymes. Specifically, the alanine aminotransferase (ALT) and aspartate aminotransferase (AST) were elevated to approximately twice the upper limit of the normal values. Her total bilirubin and alkaline phosphatase were within normal limits. Her primary care physician investigated further with an abdominal ultrasound scan, which demonstrated an enlarged liver with increased echogenicity consistent with fatty infiltration. There was no evidence of gallstones or other significant pathology. She denied a history of abdominal pain, nausea or vomiting, or fatigue. Alcohol intake was reported as occasional. No new prescription drugs were prescribed within the last year. Exam findings were fairly benign, and significant only for truncal obesity out of proportion to her morbid obesity. The liver span was normal at 9 cm.

Case conclusion

Laboratory tests were negative for the presence of chronic hepatitis, Wilson's disease, haemochromatosis, α_1-anti-trypsin deficiency and autoimmune hepatitis. Her glycated haemoglobin (HbA1c) was measured at 9 per cent. Her lipid profile demonstrated normal levels of low-density lipoprotein (LDL) but low levels of high-density lipoprotein (HDL). She was given a presumptive diagnosis of NAFLD, given the absence of serological and radiological findings to suggest another aetiology for her liver disease. A liver biopsy revealed simple steatosis, confirming the diagnosis.

Management focused on glycaemic control, weight reduction and achieving a normal blood pressure. A thorough review of her dietary and lifestyle habits revealed a sedentary lifestyle. She consumed close to a litre of soda daily. Her insulin regimen was adjusted and the patient signed up for a local weight loss support group with her husband. In the 8 months that followed, the patient lost a thirty pounds with BMI transitioning her from the obese to the overweight category. Her HbA1c has decreased to 7 per cent. Repeat laboratory values do not suggest burgeoning advanced liver disease. There are no plans to repeat a liver biopsy at this time.

References

1. Ludwig J, Viggiano TR, McGill DB, Oh BJ. Nonalcoholic steatohepatitis: Mayo Clinic experiences with a hitherto unnamed disease. *Mayo Clin Proc* 1980;**55**:434–438.
2. Shaw JE, Sicree RA, Zimmet PZ. Global estimates of the prevalence of diabetes for 2010 and 2030. *Diabetes Res Clin Pract* 2010;**87**:4–14.
3. Browning JD, Szczepaniak LS, Dobbins R, et al. Prevalence of hepatic steatosis in an urban population in the United States: impact of ethnicity. *Hepatology* 2004;**40**:1387–1395.
4. Ong JP, Elariny H, Collantes R, et al. Predictors of nonalcoholic steatohepatitis and advanced fibrosis in morbidly obese patients. *Obes Surg* 2005;**15**:310–315.
5. Baumeister SE, Volzke H, Marschall P, et al. Impact of fatty liver disease on health care utilization and costs in a general population: a 5-year observation. *Gastroenterology* 2008;**134**:85–94.
6. Targher G, Bertolini L, Padovani R, et al. Prevalence of nonalcoholic fatty liver disease and its association with cardiovascular disease among type 2 diabetic patients. *Diabet Care* 2007;**30**:1212–1218.
7. Dam-Larsen S, Franzmann M, Andersen IB, et al. Long term prognosis of fatty liver: risk of chronic liver disease and death. *Gut* 2004;**53**:750–755.
8. Cortez-Pinto H, Baptista A, Camilo ME, De Moura MC. Nonalcoholic steatohepatitis – a long-term follow-up study: comparison with alcoholic hepatitis in ambulatory and hospitalized patients. *Dig Dis Sci* 2003;**48**:1909–1913.
9. Matteoni CA, Younossi ZM, Gramlich T, Boparai N, Liu YC, McCullough AJ. Nonalcoholic fatty liver disease: a spectrum of clinical and pathological severity. *Gastroenterology* 1999;**116**:1413–1419.
10. Adams LA, Harmsen S, St Sauver JL, et al. Nonalcoholic fatty liver disease increases risk of death among patients with diabetes: a community-based cohort study. *Am J Gastroenterol* 2010;**105**:1567–1573.
11. Davila JA, Morgan RO, Shaib Y, McGlynn KA, El-Serag HB. Diabetes increases the risk of hepatocellular carcinoma in the United States: a population based case control study. *Gut* 2005;**54**:533–539.
12. Jou J, Choi SS, Diehl AM. Mechanisms of disease progression in nonalcoholic fatty liver disease. *Semin Liver Dis* 2008;**28**:370–379.
13. Feldstein AE. Novel insights into the pathophysiology of nonalcoholic fatty liver disease. *Semin Liver Dis* 2010;**30**:391–401.
14. Castera L, Foucher J, Bernard PH, et al. Pitfalls of liver stiffness measurement: a 5-year prospective study of 13,369 examinations. *Hepatology* 2010;**51**:828–835.
15. Rockey DC, Caldwell SH, Goodman ZD, Nelson RC, Smith AD. Liver biopsy. *Hepatology* 2009;**49**:1017–1044.

16. Kleiner DE, Brunt EM, Van Natta M, et al. Design and validation of a histological scoring system for nonalcoholic fatty liver disease. *Hepatology* 2005;**41**:1313–1321.

17. Lazo M, Solga SF, Horska A, et al. Effect of a 12-month intensive lifestyle intervention on hepatic steatosis in adults with type 2 diabetes. *Diabet Care* 2010;**33**: 2156–2163.

18. Promrat K, Kleiner DE, Niemeier HM, et al. Randomized controlled trial testing the effects of weight loss on nonalcoholic steatohepatitis. *Hepatology* 2010;**51**:121–129.

19. Ouyang X, Cirillo P, Sautin Y, et al. Fructose consumption as a risk factor for nonalcoholic fatty liver disease. *J Hepatol* 2008;**48**:993–999.

20. Abdelmalek MF, Suzuki A, Guy C, et al. Increased fructose consumption is associated with fibrosis severity in patients with nonalcoholic fatty liver disease. *Hepatology* 2010;**51**:1961–1971.

21. Chavez-Tapia NC, Tellez-Avila FI, Barrientos-Gutierrez T, Mendez-Sanchez N, Lizardi-Cervera J, Uribe M. Bariatric surgery for non-alcoholic steatohepatitis in obese patients. *Cochrane Database Syst Rev* 2010;**(1)**:CD007340.

22. Farrell GC, Larter CZ. Nonalcoholic fatty liver disease: from steatosis to cirrhosis. *Hepatology* 2006;**43**(suppl 1):S99–S112.

23. Lutchman G, Modi A, Kleiner DE, et al. The effects of discontinuing pioglitazone in patients with nonalcoholic steatohepatitis. *Hepatology* 2007;**46**:424–429.

24. Duvnjak M, Tomasic V, Gomercic M, et al. Therapy of nonalcoholic fatty liver disease: current status. *J Physiol Pharmacol* 2009;**60**(suppl 7):57–66.

25. Sanyal AJ, Chalasani N, Kowdley KV, et al. Pioglitazone, vitamin E, or placebo for nonalcoholic steatohepatitis. *N Engl J Med* 2010;**362**:1675–1685.

26. Torres DM, Harrison SA. Diagnosis and therapy of nonalcoholic steatohepatitis. *Gastroenterology* 2008;**134**:1682–1698.

CHAPTER 4

Diabetes and the Gastrointestinal Tract

Zeeshan Ramzan and Henry P Parkman

Gastrointestinal Section, Temple University School of Medicine, Philadelphia, PA, USA

 Key points

- Gastrointestinal (GI) symptoms are more prevalent in patients with diabetes compared with the general population. These GI symptoms have a negative impact on the quality of life.

- Disordered GI motor and sensory function occur frequently in both type 1 and type 2 diabetes and can manifest in a wide variety of signs and symptoms.

- Poor glycaemic control is associated with an increased prevalence of GI symptoms.

- Gastroparesis can affect individuals with both type 1 and type 2 diabetes. Those with type 1 have a higher prevalence of gastroparesis (30–50%) than those with type 2 (10–30%).

4.1 Introduction

The prevalence of diabetes in the USA is approximately 12 per cent and is increasing every year due, in part, to the increasing prevalence of obesity and its associated complications. Gastrointestinal (GI) symptoms are more prevalent in patients with diabetes in comparison with the general population and have a negative impact on the quality of life. Disordered GI motor and sensory function occur frequently in both type 1 and type 2 diabetes;[1] they show up as a wide variety of signs and symptoms.

4.2 Epidemiology

Diabetes may have effects on the oesophagus, stomach, small intestine, colon, anorectal sphincter complex, pancreas, gallbladder and liver. The prevalence of GI symptoms in individuals with diabetes has been studied

---

Diabetes: Chronic Complications, Third Edition. Edited by Kenneth M. Shaw, Michael H. Cummings.
© 2012 John Wiley & Sons, Ltd. Published 2012 by John Wiley & Sons, Ltd.

Table 4.1 Gastrointestinal (GI) symptoms in diabetes

	Rundles (1945)[4]	Feldman and Schiller (1983)[5]	Clouse and Lustman (1989)[6]	Ko et al.[a] (1999)[3]
Abdominal pain (%)	70	30	32	16
Constipation (%)	42	60	12	28
Diarrhoea (%)	22	22	21	35
Nausea/vomiting (%)	–	29	21	–
Faecal incontinence (%)	–	20	–	–
Dysphagia (%)	–	27	–	–
More than one GI symptom (%)	>60	76	68	71

[a]Type 2 diabetes.

extensively in the past with reports of mixed results. Some studies have reported no difference in the prevalence of GI symptoms in individuals with diabetes compared with age-matched controls;[2,3] others have revealed that abdominal pain and problems with bowel function are found more often in individuals with diabetes. Approximately 70 per cent of these patients had more than one GI symptom.[3] Prevalence of GI symptoms is higher in woman with diabetes than in man. A summary of studies on GI symptoms in patients with diabetes is shown in Table 4.1.[3–6]

Many studies have shown an association between prevalence of GI symptoms and poor glycaemic control. A study by Bytzer et al.[7] evaluated a range of gastrointestinal symptoms in relation to glycaemic control. Gastrointestinal symptoms originating in multiple organs were significantly more common when glycaemic control was poor. The variability in the reported results may be due, in part, to the lack of standardized tool used to collect data. Recently, the Diabetes Bowel Symptom Questionnaire has been developed and tested in an attempt to validate the findings in epidemiological and clinical studies.

4.3 Pathophysiology

Multiple mechanisms of gastrointestinal dysfunction with a significant overlap have been identified. Some of these include autonomic neuropathy, microangiopathy and hyperglycaemia. Many mediators reported to be involved in the pathogenesis of diabetic gastroenteropathy include amylin, C-protein, glucagon, glucagons-like peptide-1 (GLP-1), pancreatic polypeptide, peptide YY, somatostatin and gastric inhibitory peptide.

Neuropathy

Abnormalities at a number of different levels of the nervous system in patients with diabetes have been identified. Diabetic gastropathy/gastroparesis has been the most extensively studied. It was initially felt that most of the detrimental effects of diabetes on the gut were secondary to vagal neuropathy, because the effects of vagotomy appeared very similar to the physiological findings in patients with gastroparesis. However, although this may be relevant in some symptomatic patients, it is not universally present. Abnormalities are present in both the parasympathetic and the sympathetic autonomic systems in gastroparetic patients, and in addition there are enteric nervous system abnormalities.

Diabetic autonomic neuropathy is a common and serious complication of diabetes, which can involve the entire autonomic nervous system (ANS), significantly impairing the survival and quality of life of patients with diabetes. There are many possible explanations of this phenomenon, including a metabolic insult to nerve fibres, neurovascular insufficiency, autoimmune damage and neurohumoral growth factor deficiency.[8] In addition to the multiple possible aetiologies to this neuropathy, there are also multiple levels at which this neuropathy could affect bowel function.

Enteric abnormalities

The role of intrinsic enteric neuropathy in individuals with diabetes has been investigated by numerous studies. Burnstock and colleagues have documented disturbances in intrinsic nerves and the protective role of gangliosides in a series of studies in the streptozotocin rat model of diabetes.[9] They have shown a deficiency of nitrergic neurons in the pyloric sphincter, as well as a decrease in inhibitory neurotransmitters and an increase in excitatory transmitters in non-sphincteric muscle. Recent studies have demonstrated abnormalities in the pacemaker cells of the stomach, the interstitial cells of Cajal, of the upper gut. A decrease in number and remodelling of interstitial cells of Cajal has been reported to cause a decrease in inhibitory innervations (neuronal nitric oxide synthase – nNOS; vasoactive intestinal peptide – VIP) in the ENS with an associated increase in excitatory innervation.[10,11]

Autonomic abnormalities

It has long been recognized that gastroparetic patients have vagal dysfunction, and several of the motor abnormalities observed in patients with symptomatic diabetes are indistinguishable from those seen in patients with other syndromes that affect postganglionic sympathetic function. Autonomic dysfunction in diabetes (diabetic autonomic neuropathy) is probably multifactorial and related to hyperglycaemia, neurovascular insufficiency, autoimmune damage and neurohormonal growth factor deficiency. A functional IgG autoantibody acting as an agonist at the L-type calcium channels of smooth muscle of the colon has been proposed to modulate the enteric neurotransmission in type 1 diabetes. Although motility disturbances are common in patients with diabetic autonomic neuropathy, they do not correlate well with the presence and severity of symptoms, suggesting that other manifestations of diabetic autonomic neuropathy may play a role in the development of symptoms.

In a rat model of diabetic diarrhoea, α_2-adrenergic tone is impaired,[12] and it is thought that this in turn leads to impaired water and electrolyte transport, resulting in diarrhoea. The degree to which gut neuropathy is associated with cardiac autonomic neuropathy is not clear.

Central abnormalities

There is an evolving understanding of the importance of central processing in the pathophysiology of diabetic gut symptoms, as is true with other functional gut disorders. Recent functional imaging studies have looked at brain structure and function in patients with type 1 diabetes. It is known that acute hypoglycaemia has an acute detrimental effect on brain function.[13] On the other hand, chronic hyperglycaemia appears to be associated with small focal white matter changes in the basal ganglia and significant cognitive disadvantage.

4.4 Oesophageal dysfunction

Patients with diabetes have been shown to have a variety of oesophageal motility abnormalities (mostly hypomotility rather than hypermotility). The motility problems mostly associated with diabetes include hypotensive lower oesophageal sphincter pressure, decreased amplitude of oesophageal contractions, and simultaneous, prolonged and failed (aperistaltic) contractions in the body of the oesophagus. Ineffective oesophageal motility (IEM), defined by >50 per cent wet swallows with low distal peristaltic amplitude (<30 mmHg), is the most common primary motility abnormality seen in individuals with diabetes. Prolonged oesophageal transit has been demonstrated on oesophageal scintigraphy and oesophageal capsule studies.

Interestingly, abnormal oesophageal manometry in individuals with diabetes is not necessarily accompanied by significant functional disturbances or symptoms. Gastro-oesophageal reflux disease (GORD) is seen more commonly in individuals with diabetes, perhaps due to hypotensive lower oesophageal sphincter and oesophageal dysmotility resulting in impaired clearance of acid in the distal oesophagus. Vagal neuropathy, partly due to demyelination and loss of Schwann cells in the parasympathetic fibres in patients with longstanding type 1 diabetes, has been implicated in the pathogenesis. Furthermore, abnormal oesophageal sensory perception in patients with diabetes has been demonstrated by showing increased cortical evoked perception to low-pressure balloon distension in the oesophagus.[14] Increased prevalence of anxiety and depression has been noted in diabetic patients with oesophageal contraction abnormalities.[15]

Dysphagia in diabetes can be due to oesophageal dysmotility or infections such as candida oesophagitis. Odynophagia, on the other hand, should suggest an infectious aetiology and warrants a thorough investigation, including oesophagogastroduodenoscopy (EGD or upper endoscopy) to rule out *Candida* species or other opportunistic infections. Pathologically, oesophageal dysmotility in diabetes has been attributed to diabetic autonomic neuropathy mediated by vagal nerve dysfunction. Nerve conduction studies may also suggest a motor neuropathy in some patients.

4.5 Gastric dysfunction

Abnormal gastric motility results in disordered gastric emptying, or gastroparesis diabeticorum, which affects as many as 30–60 per cent of patients with diabetes.[16] Individuals with type 1 diabetes have a higher prevalence of gastroparesis (30–60%) than those with type 2 (10–30%). A female predominance (approximately 2–4:1) is seen. Some risk factors that have been identified include duration of diabetes, glycaemic control and presence of autonomic neuropathy. Abnormal gastric emptying results in variable absorption of glucose, causing poor glycaemic control.

Hyperglycaemia in diabetes impairs the normal physiology of gastric emptying due to vagal nerve dysfunction. Hyperglycaemia may induce gastric dysrhythmia and abnormal relaxation of the proximal stomach. Phase 3 contractions of the migrating motor complex (MMC), which normally stimulate antral contractions, are frequently absent, resulting in poor antral expulsion of indigestible solids, predisposing to bezoars. Furthermore, maintenance of the gastroduodenal pressure gradient, as well as receptive relaxation of the stomach, is abnormal. Prolonged pyloric contractions (pylorospasm) may cause functional resistance to gastric outflow. Liquid emptying may be normal, but solid emptying is frequently delayed. Furthermore, hyperglycaemia may affect the efficacy of therapy by attenuating the effect of erythromycin.

The pathophysiology of these motor disturbances is unclear. The pathogenesis of disordered gastric emptying in patients with diabetes is multifactorial. Vagal nerve injury or dysfunction and loss of the interstitial cells of Cajal have been observed. Microangiopathy, eventually leading to ischaemia of the smooth muscle, may play a role. Neurohormonal imbalance may be seen, most significantly with NO, calcitonin gene-related peptide (CGRP), serotonin (5-HT or 5-hydroxytryptamine), substance P and neuropeptide Y. The gut peptide motilin is thought to be an important mediator in the pathogenesis of gastroparesis. This is supported by the presence of high plasma levels of motilin in patients with gastroparesis. As motilin stimulates the initiation of phase 3 activity, the elevation of this peptide in patients with diabetes and gastroparesis may, in part, be compensatory. This is consistent with the observation that the treatment of gastroparesis with prokinetic agents is associated with a fall in plasma motilin levels. An autoimmune aetiology has been reported recently, supported by observed autoantibodies against calcium-channel receptors in gastric smooth muscle cells of patients with gastroparesis.[17]

Gastroparesis presents with a wide variety of symptoms, e.g. epigastric discomfort, nausea, vomiting, early satiety, abdominal bloating and fullness. These symptoms are worse postprandially. Physical examination may reveal gastric dilatation with a succussion splash. Although many individuals with diabetes have abnormal gastric emptying, they might not display overt clinical symptoms. There is a poor correlation between symptoms and the presence of delayed gastric emptying. The gold standard for diagnosis of gastroparesis is a 4-hour radiolabelled scintigraphy, performed after an overnight fast while the patient is off anticholinergics, tricyclic antidepressants, benzodiazepines and ganglionic-blocking agents because these agents may contribute to delayed emptying in these patients. Structural lesions should be first excluded by an EGD or barium study as appropriate. In July 2006, the US Food and Drug Administration (FDA) approved a wireless motility capsule (SmartPill Capsule, SmartPill, Buffalo, NY, USA) for evaluation of gastric emptying by measurement of luminal pH, pressure and temperature.

The management of gastroparesis requires a multimodal approach. Strict glycaemic control by dietary (low-fat, low-fibre soft diet with frequent small meals) and pharmacological agents should be adequately emphasized. Antiemetics and prokinetics are the two primary classes of medical therapy for gastroparesis. Metoclopramide (10–20 mg, 30 min before each meal and at bedtime) and domperidone (10–30 mg four times a day, also given 30 min before meal and bedtime; not FDA approved) are dopamine type 2 (D_2)-receptor antagonists that increase antral contractions and decrease receptive relaxation of the proximal stomach. Metoclopramide crosses the blood–brain barrier whereas domperidone does not. This penetrance into the central nervous system (CNS) may explain the higher incidence of neurological side effects with metoclopramide than with domperidone.

The macrolide antibiotic erythromycin, a motilin agonist, has been found to be effective in accelerating gastric emptying in gastroparesis but data regarding long-term symptomatic relief are limited. Several compounds derived from erythromycin (retaining its promotility properties only) have been developed and tested. Despite the promise shown in the pre-clinical settings, they have not consistently demonstrated a long-term effect on symptoms. In a small pilot study, the infusion of ghrelin, an appetite-stimulating hormone synthesized within the stomach, was shown to improve gastric emptying.[18] Case series suggested that endoscopic therapy with injection of botulinum toxin into the pyloric sphincter resulted in improvement in both gastric emptying and subjective symptoms; however, a double-blind, randomized controlled trial showed no significant benefit.[19] In severe or refractory cases, a venting gastrostomy and feeding jejunostomy tube can be placed.

Surgical therapy had been limited to partial or complete gastric resection in medically refractory cases, with often disappointing results. Enterra (Medtronic, Minneapolis, MN, USA), a gastric electrical stimulator (GES) device, was approved in 2000 for treatment of refractory gastroparesis. This involves subcutaneous implantation of a device (approximate size of a cardiac pacemaker), comprising an impulse generator connected to two electrodes. The electrodes are placed deep into the muscularis propria 1 cm apart and about 9–10 cm from the pylorus along the greater curvature of the stomach. The electrical stimulation is set at a high frequency (12 cycles/min) and low energy levels (300 ms pulse width, 4–5 mA). In long-term follow-up of up to 5 years, GES device placement has been shown to decrease symptoms, improve glycaemic control and nutritional parameters, enhance quality of life and decrease health-care costs.[20] Some preliminary data from high volume centres seem to suggest that patients with diabetes and nausea and vomiting (not abdominal pain requiring opiate analgesics) seem to benefit the most. Total gastrectomy with a Roux-en-Y loop has been reported in some case reports. This is associated with a significant morbidity and increased incidence of long-term complications, and hence should be considered as a last resort in selected patients who are refractory to all treatment options.

Acute erosive gastritis is common in diabetic ketoacidosis and frequently accompanied by bleeding. A postulated association between diabetes and *Helicobacter pylori* has been called into question. The incidence of duodenal ulcer in diabetes is lower than expected. Autoimmune chronic gastritis and gastric atrophy also may be seen with long-standing diabetes. In type 1 diabetes, 15–20 per cent of patients have serological evidence of anti-parietal cell antibodies, and this subset of patients has an increased prevalence of autoimmune gastritis with pernicious anaemia, iron deficiency anaemia, hypochlorhydria and hypergastrinaemia.

4.6 Small intestine

The effects of diabetes mellitus on the small intestine remain uncertain due to small studies. Small bowel dysmotility has been reported to be as high as 80 per cent in patients with long-standing diabetes who had delayed gastric emptying. However, abnormalities in small intestinal motility can be seen independent of delayed gastric emptying.

Many different mechanisms causing delayed small bowel transit have been suggested. These include a lack of MMCs starting in the antrum, prolonged phasic non-propagated contractions, a decrease in the frequency and amplitude of duodenal and jejunal contractions, and the failure of the small intestine to adopt a 'fed motility pattern' after meal ingestion.

Some postprandial motor abnormalities include early recurrence of phase 3 and burst activity, which may indicate neuropathic changes in either the intrinsic or the extrinsic innervation of the gut. Manometric studies have also shown a decrease in the number and amplitude of contractions in the upper part of the small intestine. There is, however, poor correlation between these manometric findings and symptoms.

Several studies have shown that acute hyperglycaemia reduces the number and propagation of pressure waves in the proximal small intestine, resulting in slower small intestinal transit.[21] Hyperglycaemia also leads to an increase in the perception of both chemical and mechanical luminal stimuli. Long-term effects of hyperglycaemia have been more difficult to assess. Indirect evidence from pancreas–kidney transplantation has suggested that autonomic neuropathy may be reversible by return to normoglycaemia.

Small bowel bacterial overgrowth

The normal proximal small bowel contains fewer than 10^5 bacteria/ml, with concentrations rising to around 10^8 in the distal small intestine. In situations where there is prolonged proximal small intestinal transit, either due to mechanical or for dysmotility reasons, there can be an increase in bacteria to levels comparable with those found in the healthy colon, and this is termed 'small intestinal bacterial overgrowth' (SIBO).

In the healthy gut, bacterial levels are controlled in the proximal small bowel by gastric acid secretion and intestinal motility, of which the MMC ('the intestinal housekeeper') plays an important part. In diabetes, proximal small bowel dysmotility can lead to stagnation and increased colonization of bacteria. There may be a contributing role of immune abnormality, because patients with SIBO may have altered levels of secretory immunoglobulin A, and diabetes is associated with an immunoparesis.

Bacterial overgrowth can lead to symptoms of increased gas and bloating, which may occur secondary to fermentation of food products in the small intestine. Malabsorption of both macronutrients (fats and carbohydrates) and micronutrients (fat-soluble vitamins and vitamin B_{12}) can occur as well. The mechanism of action is multifactorial. In SIBO, bacteria in the proximal small intestine deconjugate the bile salts (needed for fat processing), resulting in steatorrhoea. Moreover, the bacteria can also produce free bile acids that can cause direct damage to the small bowel mucosa. This damage further limits the ability of the proximal small bowel to absorb nutrients. Fat-soluble vitamins A, D, E and K can be malabsorbed. With severe deficiencies, all of these can lead to clinical syndromes: vitamin A deficiency can lead to night blindness, vitamin D deficiency to osteomalacia and vitamin K deficiency to a coagulopathy. With treatment of SIBO and replacement of essential vitamins, these deficiencies can be corrected.

Carbohydrate absorption may also be affected. Intraluminal digestion of carbohydrate by bacteria can exacerbate damage to the mucosa and decrease disaccharidase activity, further exacerbating malabsorption syndromes. In addition to the free bile acids described above, malabsorbed carbohydrate can then exacerbate symptoms as it is broken down in the colon to produce other organic acids and stimulate a secretory and osmotic diarrhoea.

Weight loss may occur secondary to both malabsorption and the use of nutrients by bacteria. Some bacterial strains also utilize vitamin B_{12} and patients with SIBO are often vitamin B_{12} deficient, with the attendant neurological and haematological consequences. The vitamin B_{12} deficiency is offset to some extent by intrinsic bacterial production of the vitamin.

The 'gold standard' diagnostic test for SIBO is jejunal aspiration and culture, because this allows the sensitivities of the organisms to be ascertained. However, this is an invasive procedure. Most centres use a breath test as a surrogate marker for SIBO. Both the $[^{14}C]$cholylglycine and the $[^{14}C]$xylose breath test work by recording radiolabelled CO_2 in the breath in response to ingestion of a test meal containing either radiolabelled cholylglycine or xylose respectively. The former test used to be popular, but has a 30–40 per cent false-negative rate and is used less now. The $[^{14}C]$xylose breath test has up to 95 per cent sensitivity and 100 per cent specificity. The bacteria in the proximal small intestine break down the xylose and cause an early peak of radiolabelled CO_2 production; any undigested xylose is absorbed, avoiding any subsequent fermentation in the colon, thus enhancing specificity.

Another breath test, hydrogen breath test, involves the ingestion of either lactulose or glucose and the recording of hydrogen in the breath that has been liberated by bacterial breakdown. Lactulose will normally lead to hydrogen production when it reaches the colon, so this type of breath test shows a 'double peak' if bacteria are present in the small intestine, with the abnormal peak in hydrogen in the breath followed by the expected colonic peak. However, a significant proportion of the SIBO population (up to 40%) carries bacteria that do not break down lactulose, resulting in a false-negative result. This does not occur when using glucose, although the rapid absorption of glucose in the upper GI tract may bypass bacterial digestion and again lead to a false negative. The resting levels of hydrogen in the breath are also raised at baseline in up to 30 per cent of patients, making interpretation difficult.[22] The test results are affected by the ingestion of high-carbohydrate meals in the period before the test, and antibiotics and laxatives must be withheld. The hydrogen breath test does have the advantage of being a safe and non-invasive test avoiding exposure to radiation, but its low specificity and sensitivity make it unreliable.

To treat SIBO effectively, the primary cause for gut stasis and overgrowth should be treated. Improving glycaemic control in individuals with diabetes can improve upper gut dysmotility, but is unlikely to reverse all abnormalities in itself. The mainstay of treatment remains antibiotics. The choice and regimen of antibiotic need to cover both anaerobic and aerobic bacteria and should be given in short or cyclical courses. Antibiotics (e.g. amoxicillin–clavulinic acid, ciprofloxacin, doxycycline or rifaximin) for a duration of 10 days have been shown to be effective. In individuals with recurrent symptoms, these antibiotics can be used consecutively in a cyclical manner to avoid resistance.[22]

Probiotic therapy of SIBO is appealing for its safety profile and lack of risk of development of resistance. However, to date it has proved disappointing in this condition. Attempts to clear the bacteria by using a prokinetic have been successful with cisapride in a small study,[23] but there are few other data to suggest their use as first-line therapy.

Coeliac disease

Adult patients with type 1 diabetes have a six times greater prevalence of coeliac disease; in children, this prevalence is 15 times greater, suggesting a genetic linkage between these conditions. The HLA markers B8 and DR3 are common in type 1 diabetes and coeliac disease, their presence conferring more risk of developing both diseases. Coeliac disease is the most common small bowel enteropathy in the western world and classically presents with diarrhoea, weight loss and anaemia. The anaemia can be caused by malabsorption of iron, folic acid or vitamin B_{12}, and all of these levels should be monitored and supplemented as required. However, up to 30 per cent of individuals can be asymptomatic. Taken together with the prevalence data, this is persuasive evidence that there should be a low threshold for investigation of coeliac disease in patients with diabetes.

The gold standard investigation for coeliac disease is small bowel biopsies from the duodenum or jejunum, which show the pathognomonic features of subtotal villous atrophy and an increase in epithelial lymphocytes. Anti-endomysial antibodies (EMAs) are over 85 per cent sensitive and up to 100 per cent specific and can be used as a screening tool.[24] IgA deficiency should be excluded, as most laboratories test for the IgA EMA. Human recombinant transglutaminase antigen is more sensitive (91%) and as specific as the EMA test.[24]

Treatment of coeliac disease is the life-long exclusion of wheat, rye, barley and prolamins from the diet under the supervision of a dietician. Most patients normalize with strict dietary adherence. However, non-responders may need immunosuppressive therapy, initially with steroids, with addition of azathioprine in refractory cases.

Colon and anorectal sphincter function

Constipation, diarrhoea and faecal incontinence occur frequently in patients with diabetes.[1] Data about colonic function in patients with diabetes mellitus are limited. In one study, colonic myoelectrical and motor activities were recorded in 12 individuals with type 1 diabetes and constipation.[25] Diabetic patients with severe constipation were compared with diabetics with mild or no constipation. Patients with diabetes had less colonic spike and motor activity within the first 30-minute postprandial period.

Constipation

The most common GI complaint of diabetics is constipation (not diarrhoea).[26] Occasionally, severe constipation with megacolon may be encountered. Rarely, chronic intestinal pseudo-obstruction may result. Although the mechanism remains unclear, constipation in patients with diabetes is thought to be due to pelvic floor or colonic motor dysfunction. Patients with diabetes and mild constipation were found to have a delay in the colonic motor response to a meal (up to 60–90 min after eating). Patients with diabetes and severe constipation had no postprandial increase in colonic motility. Administration of neostigmine (0.5 mg i.m.) or metoclopramide (20 mg i.v.) increased colonic motor activity in all patients with diabetes, suggesting that smooth muscle function was intact and that the abnormal response to a meal was related to autonomic neuropathy.[25] Thus, autonomic dysfunction may lead to an absent postprandial gastrocolonic response.

In a study performed by Jung et al.,[27] colonic transit time was compared between patients with diabetes and healthy individuals, and correlated with the presence of cardiovascular autonomic neuropathy. The mean colonic transit time for 28 patients with diabetes (34.9 h) was significantly longer than that of healthy individuals (20.4 h).[27]

General treatments for constipation include increasing dietary fibre intake (20–30 g/day) and hydration. Other measures such as administration of osmotic laxatives (polyethylene glycol, lactulose and sorbitol) and saline laxatives (magnesium citrate, magnesium phosphate, magnesium sulphate) can be used in refractory cases. Chronic use of stimulant laxatives such as anthraquinones and bisacodyl is discouraged because of the potential for tachyphylaxis. Another potential approach involves the use of prokinetic drugs or lubiprostone. There is no evidence supporting use of one laxative over another; however, trial of monotherapy should be employed first with other agents added as needed to avoid polypharmacy.

A colonic transit study and evaluation of pelvic floor function (to rule out pelvic floor dyssynergia) are indicated for patients who do not respond to the above treatments. Biofeedback training may prove effective in cases of severe constipation due to dyssynergic defecation. In the selected and small group of patients in whom slow-transit constipation remains intractable despite extensive medical treatment, surgery may be considered.

Diarrhoea in individuals with diabetes

Diarrhoea is a common symptom of autonomic neuropathy, affecting 3.7 per cent of patients with diabetes, predominantly those with type 1 diabetes. The cause of diabetic diarrhoea is multifactorial, and includes abnormal intestinal motility, small intestinal bacterial overgrowth, meal composition, excessive loss of bile acids (controversial), pancreatic insufficiency, drugs, secretory dysfunction, lactose malabsorption, coeliac disease, hormonal dysfunction (hyperthyroidism) and anorectal dysfunction.

Diabetic diarrhoea occurs mostly in patients with poorly controlled type 1 diabetes who also have evidence of diabetic peripheral and autonomic neuropathy. It appears to be more common in men than in women. The diarrhoea is often intermittent and painless, and it may alternate with periods of normal bowel movement or with constipation. Symptoms may in particular be worse at night. Associated steatorrhoea is common and does not necessarily imply a concomitant GI or pancreatic disease.

The first step in evaluation is to obtain information on the volume, frequency and duration of diarrhoea. A high sorbitol intake or the use of other laxatives may be elicited. In patients with diabetes, studies have shown that as little as 10 g sorbitol can induce diarrhoea. Fructose may also be malabsorbed and lead to diarrhoea. Drugs including metformin are associated with diarrhoea, usually with the initiation of treatment but also late in therapy.[28] Extended-release metformin is less likely to cause diarrhoea than the immediate-release form, and may be an alternative to discontinuing metformin therapy. Acarbose, an α-glucosidase inhibitor that competitively inhibits the breakdown of oligo- and disaccharides to monosaccharides in the small intestinal brush border, may cause diarrhoea in 30 per cent of patients. It may also cause diarrhoea by an increase in colonic butyrate production, which increases prostaglandin E production, leading in turn to water and electrolyte loss.

The pathogenesis of diabetic diarrhoea is unclear. The causes include disordered autonomically mediated intestinal secretion and motility resulting in increased contractions and hence diarrhoea. Alternatively motility may be reduced, predisposing to small bowel bacterial overgrowth and possible bile salt malabsorption (seen in about 40% of patients with diabetes and chronic diarrhoea), and hence causing diarrhoea. Autoimmune diseases are more common in patients with diabetes and the presence of diarrhoea in a patient with diabetes should raise the suspicion of coeliac disease, especially if there is coexisting folate or vitamin B_{12} deficiency. Rapid small intestinal transit may cause an increase in intraluminal contents that reach the caecum. However, no significant differences in mouth-to-caecum or whole-gut transit times exist between patients with diabetes and control individuals. Sympathetic denervation of the gut is common in patients with diabetes and autonomic neuropathy. As adrenergic nerves normally stimulate intestinal absorption of fluids and electrolytes, decreased intestinal absorption, rather than intestinal dysmotility, may underlie the pathogenesis of diabetic diarrhoea. Type 1 diabetes mellitus has been found to be associated with inflammatory bowel disease in some case reports, and microscopic colitis was found to be more common in patients with diabetes in a recent large population study.

The management of diabetic diarrhoea is difficult. Strict control of blood glucose levels may help. As gastrointestinal adrenergic function is impaired in autonomic neuropathy, adrenergic agonists may stimulate intestinal absorption of fluids and electrolytes. In addition, they may partially correct the motility disturbances of diabetic autonomic neuropathy. Treatment with the α_2-adrenergic agonist clonidine reverses the diarrhoea in a rat model. Hence, clonidine 0.1–0.6 mg twice daily may be successful in the therapy of diabetic diarrhoea, presumably by reversing the peripheral adrenergic resorptive abnormalities. Its use is limited to some extent by the side effect of orthostatic hypotension, and, at high doses of 0.5–0.6 mg/12 h, the beneficial effects can be outweighed by its sedative effect.[29] It is advisable to start at a low dose and increase slowly if the drug is proving effective and well tolerated. In refractory cases, the long-acting somatostatin analogue octreotide (50–100 μg s.c., twice daily) may be used

in the treatment of refractory diabetic diarrhoea.[30] It may, however, predispose to intestinal bacterial overgrowth owing to decreased small bowel
transit time, and it may aggravate steatorrhoea by inhibiting pancreatic
exocrine function. Symptomatic measures that may be used include the
prescription of codeine sulphate (30 mg every 6–8 h), diphenoxylate with
atropine (Lomotil) or loperamide. In some patients, psyllium hydrophilic
mucilloid may be helpful.

Faecal incontinence

Faecal incontinence implies anorectal dysfunction causing inability to
maintain continence. Diabetes can cause faecal incontinence due to motor,
sensory and autonomic neuropathy. This may result from weakness of the
voluntary muscles (skeletal muscles, i.e. puborectalis and external anal
sphincter) or involuntary muscles (smooth muscles, i.e. internal anal
sphincter) and is manifested by a reduction in the sphincter pressures
needed to maintain continence. Sensory impairment can lead to a decreased
rectal sensitivity (patient is unable to detect arrival of stool).[31] Neuropathy
involving the sympathetic nervous system may be responsible for nocturnal symptoms associated with diabetic diarrhoea. Autonomic dysfunction
is thought to be responsible for the impairment of normal internal
anal sphincter resting tone and reflexive internal sphincter relaxation.
Incontinence often coincides with the onset of diabetic diarrhoea, but in
most cases the total stool volume is normal.

The evaluation of patients with incontinence should include a proctos-
copy and/or sigmoidoscopy. Other tests that are useful include anorectal
manometry, endoanal ultrasonography and defaecography. Endoanal
ultrasonography may be helpful in identifying a defect in the sphincter
ring, caused by obstetric or other trauma.

The main goal of treatment is an improvement in symptoms and quality
of life. The first line of treatment for diarrhoea is the use of antidiarrhoeals
such as lopermide, diphenoxylate and codeine phosphate. Faecal impac-
tion with overflow incontinence is usually treated with digital extraction and enemas, followed by a good bowel regimen. Biofeedback can
improve rectal sensitivity, increase the 'squeeze pressure', and improve
the coordination between rectal perception and external sphincter and
puborectalis muscle contraction. More severe cases may benefit from
surgery or sacral nerve stimulation. In some patients, incontinence
improves spontaneously.

Biliary tree and liver

Lithogenic bile composition and stasis of bile in the gallbladder in individuals with diabetes may contribute to stone formation. Hence, patients with

diabetes are more prone to develop cholelithasis, and have an increased risk of complications related to gallstones, e.g. cholecystitis, cholangitis, biliary sepsis from common as well as unusual gas-producing organisms and rare abscesses due to *Yersinia enterocolitica*. Despite the increased risk of complications of gallstones, prophylactic cholecystectomy is not recommended in patients with diabetes and asymptomatic cholelithiasis. There is an increased incidence of sclerosing cholangitis and non-alcoholic fatty liver disease in patients with diabetes.

Pancreatic disease

Pancreatitis, both acute and chronic, can lead to a diabetic state. On the other hand, hypertriglyceridaemia in uncontrolled diabetes can cause acute pancreatitis. Acute pancreatitis causes increased levels of glucagon and adrenaline, resulting in hyperglycaemia. This in turn can cause many gastrointestinal symptoms related to hyperglycaemia, such as nausea, vomiting. In chronic pancreatitis, chronic fibrosis of the whole organ leads to islet cell damage (causing a decrease in insulin production) and acinar cell damage (leading to inability to produce pancreatic enzymes, causing exocrine insufficiency). Pancreatic exocrine dysfunction is found in 65–80 per cent of patients with diabetes. However, steatorrhoea (marker of severe exocrine insufficiency) is uncommon due to large functional reserve of pancreatic enzymes.

Diabetes is a risk factor of pancreatic cancer and associated with increased mortality rate.[32] Diabetes of new onset in elderly person may also be an early sign of pancreatic cancer. Pancreatic carcinoma is more frequent in diabetics according to a meta-analysis (pooled relative risk of 2.1 compared with non-diabetics).[33]

Diabetic ketoacidosis (DKA) caused by acute pancreatitis carries a high mortality rate. Non-specific elevations (less than three times the upper limits of normal) in serum amylase and lipase may occur in 16–25 per cent of cases of DKA without acute pancreatitis.[34]

Unexplained abdominal pain

Diabetic radiculopathy or diabetic plexus neuropathy of thoracic nerve roots may cause otherwise unexplained upper abdominal pain in patients with diabetic neuropathy. Other symptoms may include decreased appetite, postprandial fullness/pain and weight loss. The diagnosis may be supported by an abnormal electromyogram (EMG) of the anterior abdominal wall muscles when compared with an EMG of the thoracic paraspinal muscles.[35]

Case study

A 33-year-old white man with type 1 diabetes mellitus since age of 13 has been having worsening nausea and vomiting over past 5 years. His nausea and vomiting are primarily in the morning. His vomiting starts initially as clear fluid and then becomes thick and green. His oral intake has been extremely poor over the last 3–4 months. He has required multiple hospitalizations for his persistent symptoms and s need for glucose control and rehydration. A prior gastric emptying was normal although the duration of the test was only 1 hour and he was taking metoclopramide at the time. A prior upper endoscopy showed candida oesophagitis, which was treated with fluconazole. A follow-up endoscopy was negative.

His past medical history consists of diabetes mellitus with complications of retinopathy, nephropathy and neuropathy. Current medications include insulin, enalapril, ondansetron and levothyroxine. He has had side effects to metoclopramide used previously to treat his gastroparesis.

Due to his persistent symptoms, he was transferred to Temple University Hospital. Blood work showed a glucose level of 250 mg/dl and glycated haemoglobin (HbA1c) of 9.2 per cent. A gastric emptying scintigraphy showed markedly delayed gastric emptying with 83 per cent retention of solids at 2 hours (normal <60%) and 76 per cent retention of solids at 4 hours (normal <10%). An enteroscopy showed inflammation of the lower oesophagus, multiple antral erosions and normal appearing duodenal mucosa. Biopsies of the duodenum were normal and biopsies of the oesophagus showed oesophagitis. Antroduodenal manometry showed that most phase III migrating motor complexes (MMCs) started in the small intestine rather than the stomach. In addition, there were anterograde and retrograde transmissions of MMCs combined with gastroparesis and neuropathic disorder of the small intestine. He was treated with oral domperidone 10 mg four times daily, oral Prilosec (omeprazole) 20 mg twice daily and oral Zofran (ondansetron) 8 mg every 12 h as needed for nausea. Unfortunately, he failed to improve on this medical regimen.

The Enterra gastric electric stimulator therapy was subsequently implanted. At his last follow-up visit, 1 year after implantation, he was much better, although still with some morning nausea and vomiting. His blood glucoses are better controlled and repeat HbA1c was 7.2 per cent.

References

1. Horowitz M, Sansom M, eds. *Gastrointestinal Function in Diabetes Mellitus.* Chichester: John Wiley & Sons, 2004.
2. Abid S, Rizvi A, Jahan F, et al. Poor glycemic control is the major factor associated with increased frequency of gastrointestinal symptoms in patients with diabetes mellitus. *J Pak Med Assoc* 2007;**57**:345–349.

3. Ko GT, Chan WB, Chan JC, Tsang LW, Cockram CS. Gastrointestinal symptoms in Chinese patients with type 2 diabetes mellitus. *Diabet Med* 1999;**16**:670–674.
4. Rundles RW. Diabetic neuropathy: general review with report of 125 cases. *Medicine* 1945;**24**:111–160.
5. Feldman M, Schiller LR. Disorders of gastrointestinal motility associated with diabetes mellitus. *Ann Intern Med* 1983;**98**:378–384.
6. Clouse RE, Lustman PJ. Gastrointestinal symptoms in diabetic patients: lack of association with neuropathy. *Am J Gastroenterol* 1989;**84**:868–872.
7. Bytzer P, Talley NJ, Hammer J, Young LJ, Jones MP, Horowitz M. GI symptoms in diabetes mellitus are associated with both poor glycemic control and diabetic complications. *Am J Gastroenterol* 2002;**97**:604–611.
8. Vinik AI, Maser RE, Mitchell BD, Freeman R. Diabetic autonomic neuropathy. *Diabet Care* 2003;**26**:1553–1579.
9. Soediono P, Belai A, Burnstock G. Prevention of neuropathy in the pyloric sphincter of streptozotocin-diabetic rats by gangliosides. *Gastroenterology* 1993;**104**: 1072–1082.
10. Ordog T, Takayama I, Cheung WK, Ward SM, Sanders KM. Remodeling of networks of interstitial cells of Cajal in a murine model of diabetic gastroparesis. *Diabetes* 2000;**49**:1731–1739.
11. He CL, Soffer EE, Ferris CD, Walsh RM, Szurszewski JH, Farrugia G. Loss of interstitial cells of Cajal and inhibitory innervation in insulin-dependent diabetes. *Gastroenterology* 2001;**121**:427–434.
12. Chang EB, Fedorak RN, Field M. Experimental diabetic diarrhea in rats. Intestinal mucosal denervation hypersensitivity and treatment with clonidine. *Gastroenterology* 1986;**91**:564–569.
13. Rosenthal JM, Amiel SA, Yaguez L, et al. The effect of acute hypoglycemia on brain function and activation: a functional magnetic resonance imaging study. *Diabetes* 2001;**50**:1618–1626.
14. Rayner CK, Smout AJ, Sun WM, et al. Effects of hyperglycemia on cortical response to esophageal distension in normal subjects. *Dig Dis Sci* 1999;**44**:279–285.
15. Clouse RE, Lustman PJ, Reidel WL. Correlation of esophageal motility abnormalities with neuropsychiatric status in diabetics. *Gastroenterology* 1986;**90**(5 Pt 1): 1146–1154.
16. Samsom M, Vermeijden JR, Smout AJ, et al. Prevalence of delayed gastric emptying in diabetic patients and relationship to dyspeptic symptoms: A prospective study in unselected diabetic patients. *Diabet Care* 2003;**26**:3116–3122.
17. Jackson MW, Gordon TP, Waterman SA. Disruption of intestinal motility by a calcium channel-stimulating autoantibody in type 1 diabetes. *Gastroenterology* 2004; **126**:819–828.
18. Murray CD, Martin NM, Patterson M, et al. Ghrelin enhances gastric emptying in diabetic gastroparesis: A double blind, placebo controlled, crossover study. *Gut* 2005; **54**:1693–1698.
19. Friedenberg FK, Palit A, Parkman HP, et al. Botulinum toxin A for the treatment of delayed gastric emptying. *Am J Gastroenterol* 2008;**103**:416–423.
20. Abell T, Lou J, Tabbaa M, et al. Gastric electrical stimulation for gastroparesis improves nutritional parameters at short, intermediate, and long-term follow-up. *JPEN J Parenter Enteral Nutr* 2003;**27**:277–281.
21. Russo A, Fraser R, Horowitz M. The effect of acute hyperglycaemia on small intestinal motility in normal subjects. *Diabetologia* 1996;**39**:984–989.
22. Singh VV, Toskes PP. Small bowel bacterial overgrowth: presentation, diagnosis, treatment. *Curr Gastroenterol Rep* 2003;**5**:365–372.

23. Madrid AM, Hurtado C, Venegas M, Cumsille F, Defilippi C. Long-Term treatment with cisapride and antibiotics in liver cirrhosis: effect on small intestinal motility, bacterial overgrowth, liver function. *Am J Gastroenterol* 2001;**96**:1251–1255.

24. Tesei N, Sugai E, Vazquez H, et al. Antibodies to human recombinant tissue trans-glutaminase may detect coeliac disease patients undiagnosed by endomysial anti-bodies. *Aliment Pharm Ther* 2003;**17**:1415–1423.

25. Battle WM, Snape WJ, Alavi A, et al. Colonic dysfunction in diabetes mellitus. *Gastroenterology* 1980;**79**:1217–1221.

26. Chandran M, Chu NV, Edelman SV. Gastrointestinal disturbances in diabetes. *Curr Diab Rep* 2003;**3**:43–48.

27. Jung H-K, Kim D-Y, Moon I-H, Hong Y-S. Colonic transit time in diabetic patients-comparison with healthy subjects and the effect of autonomic neuropathy. *Yonsei Med J* 2003;**44**:265–272.

28. Bytzer P, Talley NJ, Jones MP, Horowitz M. Oral hypoglycaemic drugs and gastrointestinal symptoms in diabetes mellitus. *Aliment Pharmacol Ther* 2001;**15**:137–142.

29. Fedorak RN, Field M, Chang EB. Treatment of diabetic diarrhea with clonidine. *Ann Intern Med* 1985;**102**:197–199.

30. Meyer C, O'Neal DN, Connell W, et al. Octreotide treatment of severe diabetic diar-rhoea. *Intern Med J* 2003;**33**:617–18.

31. Wald A, Tunuguntla AK. Anorectal sensorimotor dysfunction in faecal incontinence and diabetes mellitus. Modification with biofeedback therapy. *N Eng J Med* 1984;**310**: 1282–1287.

32. Everhart J, Wright D. Diabetes mellitus as a risk factor for pancreatic cancer. A meta-analysis. *JAMA* 1995;**273**:1605–1609.

33. Wideroff L, Gridley G, Mellemkjaer L, et al. Cancer incidence in a population-based cohort of patients hospitalized with diabetes mellitus in Denmark. *J Natl Cancer Inst* 1997;**89**:1360–1365.

34. Yadav D, Nair S, Norkus EP, Pitchumoni CS. Nonspecific hyperamylasemia and hyperlipasemia in diabetic ketoacidosis: Incidence and correlation with biochemical abnormalities. *Am J Gastroenterol* 2000;**95**:3123–3128.

35. O'Connor RC, Andary MT, Russo RB, DeLano M. Thoracic radiculopathy. *Phys Med Rehabil Clin North Am* 2002;**13**:623–644.

CHAPTER 5

Diabetes and Foot Disease

Kate Marsden, Sharon Tuck and Darryl Meeking

Academic Department of Diabetes and Endocrinology, Queen Alexandra Hospital, Portsmouth, UK

 Key points

- Care of the diabetic foot requires input before, during and after the development of complications. Prevention of foot ulceration can be optimized by educating patients with diabetes about the use of appropriate footwear and by regular reinforcement of foot-care advice. The annual, thorough inspection of feet is an essential part of a diabetic examination. Standards should be in place to help identify at-risk feet. In particular the feet of patients with diabetes should be carefully examined for the presence of deformities, callus, reduced blood supply and nerve damage.

- Ulceration of the diabetic foot depends on the presence of neuropathy and/or impaired blood supply. It is particularly likely to occur where high-pressure areas develop. This can be due to the neuropathic process and/or areas of foot deformity. The development of excessive callus is frequently a predictive factor and can break down and lead to secondary ulceration.

- Impaired blood supply is due to atherosclerosis involving large vessels of both legs. This is frequently distal and multisegmental, involving tibial and peroneal blood vessels.

- Nerve damage leads to reduction in heat and pain sensation. It also affects blood supply, resulting in diminished sweating. Charcot disease can be a debilitating complication.

- Damage to the peripheral nerve fibres can lead to neuropathic pain. This can be a difficult condition to treat. Patients must be educated about its cause and the natural history of the condition. They should receive detailed information about treatment options and their likely effectiveness. Systems should be put in place to enable medication to be altered and optimized quickly and effectively.

Diabetes: Chronic Complications, Third Edition. Edited by Kenneth M. Shaw, Michael H. Cummings.
© 2012 John Wiley & Sons, Ltd. Published 2012 by John Wiley & Sons, Ltd.

Therapeutic key points

- A good system of foot care should mean that the identification of an at-risk foot triggers the involvement of other health-care professionals (orthotist, podiatrist, nurse and doctor) so that the risk of progression to a diseased foot is minimized.

- Optimal care of the diabetic foot is essential and can be achieved only through close collaboration of podiatrist, orthotist, nurse, physician and surgeon. This can most easily be carried out in a dedicated multidisciplinary foot clinic. Alternatively, there needs to be a system in place that enables easy dialogue and access between these different specialties. The development of an efficient system of care requires the involvement of a dedicated group of individuals representing each specialty. This allows for the development of local care pathways and systems to support the patient with diabetic foot disease. Support networks should transcend any primary/secondary care boundaries.

5.1 Epidemiology

No discussion of diabetic foot disease can be complete without acknowledging the significant impact that this complication has in terms of its cost to the health economy and its effects on the mortality and morbidity of those with diabetes. Foot ulceration in diabetes is common. In the UK diabetic population, its prevalence is likely to be between 5 and 7.4 per cent. Despite this, diabetic foot disease is an area that has been poorly studied. As a consequence, there is a lack of agreement, let alone consensus, on how best to prevent, investigate and manage the major diabetic foot conditions.

5.2 Pathophysiology

Diabetic foot ulceration

There are a number of factors associated with the development of diabetic foot ulceration. It is caused by one or more of three major risk factors: abnormal foot shape, nerve damage (neuropathy) and impairment of blood supply.

Abnormal foot shape

Deformities in the diabetic foot may be due in part to limitation of joint mobility. There is abnormal glycosylation of connective tissue which in turn leads to limitation of joint movement and functional foot problems. There is reduced ankle joint range of motion – ankle equinus leads to increased pressures beneath the forefoot and is thought to be a contributing factor in the development of forefoot plantar ulceration. Diabetic peripheral neuropathy can lead to wasting of the intrinsic and extrinsic foot muscles – this imbalance can lead to digital deformities. Motor neuropathy contributes to the paralysis of small muscles in the feet, which in turn may exacerbate structural abnormalities. The classic example of this is clawing of the toes, which leads to prominent metatarsal heads and accompanying high-pressure zones.

Charcot disease deformities, nail abnormalities, peripheral oedema and deformities secondary to surgical procedures all increase the risk of foot ulceration.

There is good evidence that foot pressures in patients with diabetes and peripheral neuropathy are greater than those in those patients with diabetes who have no neuropathy. In the neuropathic foot, elevated local pressure increases the likelihood of hyperkeratosis and subsequent callus or corn formation. Callus formation causes a further elevation in plantar pressure and this can eventually lead to ulceration. These high-pressure areas are highly predictive of subsequent foot ulceration. Where the blood supply to the foot is impaired, excessive pressures can lead directly to foot tissue damage and subsequent ulceration.

Neuropathy

Diabetes may affect both central and peripheral nerves. It can affect single or multiple nerves, sensory, motor or autonomic nerves. The most common risk factor for the development of foot ulceration is, however, chronic sensorimotor neuropathy. This may occur with or without symptoms (painless or painful) and can be seen in the presence or absence of pedal foot pulses (neuropathic or neuroischaemic foot). The prevalence of chronic sensorimotor neuropathy may approach 30 per cent in the UK diabetic population. Its prevalence increases with age and duration of diabetes and its importance here is the magnifying effect that it has on the risk of developing diabetic foot ulceration.

Peripheral neuropathy in the foot is initially characterized by small fibre changes – a loss of pain and heat sensation. Later, a mixed fibre neuropathy develops, with small and large myelinated nerve fibres affected. There is then an additional loss of touch, vibration and proprioception sense. This can lead to weakness and wasting of the intrinsic foot muscles with subsequent deformities of the toes. Dryness and fissuring of skin are a frequent feature of diabetic neuropathy, probably as an effect of reduced sweating related to impaired autonomic function. Cracks in the skin provide an entry site for secondary infection. Symptoms are discussed later in the section on neuropathic pain.

The National Institute for Clinical Excellence (NICE) recommends the application of a 10 g monofilament to the skin at a variety of sites because it is a validated technique, or use of a calibrated tuning fork, for assessing pressure sensation. The neurothesiometer is an alternative validated device used to deliver vibrations of varying amplitude. This enables the calculation of a vibration perception threshold.

Other simple examinations methods include a tendon hammer, pin and cotton-wool swab to assess reflexes, pain and light touch sensation. Assessing for peripheral neuropathy is aimed at identifying those patients at high risk of developing subsequent foot ulceration.

Neuropathic ulceration occurs primarily because of a reduction in pain sensation. Loss of pain awareness enables the development and progression of foot lesions to proceed unchecked. The common triggers for the development of foot ulceration include callus formation, direct trauma, excessive heat, chemical trauma and local infection. Neglected callus formation can occur as a result of increased vertical and shear forces beneath the metatarsal heads or excessive friction at the tips of the toes as a result of walking, and recurrent trauma of the toe against footwear. Repetitive friction or pressure leads to cell damage, microscopic haemorrhage and callus formation. Tissue damage and necrosis beneath the callus lead to the development of small cavities which can fill with serous fluid and erupt on to the surface of the foot as an ulcer.

Ulceration may also develop from more direct trauma such as treading on sharp objects or from debris or irregular surfaces within footwear. Some foot ulcers originate from direct heat trauma. Typical causes include placing feet directly in front of fires and radiators, bathing feet in excessively hot water or placing them against hot water bottles. Loss of pain awareness prevents the person moving his or her feet away from these stimuli, and direct damage to the epithelium then occurs.

Secondary infection frequently contributes to the persistence and worsening of foot ulceration. Typically the organisms involved are the local skin commensals staphylococci and streptococci. These secrete necrotizing toxins and other enzymes that act directly on local small blood vessels to spread infection and cause local thromboses. Spreading cellulitis can develop in surrounding skin or in deeper tissues. A range of tissues including tendons, joints and bones can also become infected. Bacteria and toxins may invade systemically to cause a bacteraemia. Other complications of infection include local necrosis and gangrene. These can result from damage to microcirculation even when major foot pulses are present.

A wide spectrum of bacteria may contribute to persisting infection. These include anaerobic organisms, Gram-negative bacilli and cocci in addition to gas-forming organisms including clostridia, *Escherichia coli* and *Bacteroides* species.

Impairment of blood supply

Diabetes is partly characterized by its effects on the macro- and microcirculation. The circulatory disease of the leg seen in diabetes is different from that seen in someone who does not have diabetes, with a higher incidence of disease in the arteries distal to the popliteal artery. Small vessel disease can lead to impaired local blood supply in diabetes and inhibit healing of damaged skin. In macrovascular disease of the diabetic leg, atherosclerosis tends to be 'multisegmental' rather than involving a single region of arterial wall.

Examination of the diabetic foot for the absence of dorsalis pedis and posterior tibial pulses can indicate the presence of macrovascular disease. Intermittent claudication and rest pain may be presenting symptoms of major vessel disease. Arterial calcification is commonly observed in radiographs of diabetic feet and hands due to calcification of the media in muscular arteries. Its importance in determining blood flow is not clear, but its effects are probably not significant.

Investigations for peripheral arterial disease commonly undertaken in primary care are clinical examination including palpation of peripheral pulses, listening to the sound produced by the arterial flow with a hand-held Doppler and calculating the ratio of the ankle:brachial systolic pressure index or ABPI. This process can, however, be unreliable in patients with significant arterial wall calcification – a common finding in diabetes. Investigations carried out in secondary care most commonly include non-invasive duplex ultrasonography, which demonstrates in more detail the velocity of blood flow to map stenotic disease. Digital subtraction arteriography has more recently been replaced by the advances in magnetic resonance (MR) angiography and computed tomography (CT) angiography. MR and CT angiography give a three-dimensional image of the arterial tree using a single injection of contrast. These vascular imaging techniques give vascular surgeons preoperative information about the distribution of vascular disease in given individuals.

Arterial calcification is commonly observed in radiographs of diabetic feet and hands, due to calcification of the media in muscular arteries. Its importance in determining blood flow is not clear, but its effects are probably not significant. However, atherosclerotic disease may appear more commonly in calcified vessels.

Ulceration is a common feature of the neuroischaemic foot. Minor trauma is often the precipitating factor for tissue damage in the ischaemic foot. Simple trauma includes pressure from ill-fitting shoes or even tight socks. Its appearance is different from that of the neuropathic ulcer. Callus is not usually present and typically there is an area of necrosis surrounded by a rim of erythema. The typical sites of ulceration are the great toe, the medial surface of the first metatarsal head and the heel. Unlike neuropathic ulceration it is frequently painful. In the ischaemic foot there is frequently blockage of the metatarsal arteries and this reduces communication between plantar and dorsal arterial arches. This lack of collateral circulation can be devastating in the presence of infection because bacteria may produce toxins that cause direct damage to local blood vessels. These can lead to obliteration of local arterial blood supply which can cause tissue necrosis and gangrene.

Charcot disease

Charcot neuroarthropathy is a progressive but self-limiting condition characterized by the presence of peripheral neuropathy and joint changes, now most commonly in association with diabetes. The incidence in diabetes is reported as between 1 and 5 per cent and can occur in patients with both type 1 and type 2 diabetes. In the past Charcot's neuroarthropathy has been considered rare but it is often misdiagnosed as cellultis, osteomyelitis, gout and deep vein thrombosis. It can present bilaterally in up to 30 per cent of people with diabetes The early changes can be asymptomatic due to the neuropathy, which may delay individuals from seeking medical advice and patients often present late with an existing foot deformity.

The mechanism of the bone damage associated with Charcot's neuroarthropathy appears to be an increase in blood flow which may be secondary to the loss of the sympathetic nerve supply associated with neuropathic disease. This causes increased osteoclast activity within bone and bone turnover is increased, leading to increased bone fragility. Susceptible bone becomes more prone to damage and fracture from minor trauma and there is subsequent destruction of the bony architecture.

The patient frequently presents with a hot, swollen foot that may be painful. Complaints may include noises 'like bones cracking' or odd, uncomfortable sensations 'like stones rubbing against each other inside my feet'. The typical affected sites are the tarsal–metatarsal region or the metatarsophalangeal joints. Most patients remain mobile and usually walk into the consulting room. Trauma may be the trigger for the development of Charcot foot; however, this is not universally reported and in the patient who is profoundly neuropathic the trauma may go unnoticed. Radiographic imaging, isotope bone scans and MR imaging (MRI) can assist in diagnosis, but this can still prove difficult in the early stages.

As the disease progresses, the structure of the foot is destroyed. Joint dislocations and fractures occur. These are often in the mid-foot, leading to the collapse of the arch. This can result in a rocker-bottom deformity due to displacement and subluxation of the tarsus, or medial convexity due to the talonavicular joint or tarsometatarsal dislocation. Some patients may present with foot ulceration and acute Charcot foot simultaneously if it has not been diagnosed and immobilized.

Nerve damage and painful diabetic neuropathy

There are different forms of diabetic neuropathy.

Mononeuropathies – damage to one nerve

Peripheral or cranial mononeuropathies are fairly commonplace. They may be spontaneous or secondary to entrapment or external pressure. Carpal tunnel syndrome can occur in up to 30 per cent of patients with diabetes, with symptoms occurring in 10 per cent. Patients complain of pain in the hands or forearm, typically worse at night and early morning. Nerve conduction studies should be used to confirm the diagnosis. Although overnight wrist supports may be helpful in alleviating symptoms, definitive treatment requires surgical decompression. Entrapment of the common peroneal nerve of the thigh is seen more commonly in patients with diabetes. This can give pain and paraesthesia in the outer third of the thigh.

Spontaneous neuropathy occurs in the common peroneal nerve and leads to foot drop. Full recovery is unusual and there is no definitive therapy. The most common cranial nerves affected are the third and sixth. CT or MRI is required in cranial nerve palsies to exclude raised pressure secondary to local aneurysm formation or a space-occupying brain lesion. Axillary, ulnar and other nerves can be damaged by external pressure – occasionally wrist drop can occur in patients who are unconscious from hypoglycaemia or after an alcohol binge.

Polyneuropathies

In these more than one individual nerve is affected or damaged.

Distal symmetrical polyneuropathy

This is sometimes referred to as 'diabetic neuropathy', 'sensory neuropathy' or 'chronic distal sensorimotor polyneuropathy'; it is the characteristic neurological impairment in diabetes where foot sensation is predominantly affected and was discussed earlier. However, when considering this common diagnosis it is important to consider the alternative causes of peripheral neuropathy:

- *Metabolic*: diabetes, uraemia, amyloidosis, myxoedema and porphyria
- *Nutritional*: vitamin B_{12}, vitamin B_6, nicotinic acid or thiamine deficiencies
- *Drug/chemical*: nitrofurantoin, vincristine, chlorambucil, isoniazid, phenytoin
- *Neoplasia*: bronchogenic carcinoma, malignant lymphoma
- *Infection*: Guillain–Barré syndrome, leprosy
- *Genetic*: Charcot–Marie–Tooth syndrome
- *Organ failure*: renal and hepatic failure.

Sensory ataxia

This is a loss of proprioception, the ability to distinguish joint position. It results in a loss of balance and a resultant high incidence of falls.

Insulin neuritis

This is an acute painful neuropathy relating to a rapid alteration of glycaemic control. Sensory loss is usually mild or absent with no motor involvement. There is usually a complete resolution of symptoms within 12 months.

Acute painful neuropathy of poor glycaemic control

Ellenberg coined the phrase 'neuropathic cachexia' to describe the symptoms of neuropathic pain, poor glycaemic control and weight loss. On examination sensory loss is typically mild or even absent, ankle jerks may be absent, and nerve conduction tests are usually normal or mildly abnormal. The temperature discrimination threshold is affected (small fibres) more commonly than the vibration perception threshold (large fibre involvement). There is a complete resolution within 12 months and weight gain is usual with continued improvement in glycaemic control and the use of insulin.

Diabetic amyotrophy

This is also termed 'proximal motor neuropathy' (PMN), 'femoral neuropathy' or 'symmetrical proximal lower limb motor neuropathy'. It typically occurs in those aged less than 50 years. Patients complain of severe pain deep in the thigh or burning pain extending below the knee. They may experience difficulty in rising out of chairs, climbing stairs, etc. There may be associated weight loss. Symptoms may begin unilaterally or bilaterally. An unaffected side usually becomes involved within a few weeks. On examination there is profound wasting of the quadriceps muscles with marked weakness. Hip flexor and thigh abductor muscles can be affected. Glutei and hamstring muscles may also be involved. The knee jerk is usually absent or reduced. There may be localized sensory loss over the thigh. With this condition it is important to exclude other causes of proximal muscle wasting, including nerve root and cauda equina lesions, occult malignancy and polymyositis. Investigations should include an erythrocyte sedimentation rate (ESR), radiographic imaging of the lumbar spine and chest, and abdominal ultrasonography where indicated. Electrophysiological studies may demonstrate increased femoral nerve latency and active denervation of affected muscles. Occasionally MRI of the lumbosacral spine may be required to exclude focal nerve root entrapment. The pain usually settles within 3 months. Management of this condition is essentially supportive. Sufferers should be informed that it is likely to resolve. Physiotherapy aimed at strengthening the quadriceps muscles may be helpful.

Truncal radiculopathy or thoracoabdominal neuropathy

This condition is rare. Sufferers typically present with acute asymmetrical pain with patchy sensory loss over the thorax and/or abdomen. The onset is rapid but recovery occurs within 3–12 months. There may be associated weight loss and aching, burning or sharp pain. Other causes of nerve root compression need to be excluded.

Autonomic neuropathy

This is damage to sympathetic and parasympathetic nervous systems. The most common symptom is erectile dysfunction. Other problems include GI dysfunction, bladder dysfunction and postural hypotension. Absent or excessive (gustatory) sweating can also occur. Dryness of the feet can cause cracks in the skin and provide portals for infection.

5.3 Management

Diabetic foot ulceration

There are common principles that underpin the management of both neuropathic and neuroischaemic foot ulceration. These include local medical and surgical treatments, infection control and pressure reduction. The role of arterial surgery is restricted to those with ischaemic disease. It is probably simplest to consider the management of these two forms of foot ulceration separately.

Neuropathic ulceration

Reduction of weight bearing

It is important to reduce the pressure at the site of ulceration from repeated mechanical trauma, which inhibits healing. The trauma is usually due to walking and normal daily activities and occurs as a result of sensory loss. A variety of offloading methods can be used depending on the site, size and severity of the ulcer.

The traditional cast is the total contact plaster cast. This can be used for a short period to equalize pressure forces in the affected foot. Removable casts such as soft cast slippers are increasingly being used. Removable cast walkers such as the Aircast pneumatic diabetic walking boot is used in many centres as an alternative to the total contact casting. Half-shoes and modified temporary shoes with insoles are designed to reduce peak plantar pressures and optimise the function of the foot.

When using insoles it is important that shoes have more depth to prevent compression or abrasion of the foot. In addition, uppers should be flexible in order to respond to toe pressure. Heels should be stable and the forefoot area of the shoe wide and square. Lace-ups are essential to prevent foot slippage and resultant trauma to the ends of toes. Shoes will need to be customized individually (bespoke) where foot deformity is present and soles should be altered when cushioned insoles do not provide protection. For an ulcer situated beneath a metatarsal head, a common adjustment includes a metatarsal bar that is placed proximal to the metatarsal heads. A rocker sole can be useful for ulcers beneath the first toe because it shifts the pressure load to the mid-foot.

Local treatment

Callus surrounding a foot ulcer needs to be removed to reduce local pressure, allowing effective drainage of the wound, establishing the extent of the wound and enabling re-epithelialization of the ulcer edges. Devitalized tissue and necrotic areas are also often removed by sharp debridement with the aim of preparing the wound bed to facilitate healing. An expert, usually a specialist podiatrist, will carry out local sharp debridement and wound care. The wound and the surrounding skin should then be cleaned and covered with an appropriate sterile dressing. This procedure will need to be repeated frequently until the ulcer is healed. If ulcers are situated beneath the nail (subungual) the nail may need to be cut back or excised to allow drainage of the ulcer. When extensive surgical debridement or amputation is indicated, a surgeon will carry out these procedures and is an important part of the multidisciplinary team.

Antibiotic therapy is necessary for infected ulcers. High-dose, broad-spectrum agents should be used pending further information about organism sensitivities from wound swab cultures. The rationale for this is that tissue penetration may be poor and low doses of antibiotic may lead to inadequate levels within the target tissue. There is a wide spectrum of organisms implicated in the development of an infected foot ulcer, many of which may be opportunistic skin commensals. Typical organisms include staphylococci, streptococci, Gram-negative bacteria and anaerobes. Locally agreed guidelines for the management of diabetic foot infections suggest empirical oral regimens and microbiology advice is often needed in recurrent or difficult-to-manage infections.

It is imperative that collections of pus and abscess cavities are drained surgically. Secondary infection frequently contributes to the persistence and worsening of foot ulceration. Spreading cellulitis can develop in surrounding skin or deeper tissues. A range of tissues including tendons, joints and bones can also become infected. Bacteria and toxins may invade systemically to cause a bacteraemia.

Neuroischaemic ulceration

In addition to the management of infection and identifying and removing precipitating trauma, consideration should be given to the investigation of impaired blood supply with a view to surgical intervention where possible to improve it. Surgical management is required for the excision of necrotic tissue, which includes surgical debridement, digital amputation and major limb amputation in severe cases.

Unlike neuropathic ulceration, ischaemic ulceration is frequently painful. This can sometimes be successfully treated with simple or codeine-based therapy, but frequently responds only to regular opiate analgesia.

The vascular interventions used are angioplasty and stenting or bypass surgery. The development of new techniques of revascularization – including endovascular procedures – are minimally invasive and associated with a low risk of complications and a short duration of hospital stay. Arterial bypass therapy has traditionally been fraught with difficulty in patients with peripheral vascular disease and diabetes because of the distal and diffuse nature of the atherosclerotic disease. However, in carefully selected patients, limb salvage and graft patency are improved in distal bypass grafts to both the dorsalis pedis and posterior tibial arteries. Although this form of surgery may require repeat surgical procedures, the typical cost remains less than that of major amputation. The revascularization of feet via distal arterial reconstruction appears to provide good capillary perfusion despite the presence of diabetes.

Charcot foot

The key to treatment, and long-term preservation of the limb, is immobilization. This will prevent further joint damage and should be recommended immediately. Continued walking will inevitably lead to ulceration and more damage. Options for immobilization include crutches, wheelchair, total contact cast and removable cast walker. Immobilization is recommended whereas in the acute phases this can vary significantly from 3 months to 4 months, but can be as long as a year, depending on the activity of the disease. The foot should be reviewed and treated until the swelling has subsided and temperature returned to normal. Infrared skin thermometry is frequently used as an indicator of inflammatory destructive phase and serial radiographs are helpful to identify when there is coalescence and remodelling of bone.

When the acute phase has resolved, the foot should be reviewed and future care must be planned. The patient should be considered at high risk for ulceration. If deformity is minimal it can be managed in normal footwear with the addition of insoles or orthoses. The foot protection team should review the patient and ongoing foot support should be provided. If there is deformity that makes it difficult to obtain appropriate footwear, or if weight bearing is considered dangerous or likely to cause ulceration, then an orthotic referral for alternative footwear provision is necessary. In some cases more invasive management may be required. An orthopaedic opinion for consideration of reconstructive surgery may be useful in helping to restore normal foot shape (Figure 5.1).

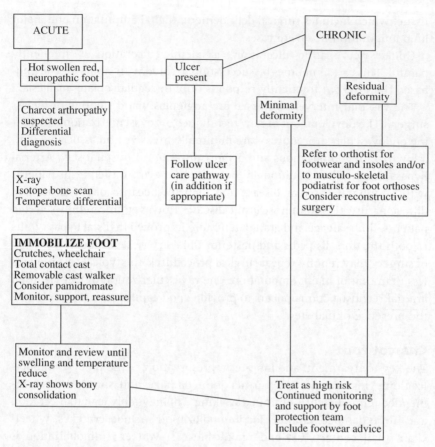

Figure 5.1 The management of Charcot foot.

Management of neuropathic pain

When assessing a patient with foot pain it is important to take a detailed history including information about the type, frequency and nature of the pain, precipitating and alleviating factors, and other associated symptoms. A detailed past medical and medication history should be sought. There should be specific questioning about the presence of back pain and bowel/bladder function. It is essential to rule out other causes of pain and peripheral neuropathy. The pain may be severe and it is important to allow patients to express their feelings and for listeners to be empathetic. An assessment of the impact of symptoms should be made.

A full physical examination should be carried out, including a clinical neurological assessment. Pain is subjective and it may be important to identify tools that enable symptoms to be quantified. Pain questionnaires are widely used to assist in the detection and measurement of severity of pain and in the evaluation of treatment.

There are a variety of treatments available for the management of neuropathic pain. However, success in alleviating all pain is unrealistic for many. Frequently the goal is an improved quality of life, improved sleep and a *reduction* in pain. A 50 per cent reduction in pain severity may be a realistic and adequate goal. The response to differing treatments will vary markedly between individuals.

Improvement in glycaemic control may help to prevent the development and progression of neuropathic pain, and it is important to target a lowering of blood glucose in those patients who have poor control as the first step in the treatment of neuropathic pain. Symptoms can, however, worsen acutely in the context of both sudden deterioration and sudden improvement in glycaemic control. The aim should therefore be a gradual improvement.

Neuropathic pain is usually a self-limiting condition but, for some patients, symptoms can last for many years. It is important to inform sufferers about the cause and natural history of the condition. This information should include a careful explanation of different treatments, their effectiveness, potential side effects and likely improvements. It is essential that support networks be put in place for patients. The authors have found that an education group involving patients, those who care for them and interested health-care professionals is one way of achieving this.

It is common for patients to require a number of different treatments, either alone or in combination. It is vital that treatment be continuously monitored and adjusted in order to maximize the beneficial effects. This may be achieved more easily by involving patients in their management through self-titration of drug therapy and agreed care protocols, and by establishing for patients an easy point of contact with a health-care professional.

Patients with sensory loss and other risk findings are at increased risk of foot ulceration and should receive increased monitoring education advice and support from an advanced podiatry team.

Medical therapies

There is now broad agreement that people with diabetic neuropathic pain should be offered the available therapies in a stepwise fashion. The 2010 NICE (National Institute for Health and Clinical Excellence) guidance on the pharmacological management of neuropathic pain in adults in non-specialist settings provides an algorithm to standardize the management of neuropathic pain, so that individual patients can receive benefit from all available treatments in an order that is most appropriate for achieving resolution of symptoms and improvement in quality of life.

Oral agents
Simple painkillers are rarely effective and their use should not be prolonged unless there is a rapid response to treatment.

Tricyclic antidepressants
These have, for many years, been a first-line systemic therapy even though they are not specifically licensed for use in this way. Several randomized controlled trials have demonstrated the efficacy of tricyclic antidepressants (TCAs) in the treatment of diabetic neuropathic pain. They block presynaptic reuptake of 5-HT and noradrenaline. Side effects of the TCA group include sedation, dry mouth, urinary retention, postural hypotension and exacerbation of glaucoma. TCA treatment for diabetic neuropathic pain should be started with a small dose of either amitriptyline or imipramine at night. The dose typically should start at 10–25 mg and be gradually titrated depending on efficacy and adverse events.

Serotonin–noradrenaline reuptake inhibitors (SNRIs)
These relieve pain by increasing synaptic availability of serotonin and noradrenaline in the descending pathways that inhibit pain impulses. Duloxetine is currently recommended by NICE as the preferred first-line treatment for diabetic neuropathic pain.

The anticonvulsants
Gabapentin (Neurontin) and pregabalin (Lyrica) are licensed as oral agents for use in painful neuropathy. The mode of action for these drugs is a blockage of neural transmission of pain pathways at the dorsal horns of the spinal cord. Inadequate dose titration of gabapentin will produce a suboptimal response. Common side effects are dizziness and drowsiness.

Pregabalin has a similar mode of action and appears to be as effective in the treatment of neuropathic pain. It may have benefits over its predecessor and is recommended after duloxetine and amitriptyline in the latest NICE guidance. Dose titration is simpler and quicker.

Opiate-based therapies
The use of opiate-based therapies is controversial in the management of any chronic pain. These therapies typically cause a degree of dependence but may be advocated in severe intractable cases. Tramadol is a centrally acting opiate derivative that is less addictive and has been shown to benefit some patients with neuropathic pain. The prolonged release formulation of the strong opiate oxycodone has also been shown to be effective in relieving neuropathic pain.

Lidocaine

Lidocaine patches are licensed for the treatment of neuropathic pain associated with post-herpetic neuralgia; however, the authors have had some success in using them to treat diabetic neuropathic pain.

Topical agents

Although not recommended in latest NICE guidance, several topical agents are frequently used to treat symptoms of neuropathic pain.

Capsaicin cream (0.075%)

This is derived from chilli pepper. It is applied three to four times daily to symptomatic areas of the foot. It is believed to work through depletion of substance P from nerve terminals.

Plaster sprays

These when sprayed directly on to the affected area give some patients dramatic cooling relief of symptoms. This therapy can unfortunately be somewhat messy, leaving a filmy residue on the skin surface that can be difficult to remove.

Flexitol cooling gel

This offers relief from the burning sensation often reported by sufferers of diabetic neuropathic pain.

Other therapies

Spinal cord stimulation

TENS (transcutaneous electrical nerve stimulation) machines may be beneficial for some, particularly those patients with pain localized to one limb only.

Spinal nerve blocks

These have been used with mixed success but can be considered after an appropriate anaesthetic assessment from within a pain team.

Psychological support

When managing the chronic pain of peripheral neuropathy it is important to consider whether psychological support may be required. Depressive symptoms are common in this group. There is a strong association between poor glycaemic control and the prevalence of depression. There is also evidence to link loss of proprioception and balance in patients with diabetes with an increased incidence of depression. Unfortunately there is a lack of appropriately trained clinical psychologists and others to deal with the psychological effects of chronic pain in diabetes teams.

5.4 The organization of foot care

People with diabetes and those caring for them should be provided with easy access to a multidisciplinary diabetic foot care team. This may take the form of the 'gold-standard' multidisciplinary foot clinic. Alternatively this may be a team of people who work closely together in settings that allow for easy communication and direct access to each other's specialist skills.

There should be an organised programme of foot care that includes:

- continuous education of patients, carers and staff
- identification of patients with feet at high risk
- provision of measures designed to reduce risk – including the correction of elevated blood glucose, avoidance of smoking, adequate nutrition and other health strategies such as anti-platelet therapy and treatment of abnormal lipid profiles
- streamlined communication between health-care professionals that crosses the boundaries of care.

A diabetes foot care team can help to provide appropriate knowledge to each other and to others who provide care outside the group. Skills should be made easily accessible to patients and other health carers. The group should produce and disseminate practical guidelines on the avoidance, identification and management of complications. There should be clear pathways between primary and secondary care.

A multidisciplinary diabetic foot care team should incorporate a number of key individuals. From the specialist setting there should be a minimum of one individual representing the following areas: specialist podiatry, specialist orthotics, diabetes nurse specialist, consultant diabetologist, vascular surgeon and orthopaedic surgeon. It may be beneficial to involve wound care/tissue viability nurses, plaster technicians and vascular/diabetes/medical admissions ward nurses. Ideally the group should cross the primary/secondary care boundary and incorporate primary care nurse, physician and podiatrist. There should also be a patient representative.

It is not feasible for all of these individuals to be involved in one multi-disciplinary foot clinic. However, crucial leaders of the team should meet regularly to enhance the development of a coordinated diabetes foot care service. The multidisciplinary foot care team should act as a focal point and resource for patients and other health-care professionals.

The team of people caring for those with diabetes is much larger than these few individuals. Extended team members include the patient carer, reception staff, pharmacist, microbiologist, physiotherapist, occupational therapist, clinical psychologist, pain specialist, radiologist and others.

To meet the needs and achieve high standards of care for the person with diabetes there needs to be continuing education for all, in addition to effective communication between all these individuals. It is the responsibility of the team to ensure that this happens.

Although foot disease is a leading cause of hospital admission and expense, its prevention may increasingly lie in educating patients and staff away from the specialist care setting. We have also therefore helped indicate the links between primary and secondary care to ensure that risk factors are recognized and acted upon and complications are managed effectively.

Case study

A 59-year-old white man with type 2 diabetes, hypertension, dyslipidaemia and history of myocardial infarction attends for routine diabetes review. His medication includes antihypertensive therapy. Blood results include glycated haemoglobin 74 mmol/mol (8.9%), total cholesterol 4.0 mmol/l, LDL 1.9 mmol/l and triglycerides 1.8 mmol/l. Blood pressure 132/80 mmHg. He is overweight with a body mass index of 27 and sedentary lifestyle as a taxis driver.

Foot examination reveals reduced protective sensation with 10 g monofilament and intact vibration sensation with calibrated tuning fork. Foot pulses are palpable and no symptoms of vascular insufficiency are reported. Minor hallux valgus deformity and callus at the medial first metatarsal head are noted bilaterally. He is wearing supportive lace-up shoes No foot problems are reported.

Discussion

The sensory, painless peripheral neuropathy and skin changes as a result of deformity and altered foot function put him at high risk of developing foot complications according to current NICE (National Institute for Health and Clinical Excellence) guidelines. Assessment and treatment by a podiatrist are indicated to optimize foot function using insoles, reduce areas of excessive callus and provide enhanced education. Despite the lack of perceived problems by the patient, ensuring an understanding of the implications of neuropathy is essential. Education is aimed at encouraging health behaviours such as daily foot inspection, regular application of emollient cream and how to access a member of the diabetes foot protection team in the event of noticing a problem.

Monitoring of vascular risk factors is required along with a review of glycaemic control. Modifying lifestyle to include regular exercise and balanced diet to optimize blood sugars and maintain peripheral blood supply should be discussed with the patient. The prophylactic use of aspirin should be considered in this patient who has several risk factors for circulatory disease. Enquiries should be made as to his smoking status with help offered for smoking cessation if required. His lipid profile appears to be at a target level of cholesterol under current recommendations.

Managing all the risk factors is key to reducing the risk of neuropathic foot ulceration in this man. Despite the feet not presenting with perceived severe problems, expert assessment is indicated to work together with the patient to maintain foot health and optimize blood glucose levels.

Bibliography

Bansal D, Bhansali A, Hota D, Chakrabarti A, Dutta P. Amitriptyline vs pregabalin in painful diabetic neuropathy: a randomized double blind controlled trial. *Diabet Med* 2009;**26**:1019–1026.

Benbow SJ, Daousi C, MacFarlane A. Diagnosing and managing chronic painful diabetic neuropathy. *Diabetic Foot* 2004;**7**:34–46.

Boulton AJM. Understanding painful symptomatic diabetic neuropathy. *Pract Diabet Int* 2004;**21**:157–161.

Cavanagh PR, Ubrecht JS. Clinical plantar pressure measurements in diabetes: rationale and methodology. In: Boulton AJM, Connor H, Cavanagh PR (eds), *The Foot in Diabetes*. Oxford: Blackwell, 1994.

Cheshire NJW, Wolfe JHN. Critical leg ischaemia: amputation and reconstruction. *BMJ* 1992;**304**:312–315.

Gimbel JS, Richards P, Portenoy RK. Controlled-release oxycodone for pain in diabetic neuropathy: a randomized controlled trial. *Neurology* 2003;**60**:927–934.

Goldstein DJ, Lu Y, Detke MJ, et al. Duloxetine vs. placebo in patients with painful diabetic neuropathy. *Pain* 2005;**116**:109–118.

Harati Y, Gooch C, Swenson M. et al. Double-blind randomized trial of tramadol for the treatment of the pain of diabetic neuropathy. *Neurology* 1998;**50**:1842–1846.

Holland E, Bradbury R, Meeking D. Using a team approach to set up a diabetic foot referral pathway. *Diabetic Foot* 2002;**3**:106–110.

Holland E, Land D, McIntosh S, Meeking D. Development of diabetic foot service since the introduction of a multidisciplinary diabetic foot referral pathway. *Pract Diabet Int* 2002;**19**:137–138.

Max MB, Lynch SA, Muir J, et al. Effects of desipramine, amitriptyline, and fluoxetine on pain in diabetic neuropathy. *N Engl J Med* 1992;**326**:1250–1256.

National institute of Health and Clinical Excellence. *Clinical Guidelines for Type 2 Diabetes: Prevention and management of foot problems*. Clinical Guideline 10. London: NICE, 2004.

National Institute for Health and Clinical Excellence. *Neuropathic Pain: The pharmacological management of neuropathic pain in adults in non-specialist settings*. Clinical guidelines 96. London: NICE, 2010.

Raskin J, Pritchett YL, Wang F, et al. A double-blind, randomized multicenter trial comparing duloxetine with placebo in the management of diabetic peripheral neuropathic pain. *Pain Med* 2005;**6**:346–356.

Scottish Intercollegiate Guidelines Network. *Diagnosis and Management of Peripheral Arterial Disease*. A National Clinical Guideline. Edinburgh: SIGN, 2006.

Tesfaye S. An update on the management of diabetic peripheral neuropathic pain. Supplement *Diab Foot J* 2010;**13**(suppl):4–7.

Wernicke JF, Pritchett YL, D'Souza ND et al. A randomized controlled trial of duloxetine in diabetic peripheral neuropathic pain. *Neurology* 2006;**67**:1411–1420.

CHAPTER 6

Diabetes and Autonomic Neuropathy

Andrew F Macleod

Royal Shrewsbury Hospital, Shrewsbury, UK

 Key points

- Diabetic autonomic neuropathy may be uncommon but its detection may be vitally important.

- Detailed clinical assessment remains the cornerstone of the diagnosis of autonomic neuropathy.

- Other (perhaps sinister and perhaps still treatable) causes of the varied symptoms and signs MUST be excluded.

- Management of blood glucose, blood ketones and overall nutrition is the keystone of management.

- Successful metabolic management may provide many years without symptoms.

- Knowledge of the presence of autonomic neuropathy is important when deciding on drug treatment, and for safe perioperative management.

- Multiple therapies are often necessary to control symptoms.

 Therapeutic key points

Therapies that can precipitate or exacerbate diabetic autonomic neuropathy include:

- Drugs with anticholinergic action such as:

  – amitriptyline, imipramine, dosulepin

- Tranquillizers

- Diuretics

- α blockers

- Glucagon peptide-1 (GLP-1) analogues.

- Specific therapies need to be given an adequate and objective clinical trial.

- For gastroparesis, patients must be advised to continue prokinetic agents (e.g. domperidone) prophylactically, i.e. even if symptoms are absent.

Diabetes: Chronic Complications, Third Edition. Edited by Kenneth M. Shaw, Michael H. Cummings.
© 2012 John Wiley & Sons, Ltd. Published 2012 by John Wiley & Sons, Ltd.

6.1 Introduction

The autonomic nervous system is part of the peripheral nervous system and controls the involuntary functions of the body, affecting heart rate, control of blood pressure, digestion, respiratory rate, salivation, perspiration, adjustment of pupil diameter, micturition and sexual arousal. Traditionally autonomic innervation is divided into the sympathetic and parasympathetic systems. In diabetes, there can be damage to all parts of the peripheral nervous system, to ganglia, nerve axons and (more relevant to sensorimotor peripheral neuropathy) Schwann cells. Diabetic autonomic neuropathy, or damage to the autonomic nervous system, occurs in diabetes, often together with damage to the rest of the peripheral nervous system.

The diagnosis of diabetic autonomic neuropathy remains in the province of the astute and experienced clinician. It is also a 'diagnosis of exclusion' – in other words it can be made only after other conditions, which may mimic the symptoms (e.g. gastrointestinal malignancy) or affect the autonomic nervous system (e.g. Shy–Drager syndrome), have been excluded by clinical investigations.

There is no specific test to confirm the diagnosis. Autonomic function tests may be a useful aid, but must be taken in context. Tests may be 'abnormal' due to age in an elderly individual with type 2 diabetes, and a patient with type 1 diabetes may have abnormal tests but still harbour a treatable carcinoma of the caecum that is in fact responsible for the symptom of diarrhoea.

Diabetic autonomic neuropathy, however, remains a distressing condition that is often not easy to treat, may easily be overlooked and may have serious consequences for affected individuals in terms of both the quality and the longevity of their life.

6.2 Epidemiology

Widely varying estimates of the prevalence of diabetic autonomic neuropathy are published in the literature. Calculation of the prevalence of autonomic neuropathy obviously depends on the definition of the condition, the tests that are used and the population studied. The type of diabetes may also be relevant, as well as the time of the study; it would be hoped that more recent efforts to provide, for example, better glycaemic control of diabetes would reduce the prevalence. The author's anecdotal experience (and that of many of his contemporary colleagues) is that severe cases of diabetic autonomic neuropathy in type 1 diabetes are becoming less common over the last few decades, and there is some evidence to support his observation from the Pittsburgh Epidemiology of Diabetes Study. Some 900 people with type 1 diabetes diagnosed in childhood were followed for 30 years, and the study revealed a significant decrease in symptomatic autonomic neuropathy from the cohort diagnosed in the 1950s to that diagnosed in the 1980s.[1] A European study in 1993 found 16.8 per cent of patients with type 1 diabetes and 22.1 per cent of patients with type 2 diabetes to have abnormalities in three of six standard cardiovascular autonomic function tests involving heart rate variation.[2]

A French study of diabetic patients attending seven departments of diabetes (likely to have an increased prevalence of complications compared with a population-derived sample) in 2003 revealed abnormal heart rate variability in 50 per cent, even higher in those with type 1 diabetes.[3] Another French study of prevalence in 2010 of people with type 1 diabetes found that autonomic failure was confirmed in 12.3 per cent.[4] The EURODIAB study (randomly selected patients with type 1 diabetes from 31 centres in 16 European countries, published in 2001–2), examined changes in heart rate variation and blood pressure from lying to standing. An abnormality in at least one of the tests was seen in 36 per cent of patients; the heart rate variation was abnormal in 24 per cent and postural hypotension was seen in 18 per cent. Significant symptoms were seen in 18 per cent for dizziness on standing, 5 per cent for problems with bladder control and 4 per cent for nocturnal diarrhoea.[5]

In a community-based study in the UK in 1989 (mostly type 2 diabetes), the prevalence of abnormal heart rate variability tests was 16.7 per cent.[6] In the population-based Rochester study in the USA, published in 2004, the prevalence of autonomic impairment was 54 per cent in people with type 1 diabetes and 73 per cent with type 2 diabetes, compared with matched non-diabetic control participants, very similar to that reported for diabetic peripheral neuropathy. Autonomic symptoms were less prevalent although more common than in the control group. Interestingly symptoms were more common in type 2 than in type 1 diabetes, particularly for urinary problems and diarrhoea, but not for male sexual failure and syncope.[7]

Comparison of the above studies is fraught because of the varied methods of assessment and classification of the condition.

6.3 Pathophysiology

The Diabetes Control and Complications Trial (DCCT) provided evidence that improved glycaemic control was associated with both the slowing of progression and a decrease in the new development of abnormal autonomic nerve function in people with type 1 diabetes.[8] In so doing the trial confirmed the hypothesis that hyperglycaemia was a causative factor and promised that improved blood glucose control was likely to reduce the prevalence of autonomic neuropathy, as with the other chronic complications of diabetes. The EDIC study provided detailed follow-up of the same cohort of people with type 1 diabetes, 13–14 years later. There was still a significant difference in favour of the intensively treated group: prevalence of autonomic neuropathy, using a composite definition, was 29 per cent as opposed to 35 per cent in the control group, despite the fact that glycaemic control had been very similar in the two groups over the many years of follow-up. Thus the so-called 'legacy effect' of improved glycaemic control also applies to autonomic neuropathy.[9] Evidence also exists for type 2 diabetes in the Steno Type 2 Study.[10]

The association between hyperglycaemia and deteriorating autonomic nerve function is now universally accepted, but the mechanisms by which hyperglycaemia causes damage are still very much open to debate. Candidates include a direct metabolic insult to the nerve (whether neurons or ganglia) or the vasa nervorum. Possible biochemical pathways include the polyol pathway, activation of protein kinase C, increased oxidative stress, with increased free radical production, and abnormalities of nitric oxide production.[11]

The typical clinical picture of diabetic autonomic neuropathy is usually seen in type 1 diabetes. Findings of an association of the clinical picture with iritis led to the hypothesis that there might be an autoimmune component to the aetiology in this type of diabetes. The β cell is embryologically of neuroectoderm origin, and antibodies to components of the β cell are of course well recognized in type 1 diabetes. The hypothesis suggests that hyperglycaemia causes the initial damage, thus exposing intracellular components, and that an autoimmune attack against these components then accelerates the process, resulting in the clinical condition.

Antibodies directed against autonomic nerves and ganglia have been found in increased frequency in type 1 diabetes, and in increased frequency in those people with autonomic neuropathy.[12] Whether this is a causative association, or simply an unimportant by-product of autonomic nerve destruction, remains to be seen. The hypothesis is attractive because it helps to explain the finding that, although in general symptoms are more common in type 2 diabetes (see above), the most severe forms of the clinical syndrome are seen in type 1 autoimmune diabetes.

Association of diabetic autonomic neuropathy with cardiovascular risk factors have been reported in a number of studies. For example, in the EURODIAB study of people with type 1 diabetes, the presence of autonomic neuropathy was associated with cigarette smoking, total cholesterol/

HDL-cholesterol ratio, and fasting triglyceride.[13] Again, the causal mechanisms remain to be proven.

6.4 Management

Diagnosis and clinical investigations

Tests of cardiovascular autonomic function

Ewing and his colleagues in Edinburgh described a 'battery' of five tests to assess cardiovascular autonomic nerve function in the 1970s, and some or all have since been used by many for research and clinical practice.[14] They comprise: heart rate response to Valsalva's manoeuvre, deep breathing, and standing up, and blood pressure response to standing and hand grip. More sophisticated measures employing spectral analysis of variability of heart rate during normal breathing have also been used.

Two simple clinical tests that can be carried out in any hospital are the blood pressure and heart rate responses to standing (mainly sympathetic), and the 'E:I' ratio (mainly vagal).

Blood pressure response to standing

In normal individuals the blood pressure is rapidly corrected on standing by baroreflex-mediated peripheral vasoconstriction and tachycardia. There may be a slight rise in blood pressure, or at the most a fall of 10 mmHg systolic pressure. The standing pressure should be measured at least 30 seconds after standing. Postural drops often vary considerably through the day and from week to week. An agreed definition of orthostatic hypotension is a fall on standing of systolic blood pressure of ≥20 mmHg, or of diastolic blood pressure of ≥10 mmHg, accompanied by symptoms. This test assesses mainly sympathetic nerve function.

Expired:inspired heart rate ratio (E:I ratio)

The E:I ratio measures heart rate (R–R interval) from an ECG tracing during controlled deep breathing. The individual is instructed how to take a deep breath lasting approximately 5 seconds in, 5 seconds out while resting on a couch. The shortest R–R interval during inspiration (I) and the longest during expiration (E) are measured and the 'E:I' ratio calculated. A number of breaths (e.g. three) may be requested and the mean calculated. As with all tests of autonomic function, there is a decline with age: age-related normal ranges have been published.[15] This test assesses mainly parasympathetic nerve function.

The validity of the tests is affected by the metabolic status (e.g. degree of dehydration, hyperglycaemia), time of day, distance from meal and insulin, coffee intake and smoking status, and the patient's collaboration.

Table 6.1 Tests of autonomic function

	Parasympathetic	Sympathetic
Cardiovascular		
Heart rate variability	Yes (high frequency variation)	Yes (low frequency variation)
Blood pressure response to standing		Yes
Expired : inspired heart rate ratio	Yes	
The Valsalva response	Yes	
Pupillary		
Dark-adapted pupil diameter		Yes
Light reflex	Yes	
Gastric		
Scintigraphic or ultrasonographic test meal	Yes	
Peripheral		
Galvanic skin response		Yes (cholinergic)
Axon reflex		Yes
Vasoconstriction index		Yes

Other tests

Other tests of autonomic function abound in the literature, from tests that assess pupillary function to those that assess the peripheral autonomic nerves[16] (Table 6.1). Few are of use, however, in the routine clinical situation.

Clinical syndromes and their management

Sweating

Significant damage to the autonomic nerves results in reduced sweating, as seen in the dry feet of patients with severe peripheral neuropathy. Increased sweating can also occur in diabetes, particularly in the shorter nerves of the face and trunk, and is thought to be due to autonomic dysfunction. Increased sweating may also occur at night, but must be distinguished from nocturnal hypoglycaemia. Early changes in sudomotor function have been demonstrated in type 1 diabetes.[17]

This embarrassing symptom is not easy to treat but may be helped by anticholinergic agents. One widely recommended agent, poldine methyl sulphate, is currently unobtainable, but others, such as propantheline bromide, may help. Patients should be warned that such non-specific agents cause a dry mouth and can seriously exacerbate postural hypotension if present. Use can be limited to provide confidence in public situations etc.

Box 6.1 Syndromes of diabetic autonomic neuropathy

- Sudomotor
  - Abnormal sweating
  - Gustatory sweating
  - Dry warm skin
- Cardiovascular
  - Resting tachycardia
  - Postural hypotension
  - Silent myocardial ischaemia
  - Anaemia
  - ? sudden death
- Gastrointestinal
  - Oesophageal dysmotility
  - Gastroparesis
  - Diarrhoea
  - Constipation
  - Faecal incontinence
- Genitourinary
  - Neurogenic bladder
  - Erectile dysfunction
  - Retrograde ejaculation
- Metabolic
  - Hypoglycaemia unawareness
  - Hypoglycaemia-associated autonomic failure
- Respiratory
  - Sleep apnoea.

Gustatory sweating

An unusual but relatively specific symptom of diabetic autonomic neuropathy is that of profuse sweating of the face brought about by eating ('gustatory sweating'). Again, anticholinergic agents may help and caution is necessary to avoid exacerbating postural hypotension.

Painful neuropathic symptoms

Painful neuropathic symptoms in diabetes do not usually correlate with the degree of histological nerve damage. There is some evidence, however, that peripheral autonomic (sympathetic) denervation may be present and may be an aetiological factor.[18]

Gastroparesis

Gastroparesis is characterized by delayed gastric emptying without any evidence of mechanical obstruction. Diabetic gastroparesis is clinically important because it may be associated with gastrointestinal symptoms, alterations in glycaemic control, impaired nutrition and changes in oral drug absorption.[19] Abnormality of gastric emptying due to diabetic autonomic neuropathy can result in symptoms of nausea, bloating and vomiting. Diabetic control then becomes difficult, and ketosis worsens. Increased blood glucose levels and ketonaemia by themselves may adversely affect gastric emptying, and then exacerbate the condition, such that a vicious circle develops. Episodes may be precipitated by intercurrent infection.

It has been estimated that 50 per cent of patients with type 1 diabetes may have problems with gastric emptying, mostly as a direct result of raised blood glucose levels.[20] However, only 5–12 per cent may be affected by classic symptoms. The interplay between the acute effect of hyperglycaemia and that of structural (and, currently, largely irreversible) nerve damage may explain why some individuals may have weeks or months of severe problems with nausea and vomiting and then long periods without a problem (see Case study 1). There is no doubt that patients with severe autonomic nerve damage may be severely and chronically affected, but control of blood glucose and ketonaemia is still of paramount importance in such cases. Gastroparesis may also be seen in a significant number of people with type 2 diabetes.[21]

On examination there is usually evidence of coexisting sensorimotor peripheral and autonomic neuropathy, and a succussion splash may be heard. Diagnosis includes gastroscopy to exclude mechanical obstruction, and tests to measure gastric emptying. Isotopic gastric scintigraphy is thought to be the most useful test, usually by taking measurements at 15-minute intervals for 4 hours after a labelled test meal.

Management starts with efforts to maximize blood glucose control, including subcutaneous insulin pumps in appropriate cases. Scrutiny of medications is necessary to exclude or replace those that may delay gastric emptying (e.g. antidepressants with anticholinergic action). First-line treatment consists of agents to increase gastric emptying, including erythromycin, metoclopramide and domperidone. Metoclopramide and domperidone seem to be equally effective, but side effects may be less prevalent with domperidone. The patient must realize that these agents need to be taken regularly to prevent nausea and vomiting, and appropriately timed before meals, rather than simply to treat the symptoms. An antiemetic (e.g. prochlorperazine) can be added.

As above, metabolic control is vital in severe cases. First the insulin regimen must both control blood glucose and adequately suppress ketone levels, but also enteral feeding may need to be enhanced. Percutaneous endoscopic jejunostomy (PEJ) tubes may be needed in selected cases, so that the gastric area is left unimpeded in case gastric stimulators (see below) need to be used.

An implantable stimulator (Enterra) has undergone trials for severe intractable symptoms as an alternative to gastrectomy. The device is installed by laparoscopic insertion. In a case series 50–92 per cent response rates have been claimed. Of more substance, a double-blind, sham-controlled trial of 33 people with gastroparesis, 17 with diabetes, revealed a reduction in vomiting when the device was switched on. There was, however, no change in total symptom scores, but patients preferred the 'on' to the 'off' period. The device was removed in 11 per cent of patients as a result of complications.[22] In a more recent multicentre study of 55 people with diabetic gastroparesis, the device was switched on for 6 weeks, then on or off in a crossover fashion for 3-month periods. There was a 57 per cent reduction in weekly vomiting frequency after the initial 6-week period, but no difference between 'on' and 'off' during the crossover period.[23] The natural history of the condition is often one of eventual improvement, so that controlled trials will be necessary to provide conclusive proof of efficacy.

Other experimental agents, including the receptor agonists to the gut hormone ghrelin and pyridostigmine, show some promise, but are not yet available for clinical use.[24] One group has advocated gastric surgery for severe chronic cases (which are rare), but evidence-based studies are lacking.[25]

A particular problem with gastroparesis may develop in pregnancy, possibly because of a combination of the autonomic dysfunction and hyperemesis of pregnancy. Good metabolic control, i.e. blood glucose and nutrition, is essential.[26]

Diabetic diarrhoea

Intermittent profuse watery diarrhoea is a well-recognized symptom of diabetic autonomic neuropathy. Symptoms can be particularly distressing (see Case study 2), and are typically worse at night. Disturbance of intestinal motility has been demonstrated, and it is suggested that small bowel bacterial overgrowth may then contribute to symptoms.[27]

Again diagnosis is essentially clinical, and other causes must first be excluded with standard tests including sigmoidoscopy and colonoscopy. A careful drug history must be taken, particularly including metformin.

The symptom may be particularly refractive to treatment, but first-line therapy includes a short course of antibiotics such as tetracycline (or doxycycline if there is evidence of renal impairment) or erythromycin. Conventional treatment with codeine phosphate or loperamide may often help. Clonidine (0.6 mg three times daily) has been shown to reduce symptoms, but side effects may limit its use. There have been anecdotal reports of improvement with the somatostatin analogue, octreotide; there are no randomized studies and one report documents a significant rise in blood pressure that necessitated stopping treatment. In extreme and refractory cases surgery with formation of a colostomy may be considered.

Anaemia

In the 1990s research drew attention to the association of anaemia and diabetic autonomic neuropathy in type 1 diabetes. The suggestion was made that there might be impairment of putative sympathetic nervous control of erythropoietin release from the kidney. Such a mechanism has been suggested in 'pure' non-diabetic autonomic failure.[28] Proof of a causative relationship in people with diabetes was made difficult by the fact that a significant proportion of patients with clinical evidence of diabetic autonomic neuropathy also had evidence of significant renal damage.[29]

There is increasing evidence of a real relationship, however,[30] and also reports of symptomatic improvement, e.g. improvement of postural symptoms,[31] after early erythropoietin replacement. A similar correlation between evidence of autonomic nerve damage and erythropoietin deficiency has been reported in patients with type 2 diabetes – in other words a blunted response of erythropoietin to anaemia in patients without advanced renal failure.[32] Use of erythropoietin must be monitored carefully in line with guidelines for its use in renal failure, to avoid the severe cerebrovascular consequences of overtreatment.

Postural (orthostatic) hypotension

The normal response to attaining the upright posture is a slight increase in systolic pressure, mediated mainly by the sympathetic nervous system. Postural or orthostatic hypotension is usually defined as a postural drop in systolic blood pressure of at least 20 mmHg, or at least 10 mmHg for the diastolic component.[33] Postural dizziness, disorientation or loss of consciousness (syncope) can be severely disabling. The symptoms are worse on rising and in the early part of the day, and are often exacerbated after a meal, presumably due to increased splanchnic blood flow. It is also possible that autonomic neuropathy adversely affects autoregulation of cerebral blood flow, and thus the postural symptoms are exacerbated.[34] Atypical symptoms, such as generalized weakness, fatigue, nausea, headache or visual blurring, may be present. In some cases, postural symptoms may remit despite little difference in the measurement of the postural drop (see Case study 3).

For affected individuals a reduction in plasma noradrenaline release with the upright posture is usually the case, but for some a paradoxical increase in noradrenaline has been reported. The authors of the report suggest that this response may be an early feature of the condition, possibly via erythropoietin deficiency (see above).[35]

Box 6.2 Causes of autonomic neuropathy

- **Primary autonomic degenerative disorders (synucleinopathies):**
  - multiple system atrophy (Shy–Drager syndrome)
  - Parkinson's disease
  - dementia with Lewy bodies
  - pure autonomic failure
- **Peripheral autonomic disorders:**
  - diabetes mellitus
  - amyloidosis
  - alcoholic neuropathy
  - uraemic neuropathy
  - immune-mediated neuropathies (including acute post-infective polyneuritis)
  - hereditary sensory and autonomic neuropathies
  - inflammatory neuropathies
  - vitamin B_{12} deficiency
  - exposure to neurotoxins (e.g. thallium, acrylamide)
  - neuropathy due to infections (including HIV, Lyme disease)
  - porphyria
  - drugs, e.g. vincristine, cisplatin, carboplatin, vinorelbine, paclitaxel, gemcitabine, amiodarone.

Supine hypertension is often also present, and may be exacerbated by treatment. Diagnosis consists of demonstrating postural hypotension (see above) and excluding other causes.

Treatment consists first of simple measures, such as advice about posture. Manoeuvres such as crossing the legs while standing, and tensing exercises of the calves and hands before standing, may help. The head of the bed should be raised as much as is feasible while sleeping. Meals should be small and frequent, to minimize meal-induced increase in splanchnic blood flow. Alcohol may exacerbate symptoms. Drugs with anticholinergic action should be stopped or changed, e.g. tricyclic antidepressants used for neuropathic pain changed to duloxetine or gabapentin/pregabalin. Care must be taken with anaesthesia and surgical procedures. Agents to increase blood pressure, such as fludrocortisone (starting with 50 µg/day), may be tried with care to try to avoid supine hypertension and oedema. Other agents such as midodrine 2.5 mg two or three times a day, pindolol, fluoxetine, desmopressin, pyridostigmine and octreotide may help in selected cases. As above there are initial reports of success with erythropoietin replacement.

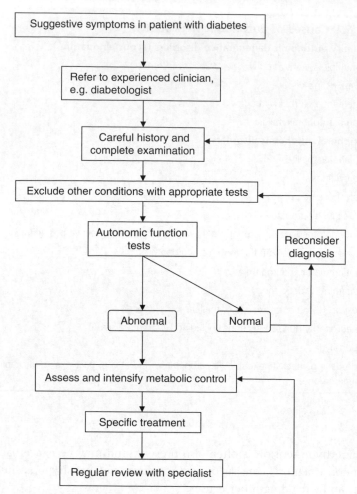

Figure 6.1 Algorithm for the diagnosis and management of diabetic autonomic neuropathy.

Silent myocardial ischaemia

It has been suggested since the 1980s that people with diabetes may not experience angina symptoms as much as people without diabetes, despite documented coronary artery insufficiency. Clearly proof is not easy, because most individuals with coronary artery disease are selected as a result of their symptoms. If the hypothesis is true, then those who are at an increased risk of coronary artery disease (CAD), i.e. those with diabetes, may present at a more advanced stage of the condition (if at all), and such patients should be screened and managed with assessment criteria that do not depend on symptoms.

Most researchers do now believe that there is an increased prevalence of silent myocardial ischaemia in people with diabetes. There is also increasing evidence that autonomic neuropathy may be a causative factor.

In a study of patients with type 2 diabetes, 81 per cent of patients with asymptomatic coronary insufficiency had evidence of autonomic neuropathy, compared with 25 per cent of those with anginal symptoms.[36] In a French study of 120 asymptomatic patients with diabetes followed for 4 years, a major cardiac event was more common in those with evidence of cardiac autonomic neuropathy. In a review of 12 studies examining the importance of autonomic neuropathy in silent myocardial ischaemia, generally measured by exercise stress testing, five studies showed a statistically significant increased frequency of silent myocardial ischaemia in individuals with, as opposed to those without, cardiovascular autonomic neuropathy.[37] The reviewers point out, however, that some authors question whether this association is causative, suggesting instead that underlying coronary disease might be a cause of both autonomic dysfunction and silent myocardial ischaemia.

Sudden death

Ewing et al.[38] reported on the natural history of diabetic autonomic neuropathy in 1981, and drew attention to the increased mortality of affected individuals. Fifty-three per cent of their diabetic patients with abnormal autonomic function tests had died at 5 years, compared with a mortality rate of only 15 per cent among individuals with diabetes and normal autonomic function tests. Half the deaths in the former group were from renal failure, but 29 per cent died suddenly. Patients with classic symptoms carried a particularly poor prognosis.

The Hoorn study examined mortality in a population-derived sample of 605 individuals aged 50–75 years. During 9 years of follow-up, 43 died from cardiovascular causes. Individuals with diabetes and evidence of autonomic impairment had an approximately doubled risk of mortality.[39] In a review of the literature in 2003, Maser et al. found 15 studies that were appropriate to include in a meta-analysis, with follow-up from 0.5 years to 16 years.[40] With the exception of one study, mortality rates in people with diabetes were higher for those with autonomic neuropathy than for those without, achieving statistical significance in 12 studies. For those studies that used two or more measures to define autonomic neuropathy, the pooled estimate for the increased relative risk of mortality for those with autonomic neuropathy was 3.45.

It has been shown that patients with diabetic autonomic neuropathy have reduced myocardial perfusion reserve capacity,[41] impaired vasodilator response of coronary vessels to sympathetic stimulation[42] and increased arterial stiffness. The exact mechanism for the increased mortality is, however, unknown. As above, renal failure is common in these severely affected individuals, which is likely to be due to the associated chronic hyperglycaemia. The increased incidence of sudden death suggests the possibility of a fatal cardiac arrhythmia. Silent myocardial ischaemia may be a factor (see above). Although Q–T interval prolongation (increased with hypoglycaemia) has been shown to be a bad prognostic indicator in type 1 diabetes,[43] there is no good evidence that this is via autonomic neuropathy.[44] Although autonomic failure may possibly precipitate hypoglycaemia (see below), and hypoglycaemia is known to produce prolongation of the Q–T interval, a study in 28 adults with type 1 diabetes revealed that patients with cardiac autonomic neuropathy were not at particular risk for abnormal cardiac repolarization during hypoglycaemia. Indeed, the authors suggest that such patients may be relatively protected, perhaps as a result of attenuated sympathoadrenal responses.[45] In the ACCORD study, where intensive therapy targeting normal blood glucose increased mortality in people with type 2 diabetes, participants with cardiac autonomic neuropathy were twice as likely to die during the 3.5-year study.[46] However there was no evidence that autonomic neuropathy was responsible for the higher mortality in the intensively treated group. A detailed postmortem study of 22 individuals with type 1 diabetes who died suddenly from 1994 to 2006 has not revealed an explanation.[47]

Hypoglycaemic unawareness, hypoglycaemia-associated autonomic failure

Severe hypoglycaemia is one of the worst fears of a person with diabetes who is treated with insulin. Being unable to detect hypoglycaemia is therefore a problem of major significance. The warning symptoms of sweating, palpitation and faintness are largely produced by increased autonomic stimulation, and it has been suggested that autonomic neuropathy might be a significant factor.

More recent studies have demonstrated that there is an acute and reversible phenomenon whereby previous hypoglycaemia lowers the threshold at which counter-regulatory responses, including catecholamines and autonomic stimulation, switch on. This has been termed 'hypoglycaemia-associated autonomic failure' (HAAF).[48] It results in both worsening of the 'hypo' as well as lack of recognition. The phenomenon can be reversed by avoidance of hypoglycaemia.[49]

Studies in patients with diabetes with and without autonomic neuropathy have failed to reveal a difference with adrenaline or symptom responses to hypoglycaemia.[50] However, data from the EURODIAB study has identified autonomic neuropathy as an independent risk factor for severe hypoglycaemia in type 1 diabetes, and in another study adrenaline responses to hypoglycaemia were reported as impaired in patients with diabetic autonomic neuropathy.[51]

It seems, therefore, that the most prevalent cause of hypoglycaemic unawareness is due to the reversible, functional phenomenon (HAAF), but that if structural damage from autonomic neuropathy is present it is likely to worsen the situation.

Hypoglycaemic unawareness is serious and of major importance to the individual with diabetes. Its presence should be checked for as part of the routine management of diabetes. When it is a problem, intensive efforts should be made to abolish hypoglycaemia[52] and, as coined by Diabetes UK, 'make 4 [i.e. a glucose value of 4mmol/l] the floor'.

Impotence

Up to 50 per cent of men with diabetes may have problems with impotence and autonomic neuropathy is a major factor[53] (see Chapter 7). Phosphodiesterase inhibitors are a major advance in this field, but the greater the evidence for clinical autonomic or peripheral neuropathy the less they are likely to provide benefit in patients.

Neurogenic bladder (diabetic cystopathy)

Damage to the autonomic nerve supply of the bladder and urethra results in impairment of bladder sensation, increased post-void residual volume and decreased detrusor contractility, all of which can be seen in diabetes. These abnormalities may produce repeated urinary infections and chronic retention of urine. The diagnosis is aided by urodynamic studies, and a urological opinion should be sought. Treatment includes bladder neck surgery, where outlet obstruction is a problem, or intermittent self-catheterization.[54]

Sleep apnoea

For many years it has been apparent that there is a relationship between diabetes and obstructive sleep apnoea. Both conditions may be exacerbated by increasing body weight, and there is evidence that regular snoring and sleep apnoea are independently associated with impaired glucose metabolism.[55] Population-based studies of sleep apnoea reveal as much as a fourfold higher prevalence of diabetes in people with significant sleep apnoea compared with those without the condition.[56] On the other hand, there is evidence that diabetes might accentuate sleep apnoea, perhaps via the presence of autonomic neuropathy. This link was first suggested in 1980, and it has been found that some 30 per cent of people with diabetes who have autonomic neuropathy may also have sleep apnoea.[57]

Screening for autonomic neuropathy

The American Association of Diabetes recommends that screening for signs and symptoms of cardiovascular autonomic neuropathy should be instituted at diagnosis of type 2 diabetes and 5 years after the diagnosis of type 1 diabetes. There is currently no specific treatment that might ameliorate diabetic autonomic neuropathy, other than intensifying blood glucose control, which is a goal of treatment in most people with diabetes. There is therefore currently no logic in screening asymptomatic patients for autonomic dysfunction.

The exception of course would be to screen for patients with asymptomatic coronary insufficiency (see above). There are no reports so far of clinical programmes being set up for this purpose. The standard exercise stress test may overdiagnose those with hypertension and underdiagnose patients with high-risk type 2 diabetes, and both research groups considered that alternative screening tests should be sought.[58] A recent randomized observational trial demonstrated no clinical benefit in routine screening of asymptomatic patients with type 2 diabetes and normal ECGs.[59] A French multicentre study has followed 370 asymptomatic people with type 2 diabetes for 3–89 months after exercise or dipyridamole myocardial perfusion imaging with thallium-201. Imaging was positive in 35 per cent pf patients, who were nearly four times as likely to have a major cardiac event if aged over 60 years.[60] The authors suggest that this test might be an appropriate screening tool in this group. A screening programme for this purpose might therefore become more relevant, especially as non-invasive tests of coronary artery structure and function become more widely available.

6.5 Conclusion

The clinical syndrome of diabetic autonomic neuropathy usually occurs in patients with long-standing and often poorly controlled diabetes. A wide variety of systems can be involved, and affected individuals often have other complications of diabetes. The condition can be at the least distressing and at the most life threatening. The diagnosis is often difficult and depends on clinical skill and experience. The management of affected patients is time-consuming and requires the full support of the multidisciplinary team.

Case studies

Case study 1
A 43-year-old man with 13 years of type 1 diabetes was admitted to hospital as an emergency. He had had increasingly severe bouts of vomiting for over 6 weeks, sometimes prolonged, resulting in prostration for 24–36 hours. Past history included a myocardial infarction 3 years previously. He was known to have background retinopathy, and had had difficulties with poor blood glucose control for years, with HbA1c estimations of 93–114 mmol/mol (10.7–12.6%) for the last 3 years despite the support of the diabetes team.

On admission he was vomiting and ketotic, with a random plasma glucose of 29 mmol/l, but normal blood pH and bicarbonate. He was treated with an intravenous insulin infusion, with saline/potassium infusion, converting to dextrose/saline when the glucose had lowered. He was given parenteral antiemetics. Symptoms improved, but worsened when initially converted to subcutaneous insulin. The intravenous insulin pump was therefore reinstated. A search for infection was negative. Eventually he was controlled on his previous multiple injection regimen, and discharged.

He was readmitted with the same symptoms 1 week later, which again settled with intensive metabolic control. He was treated with metoclopramide four times daily and low-dose erythromycin. Investigations revealed a normal abdominal ultrasound scan, oesophagogastroduodenoscopy and duodenal biopsy, and no lesions were seen on barium meal and small bowel meal, although gastric emptying was delayed. Expired: inspired beat-to-beat heart rate variation was abnormally diminished, and vibration thresholds in both great toes were abnormally increased, with absent ankle jerks, indicative of impaired autonomic and peripheral nerve function.

A diagnosis of diabetic gastroparesis was made, and he was continued on regular metoclopramide, with intensive efforts to try to improve his blood glucose control.

He has had waves of nausea since, but has had no further hospital admissions for gastroparesis for 11 years to date. Blood glucose control has improved considerably, and he remains on prophylactic metoclopramide 30 min before each meal.

Case study 2

A 40-year-old woman with type 1 diabetes of 15 years' duration presents with profuse watery diarrhoea after meals, occurring every 2 or 3 days. She also has a virtually continuous feeling of nausea. After the diagnosis of diabetes, she was admitted on a number of occasions with diabetic ketosis and ketoacidosis, and has found control difficult. HbA1c values have usually been above 86 mmol/mol (10%). She developed retinopathy 6 years after diagnosis, evidence of peripheral neuropathy at 8 years, central cataracts at 10 years and proteinuria 11 years from diagnosis.

Investigations reveal normal abdominal ultrasound scan, flexible sigmoidoscopy and biopsy, oesophagogastroduodenoscopy and duodenal biopsy, and colonoscopy with interval biopsies. Despite correcting iron and folate deficiency, her haemoglobin level is constantly below the lower limit of normal. She has mild renal impairment with proteinuria despite angiotensin-converting enzyme (ACE) inhibitors.

Treatment is started with a short course of oxytetracycline, loperamide and octreotide with no benefit. Low-dose erythromycin helps the nausea, but not the diarrhoea. She is now tolerating her symptoms and has improved her glycaemic control with the support of the diabetes team.

Case study 3

A 35-year-old woman with type 1 diabetes of 10 years' duration was seen as an emergency in the diabetes clinic. She had previously had poor blood glucose control with a number of admissions due to diabetic ketoacidosis. Her latest HbA1c was 112mmol/mol (12.4%).

For the last few weeks she had experienced increasingly distressing pains in her abdomen, and both upper and lower legs, which were burning and shooting, and kept her awake at night. She had experienced dizziness on standing, and although the pains had been helped by amitriptyline 25mg once daily the dizziness had become worse.

On examination she had hypersensitivity over the painful areas, some evidence of peripheral neuropathy and a significant postural drop in blood pressure (110/70mmHg lying, 90/60mmHg standing, with resting tachycardia and no change on standing). There was no beat-to-beat variation with breathing. A diagnosis of acute painful neuropathy and acute autonomic neuropathy was made. Amitriptyline was stopped.

Over the next few days the pains became excruciating and she was admitted to hospital. The clinical features were of a persistent postural drop in blood pressure, with severe postural dizziness, and tachycardia. Metabolic control was rapidly improved, fluids were encouraged, the head of the bed was raised and she was started on low-dose fludrocortisone. Postural hypotension and dizziness improved. Pains were treated with carbamazepine, with slight improvement. Imipramine was cautiously started, with better relief of pain (an agent such as pregabalin would be more appropriate today). Constipation became a problem and was treated with appropriate laxatives.

Over the next few weeks in outpatients her pains gradually improved, and for the first time she managed to maintain good blood glucose control. Postural symptoms had improved but blood pressure still fell from 120/80 supine to 70/50 standing. Fludrocortisone had produced ankle oedema and was phased out.

Six years later she had no pain and was fully back to work. She had minimal postural symptoms but still has a postural drop in blood pressure. She had a new relationship, but, after a number of years of good blood glucose control, HbA1c levels were back up again. A year later she was found dead by her neighbour. Postmortem examination did not reveal a definite cause of death.

Case study 4

A 48-year-old woman with type 2 diabetes was admitted as an emergency to hospital having woken at 5am feeling sweaty. She went to the toilet and collapsed with loss of consciousness for probably 5 minutes. Her husband called the ambulance. On admission she felt faint and weak. ECG showed classic changes of an inferior myocardial infarction, and cardiac enzymes were raised. She was thrombolysed and discharged on relevant medication. Exercise testing (on β blockers) showed clear evidence of ST segment depression without any pain. Coronary angiography revealed a tight stenosis of the dominant right coronary artery, and a stent was inserted with resolution of the stenosis.

She was understandably concerned that the cardiac rehabilitation advice focused on what to do when chest pain is experienced, which of course she had never had. An exercise test now showed no evidence of ischaemia, and she was somewhat reassured by the plan to arrange further tests on a 6-monthly basis, while being aggressively treated for cardiovascular protection. Such tests have remained within normal limits for 8 years.

References

1. Pambianco G, Costacou T, Ellis D, et al. The 30-year natural history of type 1 diabetes complications: The Pittsburgh Epidemiology of Diabetes Complications Study experience. *Diabetes* 2006;**55**:1463.
2. Ziegler D, Gries FA, Muhlen H, Rathmann W, Spuler M, Lessmann F. Prevalence and clinical correlates of cardiovascular autonomic and peripheral diabetic neuropathy in patients attending diabetes centers. The Diacan Multicenter Study Group. *Diabete et Metabolisme* 1993;**19**:143–151.
3. Valensi P, Paries J, Attali JR, French Group for Research and Study of Diabetic Neuropathy. Cardiac autonomic neuropathy in diabetic patients: influence of diabetes duration, obesity, and microangiopathic complications – the French multicenter study. *Metabolism: Clin Exp* 2003;**52**:815–820.
4. Pavy-Le Traon, A, Fontaine S, Tap G, et al. Cardiovascular autonomic neuropathy and other complications in type 1 diabetes. *Clin Auton Res* 2010;**20**:153–160.
5. Kempler P, Tesfaye S, Chaturvedi N, et al. Blood pressure response to standing in the diagnosis of autonomic neuropathy: the EURODIAB IDDM Complications Study. *Arch Physiol Biochem* 2001;**109**:215–222.
6. Neil HA, Thompson AV, John S, McCarthy ST, Mann JI. Diabetic Autonomic neuropathy: the prevalence of impaired heart rate variability in a geographically defined population. *Diab Med* 1989;**6**:20–24.
7. Low PA, Benrud-Larson LM, Sletten DM, et al. Autonomic symptoms and diabetic neuropathy. A population-based study. *Diabet Care* 2004;**27**:2942–2947.
8. Anonymous. The effect of intensive diabetes therapy on measures of autonomic nervous system function in the Diabetes Control and Complications Trial (DCCT). *Diabetologia* 1998;**41**:416–423.
9. Pop-Busui R, Low PA, Waberski BH, et al. Effects of prior intensive insulin therapy on cardiac autonomic nervous system function in type 1 diabetes mellitus: the Diabetes Control and Complications Trial/Epidemiology of Diabetes Interventions and Complications study (DCCT/EDIC). *Circulation* 2009;**119**:2886–2893.
10. Gaede P, Vedel P, Parving HH, Pedersen O. Intensified multifactorial intervention in patients with Type 2 diabetes mellitus and microalbuminuria: the Steno type 2 randomised study. *Lancet* 1999;**353**:617.
11. Cameron NE, Eaton SE, Cotter MA, Tesfaye S. Vascular factors and metabolic interactions in the pathogenesis of diabetic neuropathy. *Diabetologia* 2001;**44**: 1973–1988.
12. Muhr D, Mollenhauer U, Ziegler AG, Haslbeck M, Standl E, Schnell O. Autoantibodies to sympathetic ganglia, GAD, or tyrosine phosphatase in long-term IDDM with and without ECG-based cardiac autonomic neuropathy. *Diabet Care* 1997;**20**:1009.

13. Kempler P, Tesfaye S, Chaturvedi N, et al. Blood pressure response to standing in the diagnosis of autonomic neuropathy: the EURODIAB IDDM Complications Study. *Arch Physiol Biochem* 2001;**109**:215–222.

14. Ewing DJ, Martyn CN, Young RJ, Clarke BF. The value of cardiovascular autonomic function tests: 10 years experience in diabetes. *Diabet Care* 1985;**8**:491–498

15. Smith SA. Reduced sinus arrhythmia in diabetic autonomic neuropathy: diagnostic value of an age-related normal range. *BMJ* 1982;**285**:1599–1601.

16. Macleod AF, Smith SA, Cowell T, Richardson PR, Sönksen PH. Non-cardiac autonomic tests in diabetes: use of the galvanic skin response. *Diab Med* 1991;**8**: S67–S70.

17. Hoeldtke RD, Bryner KD, Horvath GG, Phares RW, Broy LF, Hobbs GR. Redistribution of sudomotor responses is an early sign of sympathetic dysfunction in Type 1 diabetes. *Diabetes* 2001;**50**:436.

18. Tack CJ, Van Gurp, Holmes C, Goldstein DS. Local sympathetic denervation in painful diabetic neuropathy. *Diabetes* 2002;**51**:3545.

19. Camilleri M. Diabetic gastroparesis. *N Engl J Med* 2007;**356**:820–829.

20. De Block CE, De Leeuw IH, Pelckmans PA, Callens D, Maday E, Van Gaal LF. Delayed gastric emptying and gastric autoimmunity in Type 1 diabetes. *Diabet Care* 2002; **25**:912–917.

21. Intagliata N, Koch KL. Gatsroparesis in type 2 diabetes: prevalence, etiology, diagnosis, and treatment. *Curr Gastroenterol Rep* 2007;**9**:270–279.

22. Abell T, McCallum R, Hocking M, et al. Gastric electrical stimulation for medically refractory gastroparesis. *Gastroenterology* 2003;**125**:421–428.

23. McCallum RW, Snape W, Brody F, et al. Gastric electrical stimulation with Enterra therapy improves symptoms from diabetic gastroparesis in a prospective study. *Clin Gastroenterol Hepatol* 2010;**8**:947–954.

24. Ejskjaer N, Dimcevski G, Wo J, et al. Safety and efficacy of ghrelin agonist TZP-101 in relieving symptoms in patients with diabetic gastroparesis: a randomised placebo-controlled study. *Neurogastroenterol Motility* 2010; **22**:1069–1281.

25. Ejskjaer NT, Bradley JL, Buxton-Thomas MS, et al. Novel surgical treatment and gastric pathology in diabetic gastroparesis. *Diab Med* 1999;**16**:488–495.

26. Macleod AF, Smith SA, Sönksen PH, Lowy C. The problem of autonomic neuropathy in diabetic pregnancy. *Diab Med* 1990;**7**:80–82.

27. Zietz B, Lock G, Straub RH, Braun B, Scholmerich J, Palitzsch KD. Small-bowel bacterial overgrowth in diabetic subjects is associated with cardiovascular autonomic neuropathy. *Diabet Care* 2000;**23**:1200–1201.

28. Biaggioni I, Robertson D, Krantz S, Jones M, Haile V. The anemia of autonomic failure: evidence for sympathetic modulation of erythropoiesis in humans and reversal with recombinant erythropoietin. *Ann Intern Med* 1994;**121**:181–186.

29. Winkler AS, Marsden J, Chaudhuri KR, Hambley H, Watkins PJ. Erythropoietin depletion and anaemia in diabetes mellitus. *Diab Med* 1999;**16**:813–819.

30. Thomas S, Rampersad M. Anaemia in diabetes. *Acta Diabetol* 2004;**41**:13.

31. Winkler AS, Landau S, Watkins PJ. Erythropoietin treatment of postural hypotension in anemic Type 1 diabetic patients with autonomic neuropathy. *Diabet Care* 2001;**24**:1121–1123.

32. Spallone V, Maiello MR, Kurukulasuriya N, et al. Does autonomic neuropathy play a role in erythropoietin regulation in non-proteinuric Type 2 diabetic patients? *Diab Med* 2004;**21**:1174–1180.

33. Freeman R. Neurogenic orthostatic hypotension. *N Engl J Med* 2008;**358**:615–624.

34. Mankovsky BN, Piolot R, Mankovsky OL, Ziegler D. Impairment of cerebral autoregulation in diabetic patients with cardiovascular autonomic neuropathy and orthostatic hypotension. *Diab Med* 2003;**20**:119–126.

35. Jacob G, Costa F, Biaggioni I. Spectrum of autonomic cardiovascular neuropathy in diabetes. *Diabet Care* 2003;**26**:2174–2180.
36. Beck MO, Silveiro SP, Friedman R, Clausell N, Gross JL. Asymptomatic coronary artery disease is associated with cardiac autonomic neuropathy and diabetic nephropathy in Type 2 diabetic patients. *Diabet Care* 1999;**22**:1745–1747.
37. Vinik AI, Maser RE, Mitchell BD, Freeman R. Diabetic autonomic neuropathy. *Diabet Care* 2003;**26**:1553–1581.
38. Ewing DJ, Campbell IW, Clarke BF/ The natural history of diabetic autonomic neuropathy. *Q J Med* 1980;**193**:95–108.
39. Gerritsen J, Dekker JM, TenVoorde BJ, et al. Impaired autonomic function is associated with increased mortality, especially in subjects with diabetes, hypertension, or a history of cardiovascular disease: The Hoorn Study. *Diabet Care* 2001;**24**:1793.
40. Maser RE, Mitchell BD, Vinik AI, Freeman R. The association between cardiovascular autonomic neuropathy and mortality in individuals with diabetes: A meta-analysis. *Diabet Care* 2003;**26**:1895–1899.
41. Taskiran M, Fritz-Hansen T, Rasmussen V, Larsson HB, Hilsted J. Decreased myocardial perfusion reserve in diabetic autonomic neuropathy. *Diabetes* 2002;**51**:3306
42. Di Carli MF, Bianco-Batlles D, Landa ME, et al. Effect of autonomic neuropathy on coronary blood flow in patients with diabetes mellitus. *Circulation* 1999;**100**: 813–819.
43. Veglio M, Sivieri R, Chinaglia A, Scaglione L, Cavallo-Perin P. QT interval prolongation and mortality in Type 1 diabetic patients: a 5-year cohort prospective study. Neuropathy Study Group of the Italian Society of Diabetes, Piemonte Affiliate. *Diabet Care* 2000;**23**:1381–1383.
44. Lee SP, Yeoh L, Harris ND, et al. Influence of autonomic neuropathy on QTc interval lengthening during hypoglycemia in type 1 diabetes. *Diabetes* 2004;**53**:1535–1542.
45. Lee SP, Yeoh L, Harris ND et al. Influence of Autonomic Neuropathy on QTc Interval Lengthening during hypoglycaemia in type 1 diabetes. *Diabetes*. 2004 Jun;**53**(6): 1535–42.
46. Pop-Busui R, Evans GW, Gerstein HC, et al. Effects of cardiac autonomic dysfunction on mortality risk in the Action to Control Cardiovascular Risk in Diabetes (ACCORD) trial. *Diabet Care* 2010;**33**:1578–1584.
47. Tu E, Bagnall RD, Duflou J, Semsarian C. Post-mortem review and genetic analysis of sudden unexpected death in epilepsy (SUDEP) cases. *Brain Pathol* 2011;**21**: 201–208.
48. Gerich JE, Mokan M, Veneman T, Korytkowski M, Mitrakou A. Hypoglycemia unawareness. *Endocrine Rev* 1991;**12**:356–371.
49. Cryer PE. Diverse causes of hypoglycemia-associated autonomic failure in diabetes. *N Engl J Med* 1994;**350**:2272–2279.
50. Kendall DM, Rooney DP, Smets YF, Salazar Bolding L, Robertson RP. Pancreas transplantation restores epinephrine response and symptom recognition during hypoglycemia in patients with long standing Type 1 diabetes and autonomic neuropathy. *Diabetes* 1997;**46**:249.
51. Meyer C, Grossmann R, Mitrakou A, et al. Effects of autonomic neuropathy on counterregulation and awareness of hypoglycemia in type 1 diabetic patients. *Diabet Care* 1998;**21**:1960.
52. Cranston I, Lomas J, Maran A, Macdonald I, Amiel SA. Restoration of hypoglycaemia awareness in patients with long-duration insulin-dependent diabetes. *Lancet* 1994;**344**:283–287.
53. Wellmer A, Sharief MK, Knowles CH, et al. Quantitative sensory and autonomic testing in male diabetic patients with erectile dysfunction. *BJU Int* 1999;**83**: 66–70.

54. Kaplan SA, Blaivas JG. Diabetic cystopathy. *J Diabet Complications* 1988;**2**:133–139.
55. Rasche K, Keller T, Tautz B, et al. Obstructive sleep apnea and type 2 diabetes. *Eur J Med Res* 2010;**15**(suppl 2):152–156.
56. West SD, Nicoll DJ, Stradling JR. Prevalence of obstructive sleep apnoea in men with type 2 diabetes. *Thorax* 2006;**61**:945–950.
57. Keller T, Hader C, De Zeeuw J, Rasche K. Obstructive sleep apnoea syndrome: the effect of diabetes and autonomic neuropathy. *J Physiol Pharmacol* 2007;**58**(suppl 5):313–318.
58. Valensi P, Pariès J, Brulport-Cerisier V, et al. Predictive value of silent myocardial ischemia for cardiac events in diabetic patients: influence of age in a French multi-center study. *Diabet Care* 2005;**28**:2722–2727.
59. Lochen ML. The Trømso study: the prevalence of exercise-induced silent myocardial ischaemia and relation to risk factors for coronary heart disease in an apparently healthy population. *Eur Heart J* 1992;**13**:728–1731.
60. Bacci S, Villella M, Villella A, et al. Screening for silent myocardial ischaemia in type 2 diabetic patients with additional atherogenic risk factors: applicability and accuracy of the exercise stress test. *Eur J Endocrinol* 2002;**147**:649–654.

CHAPTER 7

Diabetes and Sexual Health

Michael H Cummings

Academic Department of Diabetes and Endocrinology, Queen Alexandra Hospital, Portsmouth, UK

 Key points

- Erectile dysfunction (ED) represents the most common complication of diabetes.

- Diabetes, ED and cardiovascular disease are common comorbidities.

- Hypogonadism, a recognized cause of ED, affects up to a third of men with type 2 diabetes.

- The pathophysiology of ED in men with diabetes is well established and is often multifactorial.

- Neurovascular disease, and structural and functional changes in the corpus cavernosa are common abnormalities implicated in the pathophysiology of ED.

- Identification of the abnormalities of biochemical pathways at the cellular level that contribute to ED have led to the development of several successful therapeutic options.

- Although abnormalities of sexual health in females with diabetes is well recognized, the pathophysiology is poorly understood and treatment options are limited.

 Therapeutic key points

- Most men with diabetes who experience ED can be treated successfully.

- The presence of cardiovascular disease should be sought because this may affect management strategy and therapeutic options.

- Weight loss and smoking cessation can result in spontaneous improvement in erections.

- Oral phosphodiesterase type 5 (PDE-5) inhibitors remain the first-line treatment for most men with diabetes and ED. If PDE-5 inhibitors are unsuccessful, urethral pellets or intracavernosal injections of prostaglandin E_1 are effective pharmacological alternatives.

- Testosterone supplementations should be considered only in proven cases of hypogonadism.

- Non-pharmacological approaches to the management of ED in diabetes include vacuum devices, psychosexual therapy and penile implants.

- Management of female sexual dysfunction include therapeutic options to address reduced vaginal lubrication, absent genital sensation, dyspareunia, anorgasmia and diminished libido.

Diabetes: Chronic Complications, Third Edition. Edited by Kenneth M. Shaw, Michael H. Cummings.
© 2012 John Wiley & Sons, Ltd. Published 2012 by John Wiley & Sons, Ltd.

7.1 Introduction

It is now recognized that diabetes can have a profound effect on sexual health, which has been demonstrated to have a detrimental effect on quality of life. Fortunately, there have been significant advances in our understanding of the pathophysiology and management of diabetes-related sexual health problems. However, predominantly this applies to male erectile dysfunction (ED) where the mechanisms leading to its development are now better understood. It is also recognized that there is an integral link of ED, diabetes and cardiovascular disease – the presence of one of these disorders should alert clinicians to the possibility of these other comorbidities. In contrast, although it is recognized that diabetes can have a dramatic effect on sexual function in women, there is a paucity of research examining pathophysiology and treatment, and this area requires further evaluation.

7.2 Male erectile dysfunction

Definition

Erectile dysfunction is defined as the inability to achieve or maintain an erection satisfactory for sexual intercourse. In patients who present with ED, it is important to ascertain their perception of the problem for two reasons. First, the patient may use the term inappropriately (e.g. equating it to painful sex or infertility) and, second, treatment may differ depending on whether the achievement or maintenance of an erection is the main problem.

Prevalence

Diabetes represents the most common cause of ED (up to 40% of cases) and may be present in one to eight men presenting with ED hitherto unknown to have this metabolic condition.

In the largest study to investigate ED in men with diabetes, of 541 patients interviewed, the overall prevalence of the disorder was 35 per cent. The frequency of ED increased with age: 5.7 per cent of men aged 20–24 years with diabetes were impotent, increasing to 52.4 per cent in the group aged 55–59 years. This population was re-interviewed 5 years later.[1] In the group of patients who were originally potent, 28 per cent had subsequently become impotent. Five factors were identified as independently predictive of the subsequent development of ED: age, alcohol intake, initial glycaemic control, intermittent claudication and retinopathy. Only 9 per cent of those patients who were originally impotent had regained potency, indicating the progressive nature of the disorder.

In other studies of men with diabetes, the prevalence of ED has been greater than the above study, ranging up to 75 per cent.[2] Thus, ED is much more common in the diabetic compared with the non-diabetic population, where the prevalence has been reported to range between 0.1 and 18.4. per cent.[3] There are relatively few studies that have specifically examined ED in the type 1 diabetic population but broadly speaking the prevalence seems to be similar to that of men with type 2 diabetes, although a vascular aetiology is more common in the former.

Aetiology

Table 7.1 shows the potential causes of ED in men with diabetes. The factors that are most commonly linked to its development in diabetes are abnormalities of the neurovascular supply to the penis or functional and structural changes within the penile tissue itself. More recently, hypogonadism has been shown to be far more common in type 2 diabetes and should be actively screened for. In many instances, patients have a multifactorial basis to their ED.

Studies of men with diabetes and ED have suggested that neurological abnormalities may be present in up to 80 per cent of cases. The principal abnormality lies within the parasympathetic (autonomic) nervous system

Table 7.1 The aetiology of erectile dysfunction

Cause	Examples
Vascular	Arterial insufficiency
	Venous leakage
Neurological	Autonomic neuropathy
	Spinal cord lesions
Penile tissue abnormalities	Fibrosis of penile tissue
	Abnormalities of smooth muscle relaxation or constriction
Psychological	
Endocrine	Primary or secondary hypogonadism
	Thyroid disorders
	Hyperprolactinaemia
Renal	Renal failure and dialysis
Pharmacological	Alcohol
	Drugs
Others	Peyronie's disease
	Penile/pelvic trauma
	Phimosis
	Balanitis
	Post-inflammatory penile fibrosis
	Penile tumour
	Congenital deformity of penis

responsible for tumescence, whereas the sympathetic and sensory nervous systems are largely unaffected. It must be recognized, however, that this represents a microvascular complication of diabetes linked in part to tissue hypoxia.

Aberrant blood flow to the penis in diabetes may be present in various forms. Diffuse atherosclerosis is a common finding in diabetes, which may affect the penile vasculature as well as other circulatory beds in the heart, brain and lower limbs. This observation supports the concept of examining other organs susceptible to vascular disease in the individual with diabetes and ED. Alternatively, there may be discrete narrowings in the external iliac artery that divert blood supply away from the penile circulation (so-called 'pelvic steal' syndrome). However, most interest has focused around the inability of the penile blood vessels to dilate in response to the appropriate vasodilatory signals (known as endothelial dysfunction), which has been demonstrated in up to 95 per cent of men with ED.[4]

The penile organ itself is susceptible to fibrosis within the cavernous smooth muscle, nerve fibres and blood vessels. The discovery that a large number of chemical mediators are involved in the process of smooth muscle relaxation that facilitates accumulation of blood within the penis and tumescence (Figure 7.1) has led to much interest in pharmacological approaches that may correct these biochemical abnormalities. Table 7.2 highlights those mediators that have been demonstrated to be abnormal in concentration or effect within the penile tissue of men with diabetes and ED or rat models, and form the basis of therapeutic options used in clinical management today.

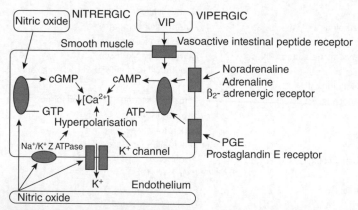

Christ GJ. Urol Clin North Am 1995;22:727–745.
Reproduced and adapted with permission of WB Sounders Company.

Figure 7.1 The biochemical pathways and receptors involved in penile smooth muscle relaxation. (Adapted, with permission, from Christ GJ. The penis as a vascular organ: the importance of corporal smooth muscle tone in the control of erection. *Urol Clinic North Am* 1995;22:727–745.)

Table 7.2 Chemical mediators enabling smooth muscle relaxation/constriction that may be affected in diabetic men with erectile dysfunction

Relaxant	Contractile
Neuronal release	
Nitric oxide	Noradrenaline
Acetylcholine	
Vasoactive intestinal polypeptide	
Local release	
Nitric oxide	Endothelin-1
Vasodilator prostanoids	Vasoconstrictor prostanoids
Adenosine triphosphate	

Many drugs are associated with the development of ED and Table 7.4 is by no means exhaustive. In particular, the use of drugs that treat common cardiovascular conditions, lipid-lowering drugs and painful peripheral neuropathy are common culprits in men with diabetes and ED. In general, modifying or stopping a potential causative drug is effective in restoring tumescence only if there is a clear acute temporal relationship between its introduction and the development of ED.

Hypogonadism may be present in up to a third of males with diabetes.[6] Commonly, hypogonadism occurs in the presence of normal gonadotrophin levels (normogonadotrophic hypogonadism). This is thought to arise from increased abdominal obesity, which promotes enhanced aromatase activity (converting more testosterone to estradiol) and the inhibitory effect of leptin, estradiol and possibly adipocytokines (interleukin-6 and tumour necrosis factor α) on the hypothalamopituitary axis suppressing luteinizing hormone (LH) production.[6]

Balanitis is more common in diabetes in the presence of hyperglycaemia, but other conditions such as Peyronie's disease and venous leaks are present only to the same degree as in the non-diabetic population.

The majority of cases of ED in diabetes have an overt organic aetiology and this is supported by the observation that the condition rarely spontaneously improves.[1] However, it is not uncommon for patients to have a concomitant secondary psychological element to their ED, e.g. performance anxiety and the fear of failure. Occasionally men with diabetes have a clear psychological or psychiatric condition precipitating ED, which may be elicited from the consultation (see Assessment below).

Assessment of the man with diabetes and ED

An accurate history, careful examination and some simple investigations should elicit the cause of ED and/or appropriate treatment in most patients

Table 7.3 The International Index of Erectile Function (IIEF) domain score used to assess the severity of erectile dysfunction[5]

IIEF domain score	Score range
1. Over the past 4 weeks, how often were you able to get an erection during sexual activity?	0–5
2. Over the past 4 weeks, when you had erections with sexual stimulation, how often were your erections hard enough for penetration?	0–5
3. Over the past 4 weeks, when you attempted sexual intercourse, how often were you able to penetrate (enter) your partner?	0–5
4. Over the past 4 weeks, during sexual intercourse, how difficult was it to maintain your erection after you had penetrated (entered) your partner?	0–5
5. Over the past 4 weeks, during sexual intercourse, how difficult was it to maintain your erection to completion of intercourse?	0–5
15. Over the past 4 weeks, how do you rate your confidence that you can keep your erection?	1–5
Total range	**1–30[a]**

[a]A higher score equates to better erectile function.

with diabetes without resorting to more complicated investigative procedures. It should be stressed that most of the assessment as to the cause of ED should be part of the regular examination of the patient with diabetes. Moreover, ED should alert the health-care professional to the possibility of underlying pathology elsewhere, e.g. the patient may also have coronary artery disease as part of widespread vascular pathology which was not necessarily previously detected.

History
Initial useful questions may include:
- What is the problem?
- Why is it a problem?
- What is the partner's attitude to the problem?
- What does the patient hope to achieve as a result of reporting the problem?

These general questions will provide an overview of the problem. Use of a validated questionnaire such as the International Index of Erectile Function (IIEF, see Table 7.3)[5] can help identify the severity of ED and response to treatment.

Specific questions about the nature of erectile failure may help elucidate a cause. Typically (but not exclusively), psychological erectile failure often presents acutely and is intermittent, whereas organic impotence has a more insidious onset and is complete. The inability to obtain an erection at times other than for sexual intercourse often implies a psychological origin to the problem. Nocturnal erections have been shown to be resistant to the effects of stress and are not suppressed by psychological means alone.

As many cases of erectile failure in men with diabetes are of neurological or vascular origin (or both), detailed assessment of the patient's neurovascular systems may provide clues as to the aetiology. The nerve supply to the bladder and the penis has the same origin (S2–4). Thus, bladder symptoms may indicate a neurological cause of ED. Evidence of autonomic neuropathy elsewhere should be sought, e.g. postural dizziness, excessive sweating, symptoms of oesophageal dysmotility or intermittent diarrhoea. Symptoms of a peripheral neuropathy, e.g. paraesthesia in a stocking distribution, may also suggest a neurological aetiology. An enquiry about the presence of symptoms arising from lesions in the cerebral cortex, e.g. a cerebrovascular accident, or spinal cord, e.g. demyelination, should also be made.

The presence of micro- or macroangiopathic complications may suggest that vascular insufficiency is implicated in the cause of the patient's ED. Thus, the patient should be questioned about the presence of angina, intermittent claudication or a past history of ischaemic heart disease, peripheral vascular disease, hypertension, renal disease or retinopathy. ED in men who have two or more of the main vascular risk factors (diabetes, smoking, hyperlipidaemia and hypertension) is very likely to be due to atherosclerosis.[7]

Metabolic factors contributing to ED should be sought. Transient ED may occur during periods of uncontrolled diabetes and improves after improvement in glycaemic control.[8] Although the classic findings of severe hypogonadism are well recognized (ED and loss of libido, loss of secondary sexual hair, gynaecomastia and small testes), many cases of mild hypogonadism exist in which patients report non-specific symptoms such as fatigue, low mood and irritability, and impaired cognitive function.[5] Patients should be questioned about the presence of symptoms that may suggest thyroid disease (ED may be associated with hypothyroidism and thyrotoxicosis) and hyperprolactinaemia.

Transient impotence may also follow an acute illness,[8] e.g. infection or myocardial infarction, and this is more often linked to a psychological origin. Enquiry about the introduction of any drug coinciding with the time when ED was first noted (typically within a 2-week time frame) should be made (Table 7.4). The patient should be questioned about alcohol intake because an excess of 40 units per week is a common precipitant of ED.[1]

Psychological assessment is best undertaken in the presence of both the patient and the partner if they are agreeable. The assessment should focus on five main areas:[9] misconception about normal sexual practice; poor

Table 7.4 Drugs known to cause erectile dysfunction

Drug class	Examples
β Blockers	Including eyedrops. Propranolol possibly the worst, labetolol the least likely to cause erectile dysfunction
Diuretics	Particularly thiazides and spironolactone
Alcohol	
Antipsychotics	Phenothiazines especially thioridazine, lithium. Less likely with haloperidol or pimozide
Antidepressants	Tricyclics and monoamine oxidase inhibitors.
Antiarrhythmics	Verapamil, disopyramide, flecainide, digoxin, propafenone.
Lipid-lowering agents	Statins, gemfibrozil, clofibrate
Other hypotensive agents	Hydralazine, methyldopa, prazosin, clonidine
Opiate addition	
Others	Anticonvulsants, allopurinol, anabolic steroids, baclofen, bromocriptine, cimetidine, gabapentin, ketoconazole, metoclopramide, non-steroidal anti-inflammatory drugs, oestrogens, acetazolamide

self-esteem and self-image; marital disharmony; and anxiety over sexual performance. The temporal relationship of a specific stress to be the commencement of ED may be elicited.

Physical examination

The genitalia should be inspected for congenital deformities, balanitis and phimosis. Plaques deposited along the shaft of the penis may suggest Peyronie's disease or intracorporeal fibrosis. The testes should be felt to establish normal size and consistency.

Neurological innervation can be tested by assessing the bulbocavernosal reflex (S2–4); pinching the glans should result in contraction of the anal sphincter. Absence of this reflex has been observed in a substantial percentage of men with primary impotence who were unable to ejaculate.[10]

Evidence of hypertension, ischaemic heart disease, peripheral vascular disease (diminished or absent peripheral pulsations, bruits, poor capillary perfusion) or cerebrovascular disease may indicate a generalized atherosclerotic process contributing to the aetiology. Postural hypotension suggests the presence of autonomic neuropathy.

A full neurological assessment should be conducted but, in particular, the lower limbs should be assessed for the presence of a peripheral neuropathy. Impaired pain and temperature sensation may be the earliest signs of neuropathy. The presence of autonomic neuropathy can be best assessed by examining the blood pressure response to standing and sustained handgrip, the immediate heart rate response to standing, the heart rate response to Valsalva's manoeuvre and heart rate variation during deep breathing. These simple tests are described in detail elsewhere.[11] Hypothyroidism may be suspected if the reflexes are slow relaxing.

The absence of secondary sexual characteristics suggests hypogonadism. Evidence of hypopituitarism should then be sought to determine if the aetiology is of a primary or a secondary nature. There may be evidence of thyrotoxicosis or hypothyroidism. Hyperprolactinaemia may be suspected by the finding of gynaecomastia.

Investigations

There is no universal agreement as to the extent of investigation that should be undertaken before initiating treatment for ED. Our local policy has been to adopt a limited and pragmatic approach. Assessment of current and previous glycaemic control through measurement of a glycated haemoglobin or fructosamine level may help to identify those patients at risk of organic disease, and be a focus of future management strategies to reduce subsequent vascular risk. However, reversal of poor chronic glycaemic control is not generally associated with improvement in erectile performance. Measurement of serum total testosterone alone may miss cases of hypogonadism. Ideally, a 9am measure (given its circadian production) of free testosterone or another surrogate measure of free testosterone such as the free androgen index (determined from simultaneous total testosterone and sex hormone-binding globulin [SHBG] concentrations) or the derived free testosterone value should be undertaken. This should be combined with checking serum LH and prolactin concentrations. A prostate-specific antigen (PSA) level may be measured if clinical assessment suggests underlying prostatic disease or if testosterone replacement is contemplated. Physical examination may lead to initiation of other investigations that are particularly relevant to the cardiovascular status, which may affect the appropriateness and type of treatment.

Urology departments commonly use a Doppler ultrasound technique or intracavernosal test dose of prostaglandin E_1 to assess the adequacy of local penile blood flow and the likelihood of response to the latter. In the main, this applies to patients who are referred for further investigation and management if there has been a failure to respond or a contraindication to oral therapy. A large number of other investigations are available to the health-care professional to further assess the nature of ED in the man with diabetes, as follows:

- Physiological tests of the autonomic nervous system (most commonly testing cardiovascular reflexes)
- Detailed psychosexual assessment
- Nocturnal penile rigidity studies
- Cavernosography (for the possibility of veno-occlusive leakage)

- Arteriography (usually only if arterial reconstruction is being considered)
- MRI of the pituitary (if prolactinoma or secondary hypogonadism is suspected)

However, it is rare that these investigations alter clinical practice and their use tends to be restricted to specialist centres or for research purposes.

Discussion and counselling

All health-care professionals should at least be prepared to discuss the problem or let the patient talk about it. Simple, although perhaps obvious, questions should be a normal part of discussion and are essential for initial assessment:

- What exactly is the problem?
- Why is it a problem?
- What is your partner's attitude?
- What would you like done about it?

These questions are important in determining whether people really have erectile failure rather than some other problem such as:

- false perceptions of normality
- pain from phimosis
- Peyronie's disease
- premature ejaculation, etc.

This is important in determining not only what the problem is, but also whether it will be necessary to refer to others and, if so, to whom. In our experience some men may not wish to pursue physical treatment methods (as currently available) but are pleased to have had the chance to discuss the problem, have it explained and put into perspective. Reassurance or advice about general health and sexual practices is appreciated and many men will come to terms with the problem.

Management of ED in the man with diabetes

Figure 7.2 outlines an algorithm that may be used in the approach to management of men with diabetes and ED.

In contrast to chronically poor glycaemic control, if ED is associated with acute metabolic deterioration, tumescence may improve with resolution of normoglycaemia. Altering or stopping causative drug treatment is a relatively uncommon therapeutic option. Testosterone should be reserved for men with proven hypogonadism. The option for treating conditions such as balanitis or corrective surgical intervention is rare.

Weight loss (14.5 per cent of original body weight) in obese individuals has been associated with improved erectile performance[12] as has smoking cessation.[13] Over-the-counter preparations such as red ginseng or folic acid

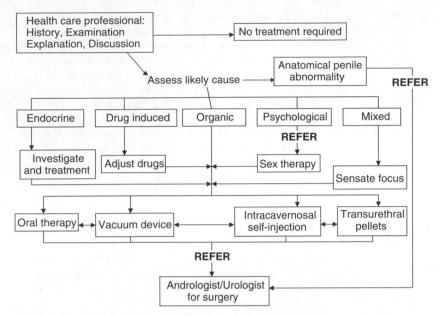

Figure 7.2 Algorithm for the management of male erectile dysfunction in diabetes.

have been promoted as improving erections but there is little scientific evidence to support this claim. Thus, many men with diabetes and ED need to give consideration to the therapeutic options discussed below. However, before embarking on these treatment options, consideration needs to be given to the presence and extent of cardiovascular disease because this impacts on the safety of individuals returning to an active sex life and the prescribing of therapeutic agents.

Cardiovascular fitness and disease

In men with diabetes and cardiovascular disease, returning to an active sex life can lead to additional anxiety. However, it has been shown that the level of exertion associated with sexual intercourse in a longstanding relationship (measured as the metabolic equivalent of the task, MET) is typically no more strenuous than walking a mile on the flat within 20 minutes.[14] Thus reassurance may be given to patients with ischaemic heart disease who are able to achieve this level of exercise without chest pain. Overall, it has been estimated that it is extremely rare for sexual activity to trigger a cardiac event (30 chances per million per hour in the 2-hour period after sexual activity).

In the presence of any form of cardiovascular disease, safety of an active sex life needs to be established. The Princeton Consensus guidelines[15] help to stratify three levels of risk (low, intermediate and high risk) when considering treatment for ED and are shown in Table 7.5. Specific therapies

Table 7.5 Approaches to the management of erectile dysfunction (ED) according to cardiovascular risk (adapted from Second Princeton Consensus Guidelines 2006[15])

Grading of risk	Cardiovascular status at presentation	Recommendation for the management of ED
Low risk	Controlled hypertension Asymptomatic and three or more risk factors for CAD Mild valvular disease Mild stable angina Post-MI (>6–8 weeks) or after successful revascularization (3–4 weeks)	Manage ED within primary care setting Review treatment options with patient and partner (where possible)
Intermediate risk	Recent MI (within 6 weeks) Asymptomatic and three or more risk factors for CAD LVD, CHF (nyha, class I, II) Non-cardiac atherosclerotic sequelae (e.g. CVA) Moderate stable angina	Specialized evaluation recommended (e.g. exercise testing or echocardiography) Place patient in high or low group based on outcome of testing
High risk	Unstable or refractory angina Uncontrolled hypertension CHF (NYHA, class III, IV) Recent MI (within last 14 days) High-risk arrhythmias Obstructive hypertrophic cardiomyopathy Moderate/severe valvular disease	Refer for specialized cardiac evaluation and management Treatment for ED to be deferred until cardiac condition stabilized and/or specialist evaluation completed

CAD, coronary artery disease; CHF, chronic heart failure; CVA, cardiovascular accident; LVD, left ventricular dysfunction. MI, myocardial infarction; nyha, New York Heart Association.

for cardiovascular disease may inhibit the use of some treatment options for ED – e.g. nitrate use precludes the use or PDE-5 inhibitors.

Oral therapy

Phosphodiesterase type 5 inhibitors

Oral PDE-5 inhibitors are now the most commonly used oral agents in the management of ED (see Cummings[16] for review). They enhance the availability of cyclic GMP (Figure 7.3), thereby facilitating smooth muscle relaxation and pooling of blood within the penis. Currently there are three PDE-5 inhibitors available: sildenafil (Viagra), tadalafil (Cialis) and vardenafil (Levitra). All three agents have been shown to be effective in treating ED in diabetes and on average two to three men respond. It is generally

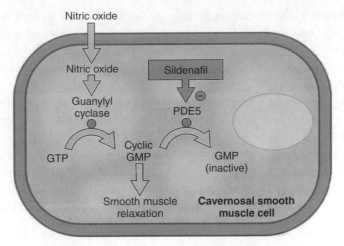

Figure 7.3 The action of phosphodiesterase type 5 (PDE-5) inhibitors.

considered that these agents are equally as effective although differ in properties (e.g. sildenafil and vardenafil have a relatively short half-life of less than 4 hours compared with tadalafil of 17.5 hours) and side-effect profiles related to their ability to inhibit other PDE isoenzymes. The most common side effects shared by all three agents include headaches, flushing and indigestion, but these are usually transient and rarely inhibit long-term use. Previously concern has arisen about the potential for increasing the risk of cardiac events with the use of PDE-5 inhibitors but meta-analysis of the use of sildenafil and the other PDE-5 inhibitors has shown this not to be the case. Indeed more recently PDE-5 inhibitors have been shown to cause a regression in microalbuminuria[17] and improve endothelial function, both surrogate markers of cardiovascular disease.

One of the most common reasons for avoiding treatment with PDE-5 inhibitors is in men with diabetes who are on concomitant therapy that may potentiate a precipitous drop in blood pressure. In particular this applies to patients who are on any form of nitrate therapy or nicorandil for angina. The need for nitrate or nicorandil therapy should be reviewed in each case, but otherwise alternative treatment options should be sought.

Practical issues that need to be considered when prescribing PDE-5 inhibitors include explaining the mode of action because many men mistakenly believe oral ingestion should automatically lead to erection or improve libido. Moreover, they need to be aware of 'the window of opportunity' to synchronize the most appropriate time to take their PDE-5 inhibitor. The effectiveness of sildenafil and vardenafil appear to be reduced if patients have recently ingested fatty foods (which are best avoided), although this does not seem to be a concern with tadalafil. We would recommend a minimum of four attempts at achieving a desired erection when determining if the dose has been effective or whether dose titration or alternative treatments should be considered. In a number of countries, low-dose tadalafil has been approved for daily use where it is anticipated that sexual activity may take place two or more times per week.

Concerns about the increase in cost for the treatment of ED since the introduction of PDE-5 inhibitors seem to be unfounded and we have demonstrated that the total costs for the treatment of ED in our district has been unchanged since their introduction.[18] Given the relatively straightforward approach to prescribing PDE-5 inhibitors and the need for limited educational input compared with more invasive treatment options, initiation and monitoring of treatment are becoming more the domain of primary health-care professionals.

Intracavernosal self-injection of vasoactive drugs

In patients who have not responded to oral therapy, this is a common second-line approach to management. When injected directly into the corpus cavernosum the drugs produce relaxation of the smooth muscle and vasodilatation. Provided that the cavernosal tissue is responsive and there is an adequate potential arterial blood supply, erection will ensue. Prostaglandin E_1 (alprostadil) is most commonly available as Caverject and is the only product actually licensed for intracavernosal self-injection within the UK. The recommended dose range is 2.5–60 µg. It is available in a dual-chamber device (powder and sterile fluid) that can be readily mixed by twisting of the chamber cap (Figure 7.4). Patients are usually taught and observed in the technique of self-injecting within the clinic setting. Evaluation of intracavernosal prostaglandin E_1 suggests that this

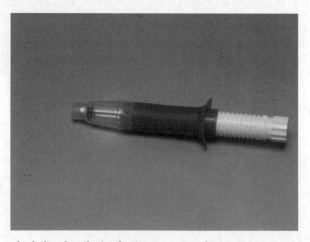

Figure 7.4 A dual-chamber device for intracavernosal injection (Caverject).

is a very effective agent for promoting tumescence in men with diabetes (up to 9 of 10 may respond) with a reduced incidence of prolonged erections and fibrosis at the injection site[19] compared with earlier injected agents such as papaverine.

Relative disadvantages include painful erections in some men although tingling is more commonly reported. Other side effects include prolonged erections and patients should be advised on what action to take in the event of priapism, ranging from simple measures that can be undertaken at home to attending A&E for aspiration of blood form the penis, injections of an antidote (such as phenylephrine) or in extreme cases shunt procedures. It should be stressed that this complication is rare provided that patients follow the appropriate advice over incremental dose adjustments and do not attempt multiple injections within a single 24-hour period. Other recognized side effects include bruising, fibrosis and scarring, infection and syncope.

Papaverine or papaverine/phentolamine combinations may be used by some specialist centres if there is insufficient response to prostaglandin E_1 although these treatments are unlicensed.

Medicated urethral system for erections ('MUSE')
An alternative to self-injection is the application of pellets of prostaglandin E_1 (MUSE) into the urethra (Figure 7.5). The active ingredient is absorbed into the penile tissue, leading to smooth muscle relaxation facilitating tumescence. As with intracavernosal therapy, time is needed to explain

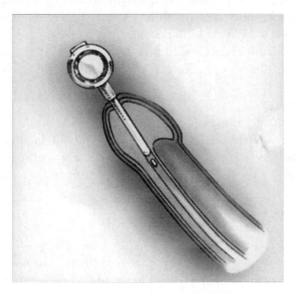

Figure 7.5 Medicated urethral system for erection ('MUSE').

the technique and dose titration is required to achieve an appropriate response. We prefer to supervise patients administrating MUSE in the clinic setting to ensure appropriate application. Although MUSE has been shown to improve erections in a subgroup of patients with diabetes within the general population,[20] most authorities regard MUSE as less effective than intracavernosal injections and associated local pain may limit its use. However, a number of men prioritize this treatment option over injection therapy, given that it is less invasive.

Testosterone replacement

Testosterone replacement in eugonadal men has not been demonstrated to improve erectile performance and has potentially dangerous long-term side effects such as sequelae of resulting polycythaemia. In hypogonadal men, testosterone replacement is a successful and relatively fast-acting therapy with recipients often noticing dramatic improvement within days of starting treatment. Given the short half-life of oral testosterone rendering it ineffective, most authorities consider replacement by other routes.[6] Intramuscular testosterone (typical given every 3 weeks with standard testosterone or every 3 months with longer-acting preparations) is well tolerated, although painful injection sites may be problematic. Topical preparations include gels, and creams and patches are also popular although practical considerations (avoiding contact with water for a period after application, the presence of sweat on the skin surface or rashes with the latter) can limit their use. Other less commonly used routes include buccal testosterone and subcutaneous implants inserted every 4–5 months. Care should be given to assess response (libido and erections) in light of achieving therapeutic replacement levels of testosterone. Other benefits of testosterone may include improved energy levels, muscle bulk and power, cognitive function, mood and bone density. It is imperative to assess for side effects such as prostatic disease and polycythaemia.

Vacuum devices

The use of vacuum tumescence devices can provide a safe and effective method of treatment for most men[21] and should be discussed and demonstrated as a potential first-line treatment particularly where patients want to avoid drug therapy or where it may be contraindicated (Figure 7.6).

The vacuum cylinder devices employ the same principle. A lubricated vacuum tube is placed over the penis with a constriction rubber band placed over the end. A battery- or hand-operated pump is then attached and a vacuum produced by pumping air out. When sufficient tumescence is produced the band is slipped off on to the base of the penis, the vacuum released and the cylinder removed. The band can safely remain in place

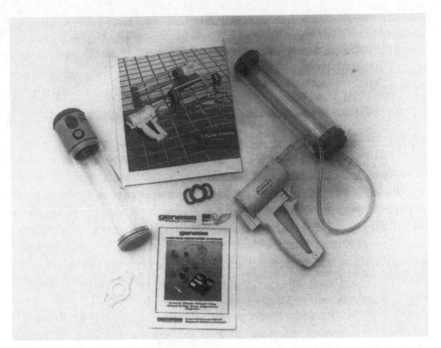

Figure 7.6 Examples of vacuum devices.

for 30 minutes. They do not produce a full erection and the base will remain flaccid with the tumescent penis hanging rather than truly erect, but the result is sufficient for sexual intercourse in 80–90 per cent of men.

Good technique is very important for success and practice may be required. Instructions should be carefully read. Most companies will provide a video instruction tape and also have a telephone helpline to guide people who are having problems. Clinicians should have available demonstration models and videos because some patients will have an initial negative view of vacuum devices as a result of the need for cumbersome equipment that appears to make it rather obtrusive. Therefore it is important to demonstrate the relative ease of this form of treatment. Within the UK, these devices have become available on state prescription and over a long period of time they are very cost-effective compared with drug therapy because it is only a single, one-off, expense.

Bruising may occur with the use of a vacuum device. Significant phimosis should be excluded before recommending use because occasionally restoration of erection may produce tearing of the foreskin. Ejaculatory failure may occur due to constriction from the retention ring. Some discomfort occurs in most patients but is usually minor. Some patients find the devices rather unnatural, obtrusive and messy. They require a sympathetic and understanding partner. The 'quality' of erection is less normal than that produced by injection therapy and, although an erection may be produced in up to 100 per cent of men, overall satisfaction rates may be as low as 50 per cent and, similar to other treatments, there is a high dropout rate over time. Constriction rings alone may be considered in men with diabetes whose predominant problem is that of maintenance of an erection.

Psychosexual therapy

In an ideal world all men should have a multidisciplinary team assessment to include specialist psychosexual advice, but unfortunately this is not possible in practice. Therefore all clinicians should have some knowledge of psychological therapies, just as sex therapists will often need to advise and instruct on physical treatments. Although most men with diabetes and ED will have an organic basis to their problem, there will be some with primary psychological problems and most with some secondary problems. Physical treatments restore only erections, not necessarily relationships, and there will always need to be some psychological input. People with overt psychological problems or frank psychiatric disease should be referred for specialist assessment and advice before embarking on the use of physical methods.

There are a large number of psychological therapies of varying complexity involving either the individual or the couple. From the physician's point of view, it is important to have, at least, a general understanding of the principles of 'sex therapy'. Predisposing, precipitating, potentiating and perpetuating factors should be explored, as a cue for both discussion and decisions on treatment. This will be helpful in improving understanding of the problem, relieving negative thoughts within the patient and directing the physician towards the most appropriate treatment.

Sensate focusing

The physician may find it helpful to be aware, in detail, of some techniques such as the modified Masters and Johnson approach based on 'couple therapy'.[22] This is a useful and logical treatment, not necessarily in the expectation of restoring erections but at least to restore the concept of physical enjoyment. It should encourage communication, discussion and understanding of the needs, likes and dislikes of the partners, and relieve performance anxiety, an important part of the treatment programme.

The suggested programme consists of staged exercises with an agreed ban on intercourse over a set period of time. Half an hour, two or three times a week, should be devoted to these exercises, which involve three phases of sensate focusing. In *phase 1* (the non-genital phase) the couple will caress/stroke and concentrate on enjoyment of touch but not of genital areas. In *phase 2* (the genital phase) stroking and caressing are allowed to include genital areas. Intercourse should not be allowed to take place even if erection occurs in either of these stages. In *phase 3* (vaginal containment phase) before allowing normal intercourse, this stage can include vaginal penetration but passively rather than with a view to orgasm or pleasing the partner.

Discussion of techniques such as the modified Masters and Johnson technique can be part of any treatment even if physical methods are to be the mainstay of therapy. Such discussion helps both the physician and the patient to take a broader view of the problem and the purpose of the treatment.

Surgical treatment

Surgical treatments may be considered in three categories: to correct penile abnormalities, vascular surgery and penile prostheses.

Surgery to correct penile abnormalities

These include:

- congenital abnormalities
- painful conditions such as a torn frenulum or phimosis
- Peyronie's disease
- trauma.

Vascular surgery

This may be considered in men with congenital or traumatic vascular insufficiency, and perhaps in men with major vessel disease in whom angioplasty or reconstruction may be of benefit. However, in general, revascularization techniques remain largely experimental and positive outcomes remain disappointing. The role of venous surgery also remains much debated. Various techniques have been used to try to overcome 'veno'-occlusive deficits' in men with proven good arterial inflow but inability to sustain erections due to 'venous leakage'. Long-term results from surgery have been disappointing and interest now lies in investigating the cavernosal muscle itself rather than venous channels. Men with such a problem may respond to vacuum devices or require a penile prosthesis.

Penile prostheses

The implantation of a penile prosthesis remains the mainstay of surgical treatment and, with careful selection of patients, is very successful in restoring the ability of an impotent man to have intercourse. It is a relatively simple operation that can be performed under general or local/regional anaesthesia.

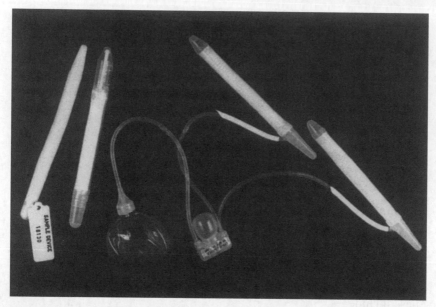

Figure 7.7 Examples of penile prostheses.

Most surgeons would reserve the operation for men who have failed to respond satisfactorily to other forms of treatment, including oral therapy, vacuum devices or intracavernosal vasoactive drugs. This most commonly occurs in men with erectile failure from a vascular aetiology but, regardless of cause, some men will require or prefer a prosthetic implant.

Prostheses are implanted as a pair and most are currently made of a silicone polymer (Figure 7.7). There are three main categories, including: malleable, inflatable and mechanical. Malleable prostheses are the cheapest and most reliable. The penis remains erect all the time but can be folded against the abdominal wall or thigh and is easily concealed. Mechanical and inflatable prostheses contain a mechanism, either intrinsic or attached to the device, whereby it can be kept flaccid or rigid as required.

Complications include infection, mechanical failure, extrusion of the prosthesis, pain and bruising but these are rarely serious, and significant in less than 5 per cent with adequate precautions and an experienced surgeon. High satisfaction rates are reported by both patients and their partners when carefully selected for this procedure.[23]

Conclusions

For the vast majority of men with diabetes who present with ED, there is now effective treatment available. Before embarking on treatment, assessment should focus on not only the aetiology (hypogonadism is now recognized as a much more common treatable cause) but also the presence of frequent comorbidities such as cardiovascular disease that influence ED management. The advent of PDE-5 inhibitors into clinical practice has had a profound impact on the management of ED in the man with diabetes. In consequence, access to treatment has improved because most primary care organizations are able to start treatment although oral treatment non-responders, or those in whom these agents are contraindicated, will still need to have access to specialist services offering other modes of treatment. Future treatments may include gene therapy and stem cell therapy, both of which hold promise in the experimental setting.

7.3 Sexual dysfunction in the female with diabetes

The nature of sexual dysfunction

The erectile tissue and neurological innervations of the female genitalia are homologous to those of the male, which may contribute to the observation that women with diabetes have more arousal phase dysfunction than their healthy spouses. The precise prevalence of female sexual dysfunction in women with diabetes remains uncertain and is quite heterogeneous in its presentation. In a recent detailed questionnaire of 270 women with diabetes (and non-diabetic control women), it was identified that there were significant differences in perceived sexual function and attitudes towards sexual health.[24] The principal findings were that of reduced lubrication/moistness in the vaginal area, painful sex, difficulty achieving orgasm, lack of interest in sex and loss of genital sensation compared with controls. A third of women with diabetes felt that their diabetes had impacted negatively on their choice and use of contraception and worry about fertility and fear of pregnancy led to sexual or relationship difficulties. Significantly increased problems of self-image and psychological concerns were also observed in women with diabetes affecting sexual function. A further review of the limited studies of sexual dysfunction in women with diabetes broadly classified the findings into four key areas.[25] Most studies identified a reduction in sexual desire, a decrease in vaginal lubrication and arousal, orgasmic dysfunction or anorgasmy, and dyspareunia.

Management

As health-care professionals, we have traditionally focused on identifying men with diabetes and ED but it is clear that we should give every opportunity for women with diabetes to express concerns about their sexual health. Although men typically complain about genital or ejaculatory response, women complain of inadequate enjoyment or interest and the impact on the quality of their relationship. It is important to take an

Table 7.6 Management strategies used in the treatment of female sexual dysfunction

Type of sexual dysfunction	Potential remedy
Reduced vaginal lubrication	Water-based vaginal lubricants, local or systemic hormone replacement therapy, clitoral stimulation aids (e.g. vacuum devices), advice on the need for extended foreplay and adequate stimulation before sex, oral therapy, e.g. sildenafil, controversial and not proven
Absent genital sensation	Psychosexual counselling incorporating arousal enhancement strategies and encouraging exploration of other erogenous zones; penetrative vibrating sex aids
Painful sex (dyspareunia)	Vaginal lubrication, arousal enhancement strategies (as above); consider and treat genitourinary disease if present; reduce focus on penetrative sex
Anorgasmia	Psychosexual therapy including arousal enhancement strategies (see above), vibrating sex aids
Diminished libido	Addressing intrapersonal, interpersonal and self-image issues, treatment of concurrent sexual problems or depressive illness, hormone therapy replacement (including low-dose testosterone)

Adapted from Meeking et al.[24]

accurate history to define the problem, given the heterogeneous nature of problems that may be affecting their sex life. Enquiry should be made about causative medication and the possibility of depression. A clinical examination should routinely be conducted and the possibility of vaginal infection and/or irritation be considered.

With knowledge of the underlying problem, there are a number of approaches to treatment that may be considered (Table 7.6). There is very limited data on the use of sildenafil and phentolamine in the general population of women with sexual dysfunction with conflicting findings.

Case study

A man with type 2 diabetes age 48 presents with a 3-year history of progressive ED. Libido is preserved. He sustained a myocardial infarction (MI) 6 months ago. He has a BMI of 38 kg/m^2 and has cut his cigarette consumption down from 40 cigarettes to 20 cigarettes per day. He has been on a β blocker and aspirin since the MI. His glycaemic control has always been stable since diagnosis (current glycated haemoglobin 6.7%). He has been in a new relationship for the last 3 months. What is the likely aetiology and how would you manage this patient?

Answer

This patient almost certainly has underlying vascular disease contributing to his ED in addition to diabetes-related failure of penile smooth muscle relaxation. His diabetes, obesity, smoking habit and established ischaemic heart disease all support this aetiology. Diabetes, cardiovascular disease and ED are integrally linked and the presence of one of these conditions should alert clinicians to consider the presence of these other comorbidities. The progressive nature of his ED makes a primary psychological cause unlikely, although the patient may express some level of anxiety about resuming a sex life after his cardiac event which may contribute to his ED. Although being overweight is associated with reduced androgen availability, preserved libido makes hypogonadism less likely.

A thorough history and examination should be undertaken as always and the presence of any cardiac symptoms should be established. If he develops angina on minimal exercise,[14] further cardiac evaluation should be sought and his condition stabilized before embarking on treatment for ED.[15] His ED preceded the introduction of β blockers and stopping this drug even if clinically safe to do so is unlikely to reverse his ED. Hypogonadism should be screened for, although was not evident in this patient on biochemical testing. Losing weight[12] and smoking cessation[13] may have some impact upon improving erections as well as his general health but is unlikely to completely resolve his erectile failure given the extent of established vascular disease.

Oral PDE5 inhibitors represent the simplest and least invasive option if his cardiovascular disease is stable. However if he uses glyceryl trinitrate (spray or sublingual tablets), an alternative approach would be the use of intraurethral pellets or intracavernosal injections. A successful outcome will also depend upon reassurance about his cardiac status in relation to resuming an active sex life and appropriate education with regard to the use of any pharmacological approach.

References

1. McCulloch DK, Young RJ, Prescott RJ Campbell IW, Clarke BF. The natural history of impotence in diabetic men. *Diabetologia* 1984;**26**:437–40.
2. Prikhozhan VM. Impotence in diabetes mellitus. *Probl Endocrinol* 1967;**13**:37–41.
3. Kinsey AC, Pomeroy WB, Martin CE. Age and sexual outlet. *Sexual Behaviour in the Human Male*. Philadelphia: Saunders, 1948: pp 218–262.
4. Jevtich MJ, Edson M, Jarman WD, Herrera HH. Vascular factors in erectile failure amongst diabetics. *Urology* 1982;**19**:163–168.
5. Rosen RC, Riley A, Wagner G, Osterloh H, Kirkpatrick J, Mishra A. The International Index of Erectile Function (IIEF): a multidimensional scale for assessment of erectile dysfunction. *Urology* 1997;**49**:822–830.
6. Jones TH. Hypogonadism in men with type 2 diabetes. *Pract Diabet Int* 2007;**24**: 269–277.

7. Virag R, Bouilly P, Frydman D. Is impotence an arterial disorder? A study of arterial risk factors in 440 impotent men. *Lancet* 1985;**i**:181–187.

8. Podolsky S. Diagnosis and treatment of sexual dysfunction in the male diabetic. *Med Clin North Am* 1982;**66**:1389–1396.

9. Fairbrun CG, McCulloch DK, Wu FC. The effect of diabetes on male sexual function. *Clin Endocrinol Metab* 1982;**11**: 749–767.

10. Brindley GS, Gillan P. Men and women who do not have orgasms. *Br J Psych* 1982;**140**:351–356.

11. Ewing DJ, Clarke BF. Diagnosis and management of diabetic autonomic neuropathy. *BMJ* 1982;**285**:916–918.

12. Esposito K, Giugliano F, Di Palo C, et al. Effect of lifestyle changes on erectile dysfunction in obese men. *JAMA* 2004 **291**:2978–284.

13. Pourmand G, Alidaee MR, Rasuli S, Maleki A, Mehrsai A. Do cigarette smokers with erectile dysfunction benefit from stopping?: a prospective study. *Br J Urol Int* 2004; **94**:1310–1313.

14. Wilson PK, Farday PS, Froelicher V, eds. *Cardiac Rehabilitation: Adult fitness and exercise testing*. Philadelphia, PA: Lea & Fabiger, 1981: pp 333–353.

15. Jackson G, Rosen RC, Kloner RA, Kostis JB. The Second Princeton consensus on sexual dysfunction and cardiac risk: new guidelines for sexual medicine. *J Sexual Med* 2006;**3**(1):28–36.

16. Cummings MH. *Managing Erectile Dysfunction*. St Albans: Altman, 2006: pp 43–49.

17. Grover-Paez F, Villegas Rivera G, Guillen Ortiz R. Sildenafil citrate diminishes microalbuminuria and the percentage of A1c in male patients with type 2 diabetes. *Diabet Res Clin Pract* 2007;**78**:136–140.

18. Ashton-Key M, Sadler M, Walmsley B, Holmes S, Randall S, Cummings MH. UK department of health guidance on prescribing for impotence following the introduction of sildenafil: potential to contain costs in the average health authority district. *Pharmacoeconomics* 2002;**20**:839–846.

19. Heaton JP, Lording D, Liu SN, et al. Intracavernosal alprostadil is effective for the treatment of erectile dysfunction in diabetic men. *Int J Imp Res* 2001;**13**:317–321.

20. Padma-Nathan H, Hellstrom W, Kaiser FE. Treatment of men with erectile dysfunction with transurethral alprostadil. *N Engl J Med* 1997;**336**:1–7.

21. Ryder RE, Close CF, Moriarty KT, Moore KT, Hardisty CA. Impotence in diabetes: aetiology, implications for treatment and preferred vacuum device. *Diabet Med* 1992;**9**:893–898.

22. Masters WH, Johnson VE. *Human Sexual Inadequacy*. London: Churchill, 1970.

23. McLaren RH, Barrett DM. Patient and partner satisfaction with the AMS 700 penile prosthesis. *J Urol* 1992;**147**:62.

24. Meeking DR, Fosbury JA, Cummings MH, Alexander WD, Shaw KM, Russell-Jones DL. Sexual dysfunction and sexual health concerns in women with diabetes. *Sexual Dysfunction* 1999;**I**:83–87.

25. Enzlin P, Mathieu C, Vanderschueren D, Demyttenaere K. Diabetes mellitus and female sexuality: a review of 25 years' research. *Diabet Med* 1998;**15**:809–815.

CHAPTER 8

Diabetes and the Heart

Miles Fisher[1] and Kenneth M Shaw[2]
[1]Glasgow Royal Infirmary, Glasgow, Scotland, UK
[2]Queen Alexandra Hospital, Portsmouth Hospitals NHS Trust, Portsmouth, UK

 Key points

- The reduction of cardiovascular risk and heart disease in people with diabetes requires a multifactorial approach comprising attention to glycaemic factors, the management of hypertension and dyslipidaemia, the use of antiplatelet drugs in suitable individuals and the correct cardiological management of patients with established heart disease.

- The approach to cardiovascular risk reduction depends on the cardiovascular status of the patient with diabetes. Patients who are free of cardiovascular disease will require a different approach to patients with stable coronary heart disease, after acute coronary syndromes or with chronic heart failure.

- For patients without heart disease, intensive glycaemic control reduces cardiovascular events on long-term follow-up, especially myocardial infarctions, with no real benefit in reducing strokes or mortality.

- For patients with established cardiovascular disease or high vascular risk, intensive glucose control, but avoiding hypoglycaemia and weight gain, reduces microvascular outcomes and does not appear to worsen macrovascular outcomes.

- The most appropriate method of controlling hyperglycaemia is not clear for patients with diabetes after acute coronary syndromes or with chronic heart failure.

Diabetes: Chronic Complications, Third Edition. Edited by Kenneth M. Shaw, Michael H. Cummings.
© 2012 John Wiley & Sons, Ltd. Published 2012 by John Wiley & Sons, Ltd.

Therapeutic key points

- For patients without heart disease metformin demonstrates benefits that are not solely explained by control of hyperglycaemia. Control of hypertension and use of statins reduce cardiovascular events, but aspirin is of no proven benefit.

- For patients with documented coronary heart disease, pioglitazone further reduces events and intensive control of hypertension will reduce further events. Angiotensin-converting enzyme (ACE) inhibitors have additional prognostic benefits, and are also of benefit for patients with normal blood pressure. High-dose atorvastatin is better than low-dose atorvastatin, and aspirin is of some limited benefit.

- After acute coronary syndromes the use of high-dose atorvastatin is mandatory, and all patients with diabetes should receive ACE inhibitors and β blockers. Dual antiplatelet therapy with aspirin plus clopidogrel will also be required.

- Chronic heart failure is common in diabetes as a consequence of previous myocardial infarction. All patients with diabetes and heart failure should receive ACE inhibitors and β blockers. Pioglitazone is contraindicated because of possible fluid retention and metformin may be the best long-term choice, but it should be discontinued during episodes of acute heart failure.

8.1 Introduction

Diabetes exerts its greatest adverse impact throughout the vascular system. This effect includes the specific microvascular complications including retinopathy, nephropathy and neuropathy, but also a predisposition to premature and accelerated macrovascular disease. The consequences of macrovascular disease contribute to significant reductions in the quality of life of a person with diabetes, and are also the most likely cause of death, and three-quarters of people with diabetes will die from cardiovascular causes. Although advanced complications from microangiopathy are potentially preventable by intensive glycaemic management in type 1 and type 2 diabetes, the careful use of multi-risk factor reduction is required to delay the ravages of large vessel disease affecting the coronary, cerebral and peripheral arterial circulations. The heart in diabetes can be affected by several pathologies, in addition to coronary heart disease, including diabetic autonomic neuropathy and a diabetic cardiomyopathy. The various clinical expressions of coronary heart disease, silent ischaemia, angina, acute coronary syndromes, heart failure and sudden death all occur more commonly with diabetes, often presenting at an earlier age.

8.2 Epidemiology

Epidemiological observations indicate geographical variation in the frequency of clinical coronary heart disease, being as low as 6 per cent prevalence in Japan, in contrast to the much higher proportion in the western world. This would suggest an environmental lifestyle effect, probably of a dietary nature, because the apparent protection is lost when a western lifestyle is adopted.

Some distinction between type 1 diabetes and type 2 diabetes seems evident from the degree of disturbed glycaemic control that correlates with the development of vascular problems. Microangiopathy seems primarily related to the degree of hyperglycaemia and its duration, with an uncertain genetic factor. This may well be similar in both type 1 and type 2 diabetes. For macroangiopathy the situation is less clear. By its very nature type 1 diabetes predominantly presents at a younger age than type 2 diabetes and so the opportunity for pre-clinical development of vascular disturbance is less. It is unusual to see serious arterial problems with teenage diabetes, or with a few years' duration. However, serious problems, including premature coronary heart disease, may present even as young as the mid-20s, and is detected increasingly during the third and fourth decades. The earlier presentation of coronary heart disease in type 1 diabetes is often evident by the fourth decade and not infrequently significant disease may present at an even younger age, including women well before the menopause.

With both types of diabetes a distinct threshold of hyperglycaemia predisposing to microangiopathy of around 11 mmol/l is apparent, whereas the threshold for large vessel disease is considerably lower. Indeed, there is now evidence that the risk of development of cardiovascular disease increases within the normal, non-diabetic range. In that regard, blood glucose can be viewed in the same way as blood pressure and serum cholesterol as a continuous variable that increases cardiovascular risk rather than there being a cut-off point at which risk suddenly rises.

Susceptibility to coronary heart disease is increased substantially in people with both type 1 and type 2 diabetes. The development of all forms of large vessel disease is accelerated with type 1 diabetes, and is often present at diagnosis in people with type 2 diabetes. It is now well established that type 2 diabetes is part of the metabolic or insulin resistance syndrome, which comprises hypertension, dyslipidaemia, central adiposity, insulin resistance, diabetes or impaired glucose tolerance, and cardiovascular disease. It is less certain whether this is a simple clustering of these factors in susceptible individuals, or whether this is a single key determinant, e.g. central adiposity or inflammation that leads to all of the other features.

With type 2 diabetes some evidence of underlying coronary disorder, be it clinical or electrocardiographic, is frequently present at diagnosis, often in association with detectable cerebrovascular and peripheral arterial disease as well. All coronary manifestations occur more frequently, and to a greater degree, although the trend towards a decline in the coronary mortality rate of the population at large is not as yet so clearly evident for people with diabetes.

Of all manifestations of coronary heart disease, much has been reported concerning myocardial infarction and acute coronary syndromes in diabetes, emphasizing the increased susceptibility to myocardial infarction and increased severity of such, with greater frequency of associated problems and higher consequent mortality, which is double the mortality in individuals who do not have diabetes.

The risk of chronic heart failure for men with type 1 diabetes increases twofold and for women fivefold, once more identifying the greater adverse effect of diabetes in the women. Similarly, with type 2 diabetes increased predisposition to angina and myocardial infarction is accompanied by greater severity of heart failure. From the cardiology perspective, a third of patients with chronic heart failure have diabetes.

8.3 Pathophysiology

The predominant large vessel disturbance of diabetes is that of atherosclerosis or atheroma. There has been considerable debate concerning whether there are specific features to diabetes, or whether it is simply an exaggeration of that seen with the non-diabetic population. Overall there is probably no major qualitative difference in the type of atherosclerosis between individuals who do and do not have diabetes; it is predominantly an increase in the amount, extent and distribution. With diabetes, atherosclerosis is observed to be more extensive throughout the circulation with more distal involvement of blood vessels.

In general, no specific arterial lesion is seen in people with diabetes, but there is evidence of more fatty streaks, intimal plaques and calcification of vessels. The process of atherosclerosis is probably similar to that observed in individuals who do not have diabetes, with smooth muscle cell proliferation, intimal thickening, excess collagen production and medial calcification leading to reduced blood flow in stable angina. Plaques appear to be more prone to rupture than in individuals who do not have diabetes, with more evidence of inflammation within the plaque, leading to acute coronary syndromes. Changes in platelet activity with increased adhesiveness and tendency to aggregation have been observed, although it is not always easy to distinguish between primary alterations as a consequence of diabetes from those changes known to occur secondarily in the presence of occlusive arterial disease.

The increased risk of acute coronary syndromes with diabetes is partly a reflection of the accelerated and more severe atherosclerotic occlusive disease process of the coronary arteries. The complications of myocardial infarction including arrhythmia, conduction disorders, cardiac failure and cardiogenic shock occur more commonly. The infarct size is not larger in people with diabetes, and there may be an adverse contribution from autonomic neuropathy and diabetic cardiomyopathy. Mortality from acute myocardial infarction is significantly worse in diabetes, with approximately twofold increased mortality risk in men, and threefold in women. The immediate mortality rate from myocardial infarction in diabetes is as high as 34 per cent compared with about 18 per cent when diabetes is not present, whereas at 6 months up to a 50 per cent mortality rate has been reported. This increased mortality is likely to reflect the greater severity of underlying coronary disease and the fact that more complications occur during the acute stages. However, recent studies from coronary care registries have shown that one reason for the increased mortality is a failure to use appropriate and proven therapies.

Acute left ventricular failure is a common consequence of acute myocardial infarction in diabetes. The degree of left ventricular dysfunction is a major determinant of outcome after a myocardial infarction, and contributes to the greater case fatality observed with diabetes, both in the immediate post-myocardial infarction period and over subsequent months.

The aetiology of chronic heart failure in diabetes is complex. Coronary artery disease significantly contributes to the development of heart failure either acutely with myocardial infarction or more insidiously in association with ventricular remodelling. In many cases, underlying myocardial ischaemia remains undetected, until heart failure presents. The diabetic myocardium may show diffuse fibrotic changes as a consequence of ischaemia. Apart from the clear effect of coronary disease, myocardial function may be impaired directly by adverse metabolic changes, such as glycoprotein deposition, and possibly in some instances by the development of microangiopathy. As a result of such observations the term 'diabetic cardiomyopathy' has been introduced, when primary myocardial disturbance is often out of proportion to the severity of the coronary disease.

8.4 Management

Primary prevention of heart disease in diabetes

Glycaemic control
Evidence that the intensive control of hyperglycaemia reduces diabetes complications comes from the Diabetes Control and Complications Trial (DCCT)[1] and the United Kingdom Prospective Diabetes Study (UKPDS).[2]

The DCCT reported on the effect of intensive treatment of diabetes on the development and progression of complications in type 1 diabetes; 1441 patients with type 1 diabetes were studied over a mean period of 6.5 years, and were divided into two groups: a primary prevention cohort without pre-existing complications and a secondary prevention cohort of patients with early complications, particularly early retinopathy. Each group was randomly assigned to either a conventional treated group or to a more intensive therapeutic regimen. The effect on microvascular complications was striking, with substantial reduction in the development of retinopathy, nephropathy and neuropathy.

The effect of intensive therapy on macrovascular disease was less marked at the end of the study. A reduction in all major cardiovascular and peripheral vascular events was observed but this did not reach statistical significance.

Most of the DCCT participants were followed in the observational Epidemiology of Diabetes Interventions and Complications (EDIC) study.[1] During the mean 17 years of total follow-up in DCCT plus EDIC there was a significant reduction in cardiovascular events in patients who had received intensive treatment in the trial, as compared with patients who had received conventional treatment. Intensive treatment reduced the risk of any cardiovascular events by 42 per cent and the risk of non-fatal myocardial infarction, stroke or death from cardiovascular disease by 57 per cent. The pathophysiological mechanisms responsible for the improvements in outcomes and for the prolonged effects of early intervention were unclear, and the authors referred to these as 'metabolic memory'.

In the UKPDS 4209 patients with newly diagnosed type 2 diabetes were studied over a 10-year period.[2] Patients with a history of myocardial infarction, current angina or heart failure in the previous year were excluded. A complex study design was followed, and there were multiple subgroups and substudies. The principal comparison was between 1138 patients who were randomly assigned to conventional treatment and 2729 patients who were assigned to an intensive therapeutic regimen based on sulfonylurea or insulin therapy. Again, the effect on microvascular disease was striking and the effect on macrovascular disease was less marked. There was a 16 per cent reduction in myocardial infarctions in the intensive treatment group compared with the conventional treatment group, but this did not quite reach statistical significance.[2]

Most of the surviving UKPDS participants were followed in post-trial monitoring for a further 10 years, and during follow-up the reduction in myocardial infarctions in the group with prior intensive glycaemic control was statistically significant, with a significant reduction in total mortality[3] (Figure 8.1). Again the pathophysiological mechanisms responsible for the

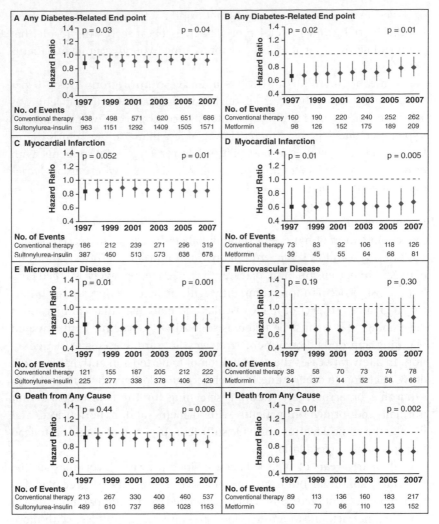

Figure 8.1 Hazard ratios for any diabetes endpoint, myocardial infarction, microvascular disease and death from any cause in the UKPDS (UK Prospective Diabetes Study) post-trial monitoring[3].

prolonged effects of early intensive intervention were unclear, and the UKPDS authors referred to these as a 'legacy effect'.

In the UKPDS a major subgroup was overweight patients, who were randomly allocated to intensive therapy with metformin in addition to randomization to either sulfonylureas or insulin:[4] 342 overweight patients were allocated to metformin, 542 to sulfonylurea therapy, 409 to insulin and 411 to the conventional treatment group. An unexpected and statistically significant 39 per cent reduction in myocardial infarctions was observed in patients treated with metformin, which was reflected by a significant reduction in total mortality. It is because of this result that metformin is the drug of first choice for treating hyperglycaemia in patients with type 2 diabetes.

The mean HbA1c in the UKPDS intensive control group was 7.0 per cent, but in the early years of the study a mean of 6.0 per cent was achieved. The main side effects of intensive control were weight gain and hypoglycaemia. A general target HbA1c of less than 7.0 per cent is therefore reasonable, with the possibility of lower targets for patients with newly diagnosed diabetes and low cardiovascular risk, where hypoglycaemia is less of a worry.

Hypertension

The combination of hypertension and diabetes poses an increased predisposition to cardiovascular morbidity and mortality. The relationship between hypertension and diabetes has been extensively studied and hypertension occurs more commonly with diabetes, its presence conferring a greater prospect of microvascular and macrovascular complications developing, and it must be taken as seriously as glycaemic control when planning appropriate treatment strategies for cardiovascular risk reduction. In a few rare cases the combination of hypertension and diabetes will draw attention to other underlying endocrine disorders such as Cushing's syndrome or acromegaly. Routine screening for these disorders is not normally performed in patients with diabetes and hypertension, and usually the clinical features provide sufficient suspicion of diagnosis to lead to appropriate investigation.

In the early years of type 1 diabetes, blood pressure levels may not be detectably abnormal, but from late adolescence onwards a degree of elevation may be observed, and when associated with microalbuminuria a complex interaction can ensue. Blood pressure inevitably rises with more advanced nephropathy, but, even in the absence of detectable renal abnormality, high blood pressure becomes more evident with longer duration of type 1 diabetes. Up to 20 per cent of type 1 patients with diabetes duration in excess of 15 years may have untreated diastolic blood pressure levels above 100 mmHg compared with 11.5 per cent of an age-matched population. With type 2 diabetes, the incidence is even greater. In the UKPDS 40 per cent of men and 53 per cent of woman recorded blood pressure levels in excess of 160/95 mmHg. Using a more modern definition of hypertension as a blood pressure >140/90 mmHg, three-quarters of patients with type 2 diabetes are hypertensive, and this increases even higher in patients with type 2 diabetes and microalbuminuria.

The presence of hypertension in diabetes is associated with reduced survival, the predominant cause of death being myocardial infarction in

40 per cent of cases. Long-term longitudinal studies show a substantial increase in mortality in the presence of both hypertension and diabetes. Furthermore, the individual increased risk of both hypertension and diabetes is not just simply doubled when the two occur together, but the combination increases the risk exponentially with the greatest risk for young adults, especially women. The effect of hypertension on the development of microvascular complications is also established in that hypertension will accelerate decline in established nephropathy, eventually contributing to end-stage renal failure, as well as eye disorders such as exudative retinopathy and retinal vein thrombosis.

Treatment of hypertension in patients with diabetes can now be based on a large body of clinical evidence. This includes many studies in patients with diabetes alone, such as the Hypertension in Diabetes Study (HDS)[5] which was part of the UKPDS, and careful examination of diabetic subgroups in other large studies, such as the Hypertension Optimal Treatment (HOT) study.[6] Initial management of the hypertensive diabetic patient should include advice on lifestyle, the patient being encouraged to reduce excessive weight, to modify diet by reducing sodium and saturated fat intake, and to limit alcohol consumption. Pharmacological treatment is usually required, and individual patients may require multiple hypotensive drugs to reach targets. Targets for the treatment of hypertension are lower than for individuals who do not have diabetes, and many guidelines set targets of <130/80 mmHg.

Most groups of drugs have been shown to be of proven benefit in people with diabetes, including ACE inhibitors, ARBs, calcium channel blockers, diuretics and β blockers. A combination of ACE inhibitor or ARB with amlodipine is suggested as a well-tolerated starting point, with diuretics as an alternative second-line drug or as a third-line drug (Figure 8.2). The α blocker doxazocin, or β blockers, should not be used as first-line treatment, but may be required in combination if the patients cannot tolerate other drugs because of side effects.

Dyslipidaemia

Although patterns may differ between type 1 and type 2 diabetes, a common basis for disturbed lipid metabolism can still be identified. Insulin deficiency is still an essential component, be it absolute (type 1 diabetes) or relative (insulin resistance/type 2 diabetes). The consequence of insulin deficiency or insulin resistance is much the same. Hypertriglyceridaemia predominates because insulin lack leads to reduced lipoprotein lipase activity, and thereby decreased clearance of circulating triglycerides and low high-density lipoprotein (HDL) levels. Increased lipolysis occurs in adipose tissue and an increase of free fatty acids is delivered to the liver, with resultant fatty change. Total cholesterol levels in people with diabetes

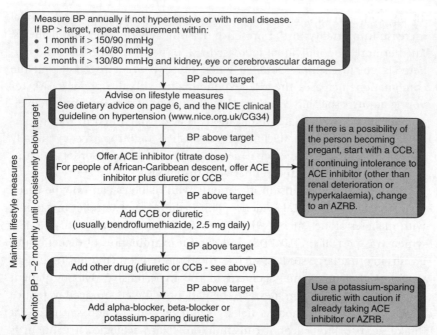

Figure 8.2 National Institute for Health and Clinical Excellence (NICE) guideline for the management of hypertension in people with diabetes. Source: National Institute for Health and Clinical Excellence (2009) Adapted from 'CG 87 Type 2 diabetes: the management of type 2 diabetes. London: NICE. Available from HYPERLINK "http://www.nice.org.uk/"www.nice.org.uk. Reproduced with permission.

are likely to reflect the pattern in the population at large with a contributory cardiovascular risk according to the precise level. However, it is important to be aware that for a given level of total cholesterol the atherogenic, small, dense low-density lipoprotein (LDL) subfraction may be a much higher percentage than in individuals who do not have diabetes.

Although a variety of drugs is available for improving abnormal lipid levels, the use of statins is preferred based on the results of many large, multicentre, randomized trials. Similar to the blood pressure studies, these have included careful examination of diabetic subgroups, e.g. in the Heart Protection Study (HPS),[7] and studies performed just in patients with diabetes, e.g. the Collaborative Atorvastatin Diabetes Study (CARDS).[8] These statin studies in diabetes have confirmed the benefit of cholesterol lowering with simvastatin and atorvastatin for patients without existing cardiovascular disease.

Protocols for the management of diabetes now include recommendations on the measurement and treatment of lipids, although the detail concerning the age to start treatment is uncertain. All patients aged >40 years should be started on a reasonable dose of a statin.

The fibrate group of drugs is pharmacologically more logical for treating the typical dyslipidaemia of diabetes, because these drugs increase HDL-cholesterol and decrease triglycerides. To date, evidence of benefit with these drugs on hard cardiovascular outcomes has been conflicting in diabetes, and appears to be of little benefit for primary prevention. There are several new lipid-lowering drugs, including ezetimibe, which lowers cholesterol by inhibiting the absorption of cholesterol. Short-term studies have shown improvements in the lipid profile of patients with diabetes using ezetimibe, but there is no evidence for a reduction in cardiovascular events when used for primary prevention. Similarly, patients with diabetes were excluded from the primary prevention JUPITER study of rosuvastatin in patients with a raised C-reactive protein.

Antiplatelet drugs

Antiplatelet therapy is of proven benefit for secondary prevention of cardiovascular events in people with diabetes, and is described below. Any possible benefit for primary prevention is unproven. Several recent meta-analyses of patients with diabetes whose sole vascular risk factor was diabetes (i.e. primary prevention) showed no evidence of benefit from antiplatelet therapy, but evidence of harm with gastrointestinal bleeding and an increase in haemorrhagic strokes. Aspirin is no longer recommended for primary prevention of vascular events in people with diabetes.

Stable coronary heart disease

Clinical presentation

The classic description of crushing central chest tightness may not always be obtained in people with diabetes, despite severe underlying coronary heart disease. Symptoms described may be much more subtle and atypical, including simple fatigue, which may obscure an accurate diagnosis. This is particularly so when the patient is young and female, and the diagnosis does not seem probable. Unusual chest symptoms, particularly with an exertional component, must be taken seriously, because 'silent' (asymptomatic) ischaemia frequently occurs, and clinically evident angina is likely to represent the tip of the iceberg phenomenon.

Investigation and cardiological considerations

A resting ECG may be helpful when angina is suspected, or as part of a review screening protocol for asymptomatic patients. ST-segment or T-wave abnormalities may be detected suggesting underlying ischaemia, and not infrequently signs of previously unsuspected old myocardial infarction may be present. Patients with suspected coronary heart disease should be referred to a cardiologist for full assessment, including stress testing. This enables confirmation of the diagnosis and stratification of the severity of the disease, which will then lead to either initial medical therapy, or invasive investigation with coronary angiography with a view to possible coronary artery bypass grafting (CABG) or percutaneous coronary intervention (PCI).

Positive exercise tests may be found in up to 25 per cent of asymptomatic patients with type 2 diabetes, and also in a significant proportion of patients with type 1 diabetes with duration of diabetes longer than 15 years. Such is the extent of potential silent coronary heart disease that could be identified by exercise testing that the need and implications of screening for asymptomatic coronary disease are hotly debated. At the moment there is no clear evidence that those without symptoms but with positive exercise ECGs are any the better managed for that knowledge, and it is doubtful whether present resources could meet the potential demand of further investigation including angiography, and its treatment consequences such as coronary interventions.

Patients with worsening angina, not responding to increasing doses of anti-anginal medication, should be re-referred to a cardiologist and considered for further investigation, including repeat stress testing and coronary angiography if necessary. Coronary angiography is likely to show more severe changes involving all three main vessels and of a more diffuse and distal nature. The latter does create greater technical difficulty for successful coronary bypass grafting, but in some instances lesions may be only proximal, and thereby amenable to either angioplasty or bypass surgery. CABG is the preferred treatment for patients with diabetes who have triple-vessel disease, because several studies have shown an improved survival compared with PCI. If the patient is suitable for PCI then a drug-eluting stent should be used because this leads to less need for re-interventions than a bare metal stent or balloon angioplasty.

Treatment of stable coronary disease

Drug therapy for angina in diabetes is similar to that given to individuals who have angina and do not have diabetes, but some extra considerations needs to be made. β Blockers can modify symptoms of hypoglycaemia and impair recovery from hypoglycaemia in insulin-treated patients if non-selective β blockers are used, so the use of cardioselective β blockers, e.g. atenolol, bisoprolol or metoprolol, is recommended. In the presence of peripheral arterial disease, claudication and cold feet can be aggravated by β blockers.

Calcium channel blockers and the potassium channel blocker nicorandil have no significantly deleterious effect in diabetes and may be used, although oral nitrates can be particularly helpful. Ivabradine, which limits heart rate through direct effects on the sinus node, may be considered for symptomatic treatment in patients unable to tolerate β blockers.

emic management

nts in the UKPDS were recently diagnosed and mostly free of cardio-
ular disease. Three recent, large trials have included patients with
standing diabetes and stable cardiovascular disease or multiple cardio-
cular risk factors, and have sought to identify the most appropriate
get HbA1c (glycated haemoglobin) for these patients.[9–11]

The Action to Control Cardiovascular Risk in Diabetes (ACCORD) trial
North American included 10251 patients with type 2 diabetes and a
hird had existing cardiovascular disease.[9] The study aimed to get patients
rapidly to an HbA1c within the non-diabetic range of <6.0 per cent. The
investigators were unable to get many patients to target because of frequent severe hypoglycaemia and marked weight gain, and the mean
HbA1c achieved was 6.5 per cent. The trial was halted prematurely when
it was clear that this very intensive approach caused an increase in mortality without any beneficial impact on cardiovascular events. An excess was
particularly seen in sudden or unexpected deaths.

The Action in Diabetes and Vascular Disease: Preterax and Diamicron
Modified Release Controlled Evaluation (ADVANCE) trial contained
11140 patients and again a third had existing cardiovascular disease.[10] The
treatment approach was much less intensive than in ACCORD. The target
HbA1c was 6.5 per cent, with slow titration of treatments, and the late
introduction of insulin. Hypoglycaemia was uncommon, and there was
very little weight gain. Benefits were obtained at the end of the 5-year
study with significant reductions in the development of microalbuminuria
and insignificant reductions in cardiovascular endpoints. As it took more
than 10 years for cardiovascular benefits to become statistically significant
in the UKPDS study,[3] it is not surprising that the reduction in macrovascular endpoints was not statistically significant in this shorter study.

Since the ACCORD study was stopped there have been several post-hoc
analyses to try to explain this excessive mortality, and the investigators
have not put forward a clear explanation. Severe hypoglycaemia was
associated with an increased mortality in both groups. As hypoglycaemia
can trigger cardiac ischaemia, myocardial infarction and arrhythmias,
hypoglycaemia is a possible explanation.

The antidiabetic drugs that were used in the UKPDS included metformin, sulfonylureas and acarbose. Sustained-release gliclazide was used
in the ADVANCE trial. Glitazones were frequently used in the ACCORD
trial, and rosiglitazone was the glitazone of choice in the intensive treatment group, but the investigators could not identify any association
between the use of rosiglitazone and increased mortality. A detailed discussion about the possible harmful effects of rosiglitazone is beyond the
scope of this chapter, and rosiglitazone has been withdrawn from use in
Europe.

Secondary prevention

ACE inhibitors do not affect anginal symptoms, b...
pril are of prognostic benefit and reduce further...
patients with diabetes and coronary heart disease....
shown similar prognostic benefit and can be used in...
inhibitor intolerant because of a cough. Low-dose a...
shown to have a slight but significant prognostic bene...
diabetes and stable coronary heart disease.

Simvastatin was one of the first treatments demonstrate...
tality in patients with diabetes and coronary heart disease....
have also been described with pravastatin and atorvastatin c...
placebo. More recent trials have compared low-dose statins w...
statins. Atorvastatin 80 mg has been shown to reduce non-fatal...
hospitalizations in patients with diabetes and proven coronary...
after coronary revascularization procedures or acute coronary sy...
(Figure 8.3). As atorvastatin will soon be available in generic form...
tatin 80 mg is preferred for secondary prevention to simvastatin...
which is recommended for primary prevention in people with diabe...

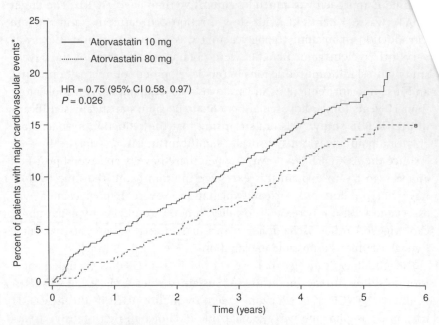

Figure 8.3 Further reductions in cardiovascular events in people treated with high-dose atorvastatin in the treating to new targets (TNT) study. CI, confidence interval; HR, heart rate. Source: Shepherd J et al. Effect of lowering LDL cholesterol substantially below currently recommended levels in patients with coronary heart disease and diabetes. The Treating to New Targets (TNT) study. *Diabetes Care* 2006; 29: 1220–1226. Page 1222 Figure 1.

There have been no parallel concerns expressed about the safety of pioglitazone. Indeed, several meta-analyses of studies with pioglitazone have shown reductions in cardiovascular events. The PROspective pioglitAzone Clinical Trial in macroVascular Events (PROactive) trial was performed in patients with diabetes and existing cardiovascular disease.[12] Nearly half had objective evidence of coronary artery disease and nearly half had previous myocardial infarction. Compared with placebo pioglitazone did not reduce the primary endpoint which included coronary, cerebrovascular and peripheral arterial events and interventions. A clear reduction was seen in a secondary composite of myocardial infarction, stroke and cardiovascular death.

Although pioglitazone can still be considered in the regimen for glycaemic treatment in selected patients with stable coronary disease, so long as they do not have chronic heart failure. The target HbA1c for these patients should be less than 7.0 per cent, avoiding severe hypoglycaemia. The European Medicines Agency (July 2011), while indicating that the benefit–risk balance remains positive for a limited population of people with type 2 diabetes, has noted reports of a small increased incidence of bladder cancer and increased forearm fractures necessitating further long-term monitoring of pioglitazone usage.

Acute coronary syndromes

Clinical presentation

As with angina the presentation of acute myocardial infarction may be very atypical, often with reduced or absent chest pain, which in turn can lead to failure to establish the correct diagnosis, delaying management and initiation of inappropriate treatment, and in particular primary PCI. Patients may present with rather vague chest symptoms, including a feeling of breathlessness rather than pain, and not uncommonly with non-specific symptoms including loss of wellbeing and tiredness. Deterioration in diabetic glycaemic control may have happened for no obvious explicable reason, and diabetic ketoacidosis may be precipitated by an otherwise silent underlying myocardial infarction. These considerations have important implications for the early management of acute myocardial infarction and so a high index of suspicion must be maintained with diabetes presenting acutely with non-specific symptoms or unexplained loss of control.

Investigation and cardiological considerations

All diabetic patients with a suspected acute coronary syndrome should have an emergency ECG performed. Patients with ST-elevation myocardial infarction (STEMI) should be considered for immediate primary

PCI, which is now the treatment of choice for patients with diabetes. Thrombolysis should be reserved for situations where primary PCI cannot be performed within 90 minutes of diagnosis. An erroneous fear is of retinal haemorrhage with thrombolytic therapy in patients with diabetic retinopathy. This is no more likely to occur in a patient with than in one without diabetes, and is exceedingly rare. Patients with non-STEMI and unstable angina should be treated with low-molecular-weight heparin. All patients with diabetes and acute coronary syndromes should receive dual therapy with aspirin plus clopidogrel. The duration of clopidogrel treatment will depend on the type of myocardial infarction and the nature of the cardiological intervention.

Glycaemic management

Hyperglycaemia, with a blood glucose in excess of 11 mmol/l, is commonly found in patients with acute coronary syndromes presenting to CCUs. In the past this was attributed to 'stress' hyperglycaemia. The precise nature of stress hyperglycaemia is still debated but in many instances observed hyperglycaemia can be a genuine indication of preceding, unsuspected diabetes. In others this is a manifestation of impaired glucose tolerance that is unmasked by the counter-regulatory hormonal response to the infarction. Of all patients leaving a CCU, a third will have diabetes, a third impaired glucose tolerance or impaired fasting glucose, and only a third will have totally normal glucose tolerance. Hyperglycaemia is associated with a more adverse outcome in proportion to the level of blood sugar. Hyperglycaemia associates with other adverse metabolic disturbance, including increased release of free fatty acids and increases in counter-regulatory hormones, which in turn may aggravate tendency to arrhythmias and impair myocardial contractility, leading to greater severity of cardiac failure.

CCU management of acute myocardial infarction complicating diabetes requires particular skilled management and locally agreed guidelines for glycaemic control should be made available. All patients should have an initial blood glucose estimation on admission to the CCU. Levels >11 mmol/l should be actively treated. In most cases, low-dose intravenous insulin infusion according to written protocols will prevent metabolic decompensation and worsening hyperglycaemia.

One study from Sweden demonstrated that a high-dose insulin infusion protocol followed by intensive subcutaneous insulin for at least 3 months reduced mortality compared with patients who were given conventional treatment.[13] A larger, multi-national study from the same researchers did not confirm these findings, and the exact role of intensive insulin therapy after myocardial infarction remains uncertain.[14] In practical terms, for patients whose blood glucose rapidly falls back to single figures, oral antidiabetic drugs may be continued, whereas for patients whose glucose remain elevated subcutaneous insulin remains the preferred therapy of choice. During convalescence review of treatment and a possible return to oral antidiabetic drugs can be made.

Secondary prevention

Two large studies including substantial numbers of participants with diabetes have demonstrated improved outcomes with the use of atorvastatin 80 mg compared with conventional dose statins after acute coronary syndromes. As the mortality after a myocardial infarction in diabetes remains high the use of atorvastatin 80 mg should be obligatory. β Blockers are of prognostic benefit but are sometimes omitted because of worries about masking symptoms of hypoglycaemia. Despite this, β blockers should not be regarded as contraindicated for people with diabetes because, in addition to providing useful control of the symptoms of angina, they also improve the long-term survival after myocardial infarction and reduce the risk of sudden death.

Other therapeutic aspects in the management of myocardial infarction should follow general principles and guidelines. The use of ACE inhibitors may have a special beneficial role with diabetes, and it is now routine practice to introduce an ACE inhibitor at an early stage of acute myocardial infarction.

Patients with diabetes who have an acute myocardial infarction may require a longer stay in hospital before discharge home, especially if they have been started on insulin. Most patients will have echocardiography and an exercise test before discharge. Treatment on discharge should include low-dose aspirin therapy, clopidogrel, a β blocker, an ACE inhibitor and high-dose atorvastatin. Eplerenone is also of benefit in patients with diabetes who have a reduced ejection fraction on echocardiography.

Chronic heart failure

Clinical presentation and investigation

In many patients with diabetes the development of heart failure is more insidious, presenting without a history of angina or infarction. Slowly developing exertional breathlessness can sometimes be difficult to distinguish from angina, when central chest tightness may be felt more as difficulty in breathing rather than as pain as such. Exertional breathlessness, particularly on walking up an incline or upstairs and on lying flat in bed at night, should raise suspicion of underlying chronic heart failure. Signs on physical examination may be deceptive initially with no clinical evidence of cardiac enlargement, while added chest sounds may be minimal or even absent.

A chest radiograph may prove unhelpful because the stiffer diabetic myocardium reduces cardiac enlargement, giving rise to an apparently normal cardiac size. An ECG may show the presence of previously unsuspected old myocardial infarction but often only non-specific abnormalities are present. If heart failure is suspected the patient should undergo echocardiography, and measurement of brain natriuretic peptide (BNP) where this is available. Echocardiography can be helpful in revealing a reduced left ventricular ejection fraction, the presence of wall motion abnormalities if there has been a previous myocardial infarction, and an overall global restriction of myocardial function. Echocardiography can also demonstrate diastolic dysfunction, which is more common in people with diabetes, and will also exclude valvular heart disease as a cause of the heart failure.

With the passage of time, heart failure becomes more manifest, often associated with relapsing bouts of acute heart failure, leading to recurrent hospital admission with severe distressing breathlessness. With prompt intravenous diuretic therapy it is remarkable how often quick return to apparent normality can be achieved once fluid overload has been relieved. The episode simply reflects the reducing capacity of the diabetic myocardium to cope with maintaining a normal cardiac output and circulation. Left ventricular dysfunction predominates during the early stages of heart failure in diabetes, but eventually features of right heart failure, particularly oedema of the legs, become increasingly apparent.

Treatment of chronic heart failure

Revascularization of the myocardium generally offers little benefit to the patient with heart failure because the coronary circulation is diffusely narrowed or occluded, and so coronary bypass surgery is unlikely to be helpful in this late situation. Occasionally, however, a single lesion can be identified that can be amenable to PCI or bypass grafting. Cardiac transplantation may be considered for severe end-stage diabetic heart failure, and indeed a number of patients with diabetes have received heart transplants. The presence of diabetes poses special difficulties, and the presence of other long-term complications or infections seriously affects outcome, such that cardiac transplantation is not always regarded as a treatment option available for the patient with diabetes.

Cardiac resynchronization therapy improves symptoms and prognosis in patients with severe, symptomatic heart failure, including patients with diabetes. The role of implantable cardiac defibrillators in patients with diabetes and heart failure is uncertain.

Pharmacological treatment of chronic heart failure in diabetes

Loop diuretics have a first-line role in the management of heart failure, either intravenously for acute episodes or as maintenance therapy for the control of symptoms once the situation is stabilized. Loop diuretics improve symptoms, but do not affect the overall poor prognosis.

The most significant development in the treatment of chronic heart failure with diabetes has been the use of ACE inhibitors and β-blocker therapies. The widespread use of these therapies has altered the natural history of heart failure, leading to longer survival and the reason why patients with chronic heart failure, interrupted by episodes of acute left ventricular failure, survive and struggle on, whereas previously they would not have done so. Most patients with diabetes and heart failure can be treated successfully with ACE inhibitor therapy. The commencement of treatment should follow the usual precautions with the first administration, namely starting with a small test dose under supine conditions. Potassium levels and urea and electrolytes should be monitored, and usually the ACE inhibitor effect is sufficient to offset the potassium-losing effect of loop diuretics. The ACE inhibitor should be discontinued if there is a significant deterioration in renal function. The main side effect of ACE inhibitor therapy is cough, and if this occurs the use of an ARB is an alternative. Indeed, some studies suggest an extra benefit if ACE inhibitors and ARBs are combined.

The potassium-sparing diuretics can be particularly prone to cause hyperkalaemia in diabetes, especially when combined with an ACE inhibitor. Spironolactone has been shown to reduce mortality in patients with moderate-to-severe heart failure. The newer aldosterone antagonist, epelerenone, has been demonstrated to reduce mortality in patients with mild heart failure, and also in patients after acute coronary syndromes with symptomatic heart failure or patients with diabetes and asymptomatic reduction in ejection fraction.

The other drug class that has transformed the management of cardiac failure is the use of β blockers, and several β blockers including carvediolol and metoprolol are of proven benefit in improving survival. A large amount of subgroup analysis shows similar mortality benefits in patients with diabetes, but data from cohort studies indicates that patients with diabetes and heart failure are less likely to be prescribed β blockers than individuals who do not have diabetes. This can be attributed to misguided concerns about hypoglycaemia.

As described earlier, ivabradine is a drug that had a different mechanism of action to β blockers to slow heart rate. In a recent trial ivabradine reduced hospitalization from heart failure and reduced deaths due to heart failure. A third of the participants had diabetes.

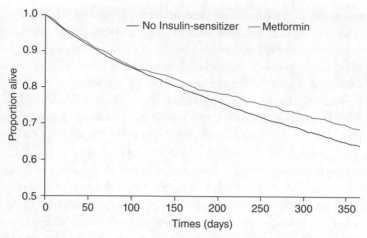

Figure 8.4 Adjusted mortality for patients hospitalized for heart failure and diabetes in patients receiving metformin and patients not treated with an insulin-sensitizing drug[15].

Glycaemic control

There is very little evidence to inform the management of glycaemia in patients with diabetes and chronic heart failure. The use of metformin has in the past been contraindicated because of concerns about the development of lactic acidosis. Results from large cohort studies, however, indicate a survival benefit for patients with heart failure treated with metformin[15] (Figure 8.4). Current practice is to use metformin unless there are renal contraindications, and to discontinue metformin during episodes of acute heart failure.

There is little information on sulfonylureas, and often these are ineffective because of the marked insulin resistance that accompanies heart failure. Pioglitazone is contraindicated because renal retention of salt and water will worsen fluid overload in heart failure. Indeed, this mechanism may unmask heart failure in a patient with asymptomatic diabetes, in which case the pioglitazone should be stopped and the patient investigated for heart failure as described above.

Cohort studies have shown a worse survival in patients treated with insulin. In some individuals insulin can cause fluid retention, worsening symptoms of heart failure. It is likely that insulin use is a marker for patients with worse heart failure and/or worse diabetes, rather than being a direct cause of increased mortality.

There is very little published information on the use of other antidiabetic drugs in heart failure, such as DPP-4 (dipeptidyl peptidase 4) inhibitors or GLP-1 (glucagon-like peptide 1) receptor agonists. Sodium–glucose transport protein SGLT-2 inhibitors cause an osmotic diuresis with a loss of sodium in the urine. This is of some theoretical advantage in patients with diabetes and heart failure and will need careful study.

Other risk factor reduction in heart failure

Patients with chronic heart failure often have a low blood pressure. The treatment of hypertension in patients with heart failure is based on the drugs that improve survival – ACE inhibitors, ARBs, β blockers and diuretics. Calcium channel blockers do not improve survival in this group of patients. Similarly, studies examining possible benefit of statins in heart failure have also been negative.

8.5 Conclusions

The reduction of cardiovascular risk and heart disease in people with diabetes requires a multifactorial approach comprising attention to glycaemic factors, the management of hypertension and dyslipidaemia, the use of antiplatelet drugs in suitable individuals and the correct cardiological management of patients with established heart disease. The exact approach for an individual patient has to take account of their cardiological status (Table 8.1).

Table 8.1 Summary of treatments for patients with diabetes depending on their cardiological status

	No known vascular disease	Stable CHD	ACS and myocardial infarction	Chronic heart failure
Glycaemia	Intensive treatment with metformin, sulfonylurea or pioglitazone	Intensive treatment, consider treatment with pioglitazone	Intensive treatment with multi-dose insulin, pioglitazone	Metformin, insulin
Cholesterol	Simvastatin 40 mg or atorvastatin 10 mg	Consider atorvastatin 80 mg	Atorvastatin 80 mg	Consider Omacor
Blood pressure	ACE inhibitor, calcium channel blocker or diuretic	β Blocker or calcium channel blocker for symptom control	β Blocker for prognosis	β Blocker for prognosis
RAS inhibition (ACE inhibitor or ARB)	For blood pressure or microalbuminuria	ACE inhibitor or ARB for prognosis	ACE inhibitor for prognosis	ACE inhibitor or ARB for prognosis
Antiplatelet drugs	None	Aspirin (or clopidogrel)	Aspirin plus clopidogrel	
Other drugs		Ivabradine	Eplerenone	Ivabradine, eplerenone

ACE, angiotensin-converting enzyme; ACS, acute coronary syndrome; ARB, angiotensin receptor blocker; CHD, coronary heart disease; RAS, renin–angiotensin system.

Case studies

Case study 1 (a typical scenario)

A 46-year-old man with no significant past medical history became aware of a vague central chest discomfort which he attributed to either muscular strain or possibly indigestion, but which later became more evident while walking outdoors in the colder weather. He recognized that he was not particularly fit, but, having reduced his cigarette smoking and restricted his trips to the pub to weekends, he did not feel unduly concerned about his health and indeed had not seen the necessity to visit his doctor for many years.

So, he was both surprised and distressed to suffer, during the early hours one morning, a more prolonged central chest pain. Despite his protestations and declared intention still to go to work that day, his wife insisted that the doctor be called to see him.

Although the doctor had no previous medical records to guide him, the history and the finding of a cold, clammy patient before him led to the strong suspicion of an acute coronary event and emergency hospital admission was advised. An ECG showed widespread ischaemic changes consistent with acute coronary insufficiency duly managed by current protocol. Urgent cardiac angiography was advised revealing diffuse coronary atherosclerotic disease and a major stenosis of the main stem coronary artery, for which a stent was inserted. An uncomplicated recovery followed.

A fuller clinical assessment soon identified significant risk features: body mass index (BMI) 35.5 (weight 96 kg); waist circumference 44 inches; BP 156/94 mmHg; random glucose 15.9 mmol/l; total cholesterol 6.1 mmol/l (HDL ratio 6.5); triglycerides 3.4 mmol/l. On enquiry, a family history of type 2 diabetes and premature coronary disease was elicited.

Comment

Type 2 diabetes is associated with increased risk of coronary heart disease. Current preventive strategies are based on identifying increased risk, and a strong family history is important in determining the need for early intervention therapies and for recognizing the nature of symptoms that might seem atypical for a relatively young age. Type 2 diabetes is frequently silent until it strikes with an acute event such as this. Diagnosis of diabetes and treatment of hyperglycaemia, which can adversely affect outcomes, at the time of acute coronary insufficiency should be an integral part of cardiac care unit (CCU) management guidelines. Audits suggest that blood glucose is still not routinely measured in the CCU. Patients with detected hyperglycaemia should receive appropriate follow-up after discharge from hospital.

Obesity is prevalent in the western population and usually not addressed until illness provides the 'wake-up call'. Ideally the diabetes should have been diagnosed well before the acute event and the triad of hypertension, dyslipidaemia and hyperglycaemia addressed. Weight reduction has to be a health management priority, but is not always easily achieved. In the pecking order of potential dividends, stopping smoking, starting statin therapy and treating blood pressure (in that order) underpin the advised treatment regimen. The relationship of good glycaemic control and reducing coronary risk is less certain, but such evidence that there is would indicate that it is the early years of diabetes control that are important in this respect. Men are known to be reluctant attenders for medical attention, but it should not be forgotten that women with diabetes appear to lose their premenopausal protection from coronary artery disease and may also present atypically.

Case study 2 (a complex scenario)

A 78-year-old woman had been on multiple medications since she was diagnosed with type 2 diabetes some 12 years earlier. She had attended the hospital clinic for many years but found the travel increasingly difficult. On discharge from hospital follow-up, she was taking a variety of prescribed medications including gliclazide, pioglitazone, furosemide, spironolactone, candesartan, nebivolol, ezitimibe and a salbutamol inhaler. Each had been introduced at different times, and although she struggled with the number of tablets to be taken each day, she persevered and did as she was advised.

However, she was feeling less well, which in part she expected as she was getting older. She was becoming more frail and less steady on her feet, much more tired and then noticeably increasingly breathless. At her next clinic appointment, she mentioned her problems to the practice nurse, who arranged for a range of blood tests to be done and the results were as follows: urea 24.8 mmol/l; K^+ 5.7 mmol/l; creatinine 209 μm/l; estimated glomerular filtration rate (eGFR) 20 ml/min per l; random glucose 3.4 mmol/l; glycated haemoglobin HbA1c 65 mmol/l (8.1%); cholesterol 6.11 mmol/l; Hb 7.5 g%, mean corpuscular volume (MCV) 80.4 fL. The nurse informed the doctor, who advised a number of changes to her treatment.

Comment

Symptomatology in elderly people is not always easily determined. Some natural symptoms with advancing years may be inevitable, but the clinician has to keep in mind the possibility of underlying disease or indeed the likely susceptibility to drug side effects. For a 78-year-old woman, an HbA1c 65 mmol/l (8.1%) is not outrageous, but, if the 'one size fits all target strategy' is followed, then more intensified glycaemic control may be pursued with increased risk of hypoglycaemia, as illustrated in this case. Rather than increasing the dose of gliclazide, it needs to be reduced if not stopped. Insulin sensitivity increases with age and also with declining renal function. This woman has significant renal impairment with implications to therapy. Risk of hyperkalaemia is increased. With both spironolactone and the angiotensin receptor blocker or ARB (candesartan) contributing to a potassium-sparing effect, the potassium will need careful monitoring and the use of these particular drugs reviewed. The anaemia appears to be of a secondary nature consequent on chronic renal impairment; it will be contributing to her tiredness and difficulty in breathing. Thiazolidinediones (pioglitazone) can be associated with fluid retention and potentially exacerbate underlying heart failure. This woman is on two diuretic agents for cause unspecified, and it is important to determine her current fluid balance status. At the moment she appears relatively fluid depleted, but it is a fine balance. The clinical message is that multiple drug regimens should be kept under regular review because the situation frequently changes with time, and therapies once appropriate may start to incur more problems than benefit.

References

1. The Diabetes Control and Complications Trial/Epidemiology of Diabetes Interventions and Complications (DCCT/EDIC) Study Research Group. Intensive diabetes treatment and cardiovascular disease in patients with type 1 diabetes. *N Engl J Med* 2005;**353**:2643–2653.

2. UK Prospective Diabetes Study (UKPDS) Group. Intensive blood-glucose control with sulphonylureas or insulin compared with conventional treatment and risk of complications in patients with type 2 diabetes (UKPDS 33). *Lancet* 1998;**352**; 837–853.

3. Holman RR, Paul SK, Bethel MA, Mathews DR, Neil HAW. 10-year follow-up of intensive glucose control in type 2 diabetes. *N Engl J Med* 2008;**359**:1577–1589.

4. UK Prospective Diabetes Study (UKPDS) Group. Effect of intensive blood-glucose control with metformin on complications in overweight patients with type 2 diabetes (UKPDS 34). *Lancet* 1998;**352**:854–865.

5. UK Prospective Diabetes Study Group. Tight blood pressure control and risk of macrovascular and microvascular complications in type 2 diabetes. UKPDS 38. *BMJ* 1998;**317**:703–713.

6. Hansson L, Zanchetti A, Carruthers SG, et al for the HOT Study Group. Effects of intensive blood-pressure lowering and low-dose aspirin in patients with hypertension: principal results of the Hypertension Optimal Treatment (HOT) randomised trial. *Lancet* 1998;**351**:1755–1762.

7. Collins R, Armitage J, Parish S, Sleigh P, Peto R, for the Heart Protection Study Collaborative Group. MRC/BHF Heart Protection Study of cholesterol-lowering with simvastatin in 5963 people with diabetes: a randomised placebo-controlled trial. *Lancet* 2003;**361**:2005–2016.

8. Colhoun HM, Betteridge DJ, Durrington PN, et al., on behalf of the CARDS investigators. Primary prevention of cardiovascular disease with atorvastatin in type 2 diabetes in the Collaborative Atorvastatin Diabetes Study (CARDS): multicentre randomised placebo-controlled trial. *Lancet* 2004;**364**:685–696.

9. The Action to Control Cardiovascular Risk in Diabetes Study Group. Effects of intensive glucose lowering in type 2 diabetes. *N Engl J Med* 2008;**358**:2545–2559.

10. The ADVANCE Collaborative Group. Intensive blood glucose control and vascular outcomes in patients with type 2 diabetes. *N Engl J Med* 2008;**358**:2560–2572.

11. Duckworth W, Abraira C, Moritz T, et al for the VADT Investigators. Glucose control and vascular complications in veterans with type 2 diabetes. *N Engl J Med* 2009; **360**:129–139.
12. Dormandy JA, Charbonnel B, Eckland DJ, et al. Secondary prevention of macrovascular events in patients with type 2 diabetes in the PROactive Study (PROspective pioglitAzone Clinical Trial in macroVascular Events): a randomised controlled trial. *Lancet* 2005;**366**:1279–1289.
13. Malmberg K for the DIGAMI (Diabetes mellitus, Insulin Glucose Infusion in Acute Myocardial Infarction) Study Group. Prospective randomised study of intensive insulin treatment on long term survival after acute myocardial infarction in patients with diabetes mellitus. *BMJ* 1997;**314**:1512–1515.
14. Malmberg K, Ryden L, Wedel H, et al. Intense metabolic control by means of insulin in patients with diabetes mellitus and acute myocardial infarction (DIGAMI 2): effects on mortality and morbidity. *Eur Heart J* 2005;**26**:650–661.
15. Masoudi FA, Inzucchi SE, Wang Y, et al. Thiazolidinediones, metformin, and outcomes in older patients with diabetes and heart failure; an observational study. *Circulation* 2005;**111**:583–590.

CHAPTER 9

Diabetes and the Brain

Iain Cranston

Academic Department of Diabetes and Endocrinology, Portsmouth NHS Trust, Queen Alexandra Hospital, Portsmouth UK

 Key points

- The brain is made up of anatomically and physiologically separate subunits with different functions that are variably impacted by diabetes and the metabolic disturbances that it can cause.

- The brain is almost completely dependent on glucose delivered in the cerebral circulation for its metabolic activity.

- Cerebral function is an amalgamation of intellect, education, development, structural integrity and interconnections modified by minute-to-minute changes in cerebral blood flow and arterial glucose concentrations.

- Cerebral function can be impaired by interruption in nutrient supply by either circulatory change or reduced glucose concentration in the blood (most commonly, stroke and hypoglycaemia).

- Cerebral development may also be impacted by such interruptions occurring either in utero or during childhood.

 Therapeutic key points

- Long-standing hyperglycaemia has a negative impact on cerebral function (as a result of both microvascular cerebral disease, which may be clinically difficult to distinguish from dementia, and macrovascular disease – stroke) and thus its avoidance should be a treatment priority.

- Acute hypoglycaemia caused by diabetes treatment can result in immediate cognitive impairment, the negative impact of which should not be underestimated by health-care practitioners offering treatment advice; chronic episodic hypoglycaemia may be associated with a degree of irreversible cognitive deficit.

- Recurrent bouts of acute hypoglycaemia associated with poorly applied treatment can result in a syndrome of impaired awareness of hypoglycaemia and impaired hypoglycaemic hormonal counter-regulation, which carries an increased risk of severe hypoglycaemia and premature death.

- Hypoglycaemia avoidance should thus also be a priority of treatment planning.
- Scrupulous avoidance of all such episodes of hypoglycaemia can reverse the syndrome of impaired awareness and counter-regulation.
- The impact of mood/emotion and their interactions with hypo-/hyperglycaemia experience on cognitive function has been difficult to establish and continues to be the focus of much clinical research activity.

9.1 Introduction

The progressive evolutionary development of the brain and higher cortical functions is the cornerstone of mammalian and particularly human survival. Unsurprisingly, therefore, mammals have developed a vast array of glucose regulatory systems in order to protect the brain from variation in supply of glucose (its primary energy source) and thus retain cerebral function under a wide variety of different circumstances. An individual's overall cerebral performance is thus a result of a complex amalgamation of cerebral anatomy, development and physiology with significant modifiers of education, mood, age, sex, blood flow and many other factors including metabolic variability (Figure 9.1). Thus cerebral function can vary widely across populations and, over time, within individuals.

Diabetes and its treatment result in far greater variability than normal in the circulating glucose levels experienced by the brain, and therefore one might expect to see disruptions in normal functioning. However, given the wide range of what is considered normal cerebral function across the population, the tools with which to record such disruptions have developed the sensitivity to demonstrate this change only in recent years. Simple measures of cognitive function testing by questionnaire has, in the last two decades, been supplemented with detailed structural imaging (magnetic resonance imaging or MRI) and functional imaging (positron emission tomography [PET] and functional MRI [fMRI]), and ever more detailed electrophysiological study and basic science animal research which have allowed our understanding of such processes and the impact of metabolic change to be measured.

Diabetes-related cerebral dysfunction may therefore theoretically be a result of diabetes-related vascular disease, chronic hyperglycaemia, episodic hyperglycaemia, hypoglycaemia episodes or simple variability in glucose levels.

In this chapter we cover the main sources of cerebral function change associated with diabetes, namely vascular disease (macro- and microvascular) associated with hyperglycaemia and cognitive deficit associated with hypoglycaemia, both acute and chronic.

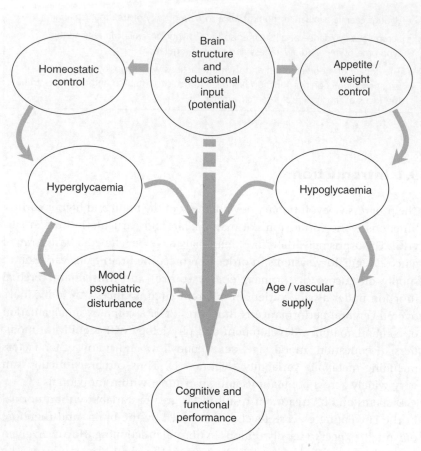

Figure 9.1 Complex interplay of some of the factors determining cerebral performance.

9.2 Cerebrovascular disease and diabetes

The acute effects of atherosclerotic cerebrovascular disease can be profound and, if survived, produce long-term defects in cerebral function, with potential loss of independence, resulting in an immense personal, social and financial burden. Worldwide there are approximately 4.5 million deaths from stroke each year, making it the second most common cause of death. In the western world between 2 and 5 in 100 adults die each year from stroke, and in the UK approximately 5 per cent of the total national health budget is consumed by stroke disease. Epidemiological studies of the prevalence of stroke reliably identify diabetes (predominantly type 2) as a risk factor for ischaemic stroke, alongside others such as smoking and hypertension; although the strength of its association is variable across studies, possibly dependent on the degree of cofactor analysis undertaken, most suggest a risk between two and three times that for the non-diabetic population. Although cofactor analysis attempts to separate risk attributable to single aspects of pathogenesis, this may actually underestimate the role of diabetes in stroke disease, as so many of the recognized risk factors coexist in the population with type 2 diabetes. Pathological examination of brain tissue from stroke victims with diabetes reveals a much higher rate of small vessel disease of the penetrating vessels supplying the thalamic and subthalamic areas, with increased rates of 'lacunar' infarction as a result. This penetrating vessel disease appears to be a specific pathological entity resulting from hypertrophy of the medial smooth muscle, with subsequent replacement by protein and vessel occlusion, known as hyaline arteriosclerosis. The large-vessel disease in patients with diabetes does not seem to differ from the large-vessel disease seen in patients who do not have diabetes. The exact frequency with which such disease affects the population as a whole is at present less clear than previously. Increased rates of high-definition cerebral imaging (with MRI particularly) are highlighting the existence of a significant level of such vascular disease, without the development of focal neurological signs that may give rise to a clinically identifiable ischaemic syndrome.

The data for stroke risk in type 1 diabetes are less clear, but those with long-standing disease would appear to have a total mortality risk of approximately 10 per cent as a result of stroke disease. Although the studies looking at haemorrhagic stroke are few, no such association has been described for diabetes as a risk factor for either intracranial or subarachnoid haemorrhage.

In addition to the greater incidence of ischaemic cerebrovascular disease seen in patients with diabetes, the outcome after such a cerebrovascular event is worse in patients with diabetes, with higher mortality, less complete and slower recovery, and higher final dependence scores for equivalent-sized infarcts occurring in the non-diabetic population. The absolute glucose level during and after an ischaemic event is an important determinant of this risk, possibly by increasing lactate-associated acidity in ischaemia-affected areas, secondary to increased anaerobic metabolic activity because of the hyperglycaemia. Animal models where focal ischaemia is induced artificially confirm this and show that hyperglycaemia present at the time of the insult increases the size of the resulting infarcted area. Indeed the presenting glucose level at the time of cerebral infarction has been shown to be an independent risk factor for the outcome of the event in a recent meta-analysis, although such associative studies cannot easily determine if the glucose is the cause of the higher morbidity, or if the more severe the insult the higher the 'stress response' glucose level. It seems likely that both these possibilities are likely to contribute a part of the total association seen, linking presenting glucose values to outcome after stroke. Although glucose levels may be the most obvious abnormality in patients with diabetes, there are other potentially important factors that also contribute to the poor outcome, such as platelet dysfunction, hyperviscosity and coagulation cascade deficits, resulting in hypercoagulability, endothelial dysfunction and decreased fibrinolytic activity. In the management of vascular risk in patients with diabetes all these factors should be taken into account and addressed if overall risk is to be reduced and outcome improved.

9.3 Primary prevention of stroke in diabetes

In order to justify an aggressive interventional approach to the primary prevention of strokes in the diabetic population (as the epidemiology would seem to indicate the need), in an ideal world one would be able to quote data from large primary prevention studies. However, one cannot at the present time quote direct diabetes-related evidence in support, because many aspects of such a multifaceted approach have proved to be of benefit only in studies excluding individuals with diabetes. It is, however, a reasonable extension of currently available data to utilize those interventions shown to be of benefit in atherosclerotic disease elsewhere (e.g. aspirin in primary prevention of ischaemic heart disease) in this population with such a high overall risk.

Recent guidelines looking into the management of vascular risk in populations with diabetes have all been in agreement that the risk level for non-diabetic patients receiving secondary preventive measures is equivalent to the primary risk level of patients with diabetes and any other vascular risk marker, even though these individuals may not have direct evidence of active vascular disease. Although this primary prevention risk case has been made most persuasively for coronary heart disease, it is also almost certainly true for cerebrovascular disease. The risk reduction strategies to prevent cerebrovascular disease will be familiar from other parts of this text; however, they can be summarized in pathway management diagrams similar to Figure 9.2.

One aspect of such multiple risk reduction strategies is particularly worthy of specific mention, namely the process of anticoagulation in individuals with non-valvular atrial fibrillation (nAF). Within the UKPDS (United Kingdom Prospective Diabetes Study) cohort, individuals with such nAF were at an eight times greater risk of developing ischaemic stroke. In the Stroke Prevention in AF trial it was shown that, if nAF is present in patients with other vascular risks (age >75, hypertension, congestive cardiac failure/left ventricular [CCF/LV] dysfunction on echocar-

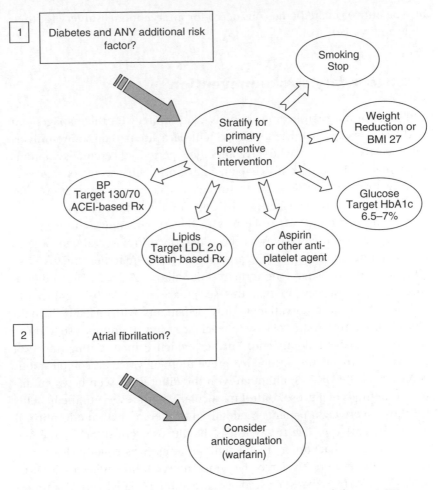

Figure 9.2 The primary prevention of cerebrovascular disease in diabetes. ACEI, angiotensin-converting enzyme inhibitor; BMI, body mass index; BP, blood pressure; HbA1c, glycated haemoglobin; Rx, treatment.

diography, previous thromboembolic disease), then warfarin should be commenced, targeting the international normalized ratio (INR) to 2.0–3.0, because it results in a 75 per cent reduction of the stroke risk. If no other risk factors exist or if the risks of anticoagulation are considered too high, then aspirin/other anti-platelet agents may be a reasonable alternative risk reduction strategy, although the evidence that they actually prevent ischaemic stroke is relatively lacking. There is, however, particularly after the recent publications relating to lack of primary prevention cardio-vascular impact in the multicentre POPADAD trial, continuing debate as to the most appropriate advice to offer with respect to aspirin use in patients with diabetes. Patients with AF and valvular disease should also be anticoagulated (and considered for interventional surgery for their abnormal valve).

9.4 Secondary stroke prevention

Although primary stroke prevention is a key strategy for the management of those at recognized risk, its component parts are perhaps more universally practised in those who have already experienced cerebral symptoms (previous stroke, transient ischaemic attack or amaurosis fugax), i.e. secondary stroke prevention. In this category specifically, there is now far more evidence from diabetes subgroups of large intervention studies. Preventing recurrence of stroke in a diabetic population is of particular importance, because diabetes has been described in observational studies as a major determinant of both early (<30 days) re-infarction (relative risk [RR] = 1.85) and later long-term re-infarction (RR = 1.7); in addition, there is some suggestion that this secondary risk can be significantly reduced, from an observational study of patients with diabetes in tight glycaemic control post-stroke, with levels seen in this group close to those of the non-diabetic population. Further evidence for the importance of glucose control in the secondary prevention of vascular complications comes from the UKPDS, although with the differences seen between different methods of glucose control (particularly with respect to the benefits for those overweight patients randomized to therapy with metformin). It is not currently possible to say if it is the glucose control or the method of achieving it that confers the benefit, although it is equally clear, from some of the more recent large glycaemia intervention studies (ACCORD/ADVANCE/VADT), that such strategies are also associated with risk unless carefully implemented, so it is encouraging that there are recent acute intervention studies that seem to describe glycaemic interventions with insulin which result in minimal hypoglycaemic risk.

Lipid therapies, particularly those lowering low-density lipoprotein (LDL)-cholesterol, have had a high profile in secondary macrovascular disease prevention since 1994, and the publication of the '4S' study using simvastatin, the diabetic cohort of this study having over 200 patients, confirmed and extended the benefits seen in the non-diabetic population. The CARE study with 588 patients with diabetes and LIPID (with 782), both using pravastatin, reported approximately 25 per cent reductions in the total atherosclerotic disease with treatment, and following on from these data there have been other numerous studies confirming the benefits. A meta-analysis and review highlighted this benefit in secondary prevention, reporting a 22 per cent risk reduction for any stroke in patients with known vascular disease treated with statins, 28 per cent for thromboembolic stroke, 23 per cent for non-fatal stroke and 2 per cent for fatal stroke, and a reduction of 6 per cent in those without known vascular disease. The recently published stroke data from the Heart Protection Study (HPS) study further confirmed this trend. Blood pressure reduction (particularly with thiazide diuretics and angiotensin-converting enzyme [ACE] inhibitors) has been shown to play a major role in the secondary prevention of stroke disease, with relative risk figures of between 0.5 and 0.7 reported across most of the larger studies where subpopulations with diabetes were involved. The UKPDS, using either captopril or atenolol as the primary therapeutic agent, showed a relative risk of 0.56 in patients with diabetes allocated to tighter hypertension control, whereas the subpopulation of HOPE, using ramipril, reported a relative risk of 0.67. Notably, the PROGRESS study, using a combination of perindopril and indapamide in secondary stroke patients with no particular blood pressure entry criteria, showed a risk reduction of 28 per cent in stroke over a 4-year period (number needed to treat for 5 years to save a life of 11), with a 16 per cent reduction in dependency/disability and a 13 per cent reduction in dementia after stroke.

Thus there is good evidence for the use of all the traditional macrovascular disease-modifying agents in diabetes for the secondary prevention of stroke and the burden of disease associated with it. In addition, there are specific protective strategies that should be considered such as antiplatelet agents. The most common of these strategies implemented in clinical practice outside a population with diabetes is of course aspirin, which in the antiplatelet trialists' meta-analysis was shown to carry a risk reduction rate of approximately 25 per cent, with equal effect in patients with and without diabetes (thus an absolute benefit that is higher in patients with diabetes who are at greater baseline risk), and re-confirmed in the 2009 systematic meta-analysis published in *Diabetes Care*. Most authors therefore agree that, for secondary prevention, anti-platelet agents in general and aspirin in particular has benefit although debate persists as to the most effective dose to recommend, with evidence for anything between 50 and 325 mg daily, and the complications data suggesting that mid- to lower-range doses may confer less risk of gastrointestinal bleeding.

There has been concern that 'aspirin resistance' may exist in patients with diabetes, although clinical studies have yet to determine any outcome benefit of higher aspirin doses, resulting in the fact that clinical practice doses remain for the most part in the 75–150 mg/day range. There are of course other antiplatelet agents with the most well publicized at present being clopidogrel for which evidence has been gathered from the CAPRIE study. The data from this study have been widely presented as showing a 0.5 per cent additional risk reduction for patients on clopidogrel as opposed to aspirin, with complications and side effects very similar to those with aspirin; however, interestingly the data from this study for true secondary stroke prevention ($n = 6400$) do not show any superiority of effect. It may, however, be prudent to use this therapy in particularly at-risk groups, e.g. where there has been a recurrent event despite aspirin in an individual who is not suitable for anticoagulation. Ticlodipine (another member of the same class) has also undergone trials with some success in stroke disease, although its side-effect profile has significantly limited its usefulness in routine clinical practice. A more traditional antiplatelet agent that has been in clinical use for many years is dipyridamole, which used in monotherapy is probably less effective than aspirin (although remains a useful alternative in those who are unable to take aspirin, with a lower gastrointestinal side-effect rate than clopidogrel, but with potential side effects of headache); however, its recent evidence base would suggest that, when used in combination with low-dose aspirin, it has a significant additive effect, almost doubling the risk reduction seen with aspirin 50 mg alone. Following on from the success of preventive strategies for embolic disease in patients with AF, formal anticoagulation with warfarin has been suggested as a potential therapy; however, for those patients in sinus rhythm, the evidence for use of warfarin is poor. The SPIRIT study of 1997 showed that full anticoagulation of patients with previous strokes resulted in dramatically increased bleeding rates, making its use inadvisable, although less aggressive anticoagulation regimens are currently being studied.

Surgical preventive therapies in stroke disease have become increasingly prevalent after the publication of papers in 1998 demonstrating the benefits of carotid endarterectomy in symptomatic patients with significant stenosis of the common or internal carotid artery. The presently accepted advice is that patients with >50 per cent stenosis and symptoms should be considered for treatment; however, despite the tenfold increased incidence of >50 per cent stenosis seen in patients with compared with patients without diabetes, the diabetes-related data with respect to this intervention were less clear in showing benefit, particularly in the group with 50–70 per cent stenosis, where there was no statistical outcome benefit seen with treatment; there was a higher complications rate, however, especially of myocardial infarction. Thus, although lesions of >70 per cent stenosis are generally referred for endarterectomy, the lower-grade stenoses may, as the techniques are perfected, be more appropriately treated with carotid angioplasty with stenting (in parallel to the data about coronary vascular disease in diabetes, where stenting has produced a much better result for patients with diabetes).

9.5 Management of acute stroke in patients with diabetes

The acute management of stroke concentrates on two main goals: (1) the overall supportive care and wellbeing of the patient and (2) minimizing the ischaemic area of brain tissue affected by the stroke in order to maximize potential recovery.

The initial supportive care of individuals with diabetes and stroke does not differ from that of patients without diabetes who experience a stroke, and consists of basic observations and investigations to determine cause and complications. Monitoring of oxygen saturation, blood pressure, pulse, temperature and respiration is vitally important, along with the provision of supplemental oxygen therapy and airway maintenance (if necessary by mechanical means). Initially oral intake should be prevented until the safety of the swallow has been assessed and assured to be stable; intravenous fluid should be commenced in order to maintain the hydration status. Diagnostic testing should include a full biochemical panel with glucose level, a full blood count, an electrocardiograph to exclude acute myocardial ischaemia (with consideration given to continuous cardiac monitoring) and an unenhanced CT scan as soon as possible. This CT scan becomes compulsory almost immediately if thrombolytic therapy is to be considered. Unless the blood pressure is severely raised, most guidelines do not recommend initial therapy for hypertension in the immediate post-stroke period, because cerebral autoregulation is usually impaired in this event and thus the ischaemic penumbra is often dependent on systemic pressure for continued circulation. The majority of elevated blood pressure after a stroke will resolve without the need for specific intervention after the first 24–48 h.

Much basic scientific work has suggested that hyperglycaemia documented in the early stages of stroke is associated with worse outcome (parallel to the observed state in cardiac disease). Hyperglycaemia is in fact a very commonly described event in acute stroke (25–50% of all patients), and animal work has suggested that insulin infusions may be able to minimize the ischaemic damage from surgically induced lesions. The management of hyperglycaemia after a stroke is then a common dilemma and one around which there is surprisingly little evidence or guidance. In contrast to myocardial infarction and cardiac surgery, where there has been extensive (and continued) research interest resulting in guidelines recommending glucose–insulin–potassium (GIK) infusions for acute therapy, the acute management of hyperglycaemia in stroke has not until quite recently received the same attention. although the practicality of GIK therapy for this group of patients has been investigated and found to be feasible, there has been no conclusive study in stroke powered to determine if such therapy is beneficial to outcome, in patients either with diabetes or previously without diabetes plus acute hyperglycaemia associated with their stroke. Indeed even the Glucose Insulin in Stroke Trial (GIST) data did not answer the feasibility question fully, because the glucose levels achieved with the infusion were not significantly different from those without the infusion. For now, hyperglycaemic management after stroke in clinical practice is often based on pragmatic rather than scientific principles. Known individuals with pre-existing diabetes are far more likely to receive intravenous insulin and glucose therapy than those presenting with acute hyperglycaemia; however, the duration and aggression of such therapies vary widely, and many patients receive one-off boluses of subcutaneous insulin, which is both untested and potentially more hazardous than more closely monitored intravenous therapy.

Another strategy that reflects parallel thinking to that for myocardial ischaemia is the area of thrombolysis in acute stroke. There is now significant clinical research on the practice which has demonstrated the benefits of early (<3 h from onset of symptoms) therapy with recombinant tissue-type plasminogen activator (rt-PA) for effective recovery at 3 months after a ischaemic stroke, with equivalent mortality data from the two groups (an early excess of haemorrhage-associated deaths in the treated group being matched by a later excess of mortality in the untreated group) such that national and international guidance for early stroke management now includes recommendations for thrombolytic therapy as early as possible. Subanalysis of studies of patients with diabetes showed a greater mortality in them, but with an equally important benefit from thrombolytic therapy. The main problem of utilizing such therapies comes from the difficulty of arranging cerebral imaging and assessment quickly enough to allow safe administration of thrombolytic within the 3- to 4-h therapeutic window.

9.6 Diabetes and cognitive function

The term 'cognitive function' includes a diverse range of mental activities such as orientation, attention/concentration, perception (processing of external stimuli), memory (of all types), language, construction, reasoning, executive function (decision-making) and control of motor skills. This range includes both basic functions common to all species and most of the skills that differentiate humans from other mammals. The changes associated with diabetes in respect of cognitive functioning are relatively modest when put into this enormously wide scope; however, they can be exceptionally important in the day-to-day functioning of individuals and their mood/character.

The 1990s were dubbed 'the decade of the brain' and, fittingly, it was during this decade that the associations of cognitive dysfunction and diabetes were first described in detail. Postmortem studies had suggested that the recurrent metabolic abnormalities associated with diabetes are also associated with degenerative structural change, but clinical studies had not focused sufficiently on associating functional disturbances with this structural change. Basic clinical observation, however, had clearly described that, although acute hypoglycaemia is associated with pronounced cognitive impairment, acute hyperglycaemia (in the absence of acidosis or ketosis) is not. The chronic effects of hypo- or hyperglycaemia have, however, been far more difficult to determine, because experimental animal data designed to look at the problem are limited by the fact that there are clear species differences in cognitive dysfunctional processes. Thus the chronic effects of diabetes became clear only with structured and large-scale observational longitudinal studies of humans.

Acute cognitive changes

Hypoglycaemia – cognitive function and counter-regulation
The first reported cognitive changes associated with diabetes were observed during acute hypoglycaemia.[30] This observed ability to affect higher cognitive functioning was of course utilized extensively by psychiatrists in the 1950s in the form of 'insulin-shock therapy' for severe psychosis and depression. More systematic study revealed that the major effects of hypoglycaemia affected primarily the following aspects of cognition at blood sugar levels <3 mmol/l: concentration, some aspects of memory, mental processing speed and fine motor coordination, coarse motor functions being left intact. Closer study of the effects of hypoglycaemia on cognition was made possible by the use of the hyperinsulinaemic glucose clamp technique, which was extensively utilized from the 1980s in experimental study design. These studies were able to determine both the hierarchy of symptom generation from experimental hypoglycaemia and the thresholds for induction of specific cognitive dysfunction. They describe in summary:
- Slowed choice-reaction times (reaction times responding to a visual stimulus with a specific action)
- Slowed mental arithmetic (e.g. serial sevens)
- Impaired verbal fluency (word finding)
- Reduced fine manual dexterity (grooved pegboard)
- Reduced hand–eye coordination
- Reduced mental flexibility (letter/number trail following tests)
- Reduced story recall (long-term memory).

Occurring at blood glucose levels between 3.1 and 3.3 mmol/l on average, but with considerable inter-individual variation, functions such as finger tapping and other simple motor functions were barely affected. Some more subtle cognitive functions could take 60–90 min to recover after hypoglycaemia.

With such widespread cognitive effect of hypoglycaemia, it is thus unsurprising that complex day-to-day cognitive tasks (such as driving a car) are significantly impaired during acute hypoglycaemia,[33] with poor steering, road positioning, swerving and spinning when tested on driving simulators during hypoglycaemia.

One important aspect of cerebral function, which is not readily observed as an issue in fit individuals who do not have diabetes, but which is particularly evident when related to patients with insulin-controlled diabetes, is the control of the counter-regulatory response to the hypoglycaemia itself. As blood glucose levels fall there are a number of physiological, predominantly hormonal mechanisms invoked, with the aim of supporting circulating glucose levels and thus maintaining cerebral (and to a lesser degree other organ) function (Figure 9.3).

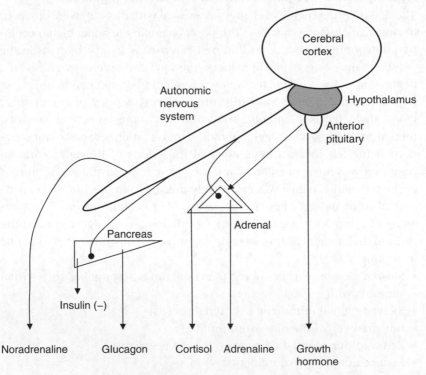

Figure 9.3 Schematic of the relationship of the hypothalamus, the pituitary and the autonomic nervous system as mediators of the counter-regulatory response.

In individuals who do not have diabetes, although this counter-regulatory response may be partially activated (primarily reduced insulin production with an accompanying glucagon surge) periodically in response to either starvation or prolonged physical activity, it is rarely if ever exposed to the state in which individuals with diabetes may frequently find themselves, where low blood glucose levels are seen at the same time as high circulating insulin levels. Such regular triggering of the counter-regulatory response tests the physiological mechanisms to the limit, in a circumstance where the primary pancreatic counter-regulatory responses are unresponsive (the insulin levels are by definition not under counter-regulatory control, and glucagon production in response to hypoglycaemia is lost because of a failure of α-/β-cell communication within the islets). Thus the autonomically generated (cerebrally controlled), hormonal, counter-regulatory responses are the primary form of defence from severe hypoglycaemia in individuals with diabetes, and this non-physiological state can result in counter-regulatory failure and hypoglycaemia unawareness.

Encapsulating this issue is the fact that the brain is both (the most important) target organ for the adverse effects of hypoglycaemia and the organ that is most important in controlling metabolic responses to protect against it. It is at risk of recurrent hypoglycaemia secondary to relative excesses, in the imperfect subcutaneous route of insulin delivered in greater quantities than actually required, alternating with periods of hyperglycaemia. It has been repeatedly observed in studies using the insulin–glucose clamp technique that cerebral adaptation to repeated episodes of hypoglycaemia exists, resulting in altered (reduced) counter-regulatory hormone responses to and symptoms of hypoglycaemia. These effects result in a reduced awareness of the onset of hypoglycaemia in those frequently exposed to it. This phenomenon has been observed in people without diabetes (those with insulinoma) and can thus be said to represent a physiological (mal)adaptation to a non-physiological state.

Although the premise that adaptation to recurrent hypoglycaemia results in delayed and diminished counter-regulatory hormone responses and symptoms of acute hypoglycaemia is widely accepted, the question of higher cortical adaptation to recurrent hypoglycaemia, such that global cognitive function may be better preserved during hypoglycaemia in those patients with recurrent episodes, remains controversial. Some investigators have indeed found that individuals in whom counter-regulatory responses are blunted to hypoglycaemia also show preservation of cognitive function to lower glucose thresholds than patients not so adapted, whereas others show deterioration of cognitive function in all individuals at consistent glucose thresholds. This apparent contradiction is perhaps partly explained by the choices of cognitive function test that best represent clinically significant cerebral dysfunction during hypoglycaemia. No consensus view is held on which of the cognitive function tests used is the most significant. Some investigators prefer to use a single well-validated quick test throughout all studies (e.g. auditory or brain-stem-evoked potentials or four-choice reaction time), whereas others use batteries of tests, which are then analysed either singly or as a grouped 'z score'. Another confounding variable may be the duration of the hypogly-caemic stimulus. It may take a finite period of time, possibly up to 40 min, for performance to be detectably affected by the hypoglycaemia,[38] so that longer tests may be confounded. Nevertheless, the probability that different tests reflect different areas of brain with different sensitivities to hypoglycaemia is likely to underlie many of the observed discrepancies.

Investigations into the levels of glucose associated with the onset of cognitive dysfunction in individuals with delayed onset of symptomatic counter-regulatory responses to hypoglycaemia have thus been controversial. In normal individuals studied after 56 h of enforced moderate hypogly-caemia (2.9 mmol/l), Boyle et al. demonstrated preservation of performance in Stroop tests and finger tapping to lower glucose levels, associated with better preservation of cerebral glucose uptake and delayed counter-regulation. These data suggest a *global* adaptation of the human brain to preceding hypoglycaemia, involving both glucose-sensing regions and the cerebral cortex. One possible mechanism is a hypoglycaemia-induced up-regulation of endothelial glucose transporters.

However, the clinical picture of defective symptomatic counter-regulatory responses, hypoglycaemia unawareness and increased risk of severe hypoglycaemia (summarized figuratively in Figure 9.4) does not fit with such global adaptive change and clinically suggests the experimen-

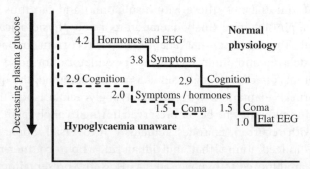

Figure 9.4 Schematic representation of glycaemic thresholds for change associated with hypoglycaemia. The solid line represents thresholds for change in normal physiology, whereas the dashed line represents individuals exposed to frequent hypoglycaemia with regional adaptation, resulting in hypoglycaemia unawareness, because cognitive function is impaired before any symptom generation.

tally supported notion that there is no preservation of cognitive function during hypoglycaemia in patients with hypoglycaemia-prone diabetes, despite substantial delay in the onset of counter-regulatory responses. Several investigators have described dissociation between the onset of counter-regulatory responses and cognitive dysfunction during acute hypoglycaemia in patients with diabetes, suggesting that the degree of adaptation of cerebral response to hypoglycaemia may vary regionally throughout the brain, the higher neocortex functions being those most susceptible to hypoglycaemic impairment. Thus, although the deleterious effects of hypoglycaemia on higher cortical cerebral function remain relatively unchanged whatever the previous experience of hypoglycaemia, the effectiveness of the counter-regulatory response may vary widely depending on previous experience of hypoglycaemia. This is described in the model proposed in 1992 by Philip Cryer, which he termed 'hypoglycaemia-associated autonomic failure', bringing together in a single model all the aspects associated with cerebral function, described in Figure 9.1.

The exact cortical mechanisms underlying the triggering of counter-regulation remain under intense investigational scrutiny, with recent studies concentrating on regional rates of change in cerebral glucose metabolism (particularly in the ventromedial nucleus of the hypothalamus) as a likely, although not yet definitively proven, source. However, despite this uncertainty in the basic physiology, there are a number of clearly observed clinical phenomena, which are able to inform the management of patients with hypoglycaemia unawareness and its concomitant increased risk of severe hypoglycaemia. Developing observations made after the successful removal of insulinomas and the effects seen on the normalization of previously abnormal counter-regulation, three separate groups of researchers observed that the strict avoidance of hypoglycaemia in day-to-day life will result in improvement towards normal of the counter-regulatory hormonal response when it has previously been blunted, regained awareness of warning symptoms for hypoglycaemia and reduced risk of severe hypoglycaemia. This is encouraging research data, particularly as the researchers in closely supervised day-to-day activity were able to achieve avoidance of hypoglycaemia without significant deterioration of overall control (and indeed in some individuals with particularly fluctuant control even an improvement in HbA1c). However, the amount of clinical input required in these studies (and indeed in those DCCT centres where improved glycaemic control was achieved without increasing the risk of incident hypoglycaemia) is perhaps at a higher level than is practical in the normal day-to-day clinical care for the vast majority of our patients; thus it is important to look for the key clinical interventions that seem to have the most impact on hypoglycaemia avoidance:

- *Insulin regimens*: over the last decade much attention has been paid to the development of analogue insulins that might be able to mimic more closely the 'physiological' insulin secretion curve and thus reduce the periods when individuals are exposed in inappropriate hyper- or hypoinsulinaemia, with resultant glucose fluctuations. Within the confines of closely regulated studies, some significant success has been achieved both with short-acting (prandial) insulin analogues (e.g. Humalog and Novorapid), which (with judicious and appropriate use) reduce the pre-meal exposure to hyperinsulinaemia, and long-acting (basal) analogues (e.g. insulin glargine and detemir), which can reduce the overnight exposure to hyperinsulinaemia at a time when physiologically the insulin secretion levels are very low. The most successful insulin regimen in studies for the avoidance of hypoglycaemia in well-motivated patients is, however, clearly the use of continuous subcutaneous insulin infusions (CSIIs) which, because of the ability to adjust basal infusion rates across the day and to infuse very small boluses frequently if so required, along with the fact that the subcutaneous 'insulin reservoir' at any given time is very small (thus resulting in more predictable absorption), provides for very precise insulin adjustment in those who monitor their glucose levels sufficiently closely to allow it. However, despite these advances, the type of insulin or method of injection will not allow hypoglycaemia avoidance reliably if used in isolation of other (often more important) aspects of daily life, or in those people whose attention to glucose fluctuations is less close than individuals used in studies.

- *Physical activity* is clearly an important part of daily routine to which attention must be addressed if hypoglycaemia is to be avoided. The type, intensity, duration and timing of exercise along with the conditions in which it is conducted (ambient temperature, underlying fitness of the individual, etc.) will all impact on the glycaemic excursion seen during and after a bout of activity. Thus, if hypoglycaemia is a problem, then activity and insulin/carbohydrate responses to it need to be carefully planned in advance with knowledge of the individual and his or her insulin sensitivity as an integral part of such planning. This is an often ignored aspect of day-to-day glucose control, especially for unplanned bouts of activity (e.g. sex), on which attention deserves to be focused more in the future.

- *Diet,* similar to activity, is obviously an important determinant of glucose excursions, particularly the carbohydrate component of diet. It is increasingly being recognized that the day-to-day variations in both the size and content of a normal healthy diet require both knowledge of glycaemic effect and planning in order to minimize glucose excursion, especially if hypoglycaemia is a problem. 'Carbohydrate counting' (usually in 10-g portions) with knowledge of the carbohydrate:insulin ratio (traditionally expressed as units of insulin/10-g carbohydrate portion) is a basic necessity if such glucose excursions are to be minimized, but in addition glycaemic index, glycaemic load and meal composition will all have significant impacts and require attention. In addition the timing of carbohydrate intake is an important consideration in the overall glucose control over 24h, particularly in the form of between-meal snacks for those individuals who, based on previous experience, have a reproducible time when the risk of hypoglycaemia is greatest.

- *'Awareness training' and continuous monitoring*: symptomatic awareness of hypoglycaemia relies on both the generation of symptoms and the correct recognition of those symptoms as a feature of impending hypoglycaemia. Over time the symptoms generated may change so that individuals fail to recognize them even when they are present. There has been some success using biofeedback techniques to improve recognition of symptoms earlier in the fall of glucose, especially when the symptoms may be idiosyncratic or atypical and otherwise missed. The appropriate use of finger-stick monitoring is clearly important for hypoglycaemia avoidance during the day, but, in addition to the goal-oriented use of such monitoring, the more detailed 'minimally invasive' continuous monitoring techniques based on continuous subcutaneous sampling techniques have over the course of the last decade significantly improved the recognition of hypoglycaemia risk periods, either when used alone or particularly in conjunction with CSIIs in specially adapted pumps that are able to suspend insulin delivery for up to 30 min when the CGM sensor detects impending hypoglycaemia (Medtronic MiniMed). Patient-oriented CGM sensors for which the glucose values are continuously displayed on a handset to the individual (and equipped with alarms as necessary) can be especially useful when the periods of hypoglycaemic risk occur at night and the individual would otherwise be unaware of them. Indeed one of the major causes of hypoglycaemia unawareness may be after recurrent unidentified nocturnal hypoglycaemic exposure with no clearly identifiable pattern of recurrent daytime hypoglycaemic experience.

- *Education programmes*: based on the pioneering work of Michael Berger and the Düsseldorf group, there has been increasing recognition worldwide over the last decade of the importance of the patient as the expert in self-management, particularly where issues of day-to-day control are involved. In addition, the traditional educational process of group learning has finally been successfully incorporated into the routine clinical practice of diabetes education with significant impact for the psychological and physical health of individuals with diabetes. Glycaemia management and hypoglycaemia avoidance form the mainstay of many of these programmes, such as the recently studied DAFNE (Dose Adjustment For Normal Eating) programme in the UK.

- *Drugs*: although a pharmaceutical product to allow continued timely recognition of hypoglycaemia has not been identified, many substances have been shown to have modulatory effects on glycaemia awareness, and the search for appropriate pharmacological intervention continues to gather pace, encouraged by experimental data using such 'everyday' compounds as caffeine. In studies of hypoglycaemia, it has been found that prior dosing with caffeine enhances hypoglycaemic awareness – albeit to a relatively mild degree.

- *Islet cell transplantation*: for those individuals with intractable hypoglycaemia problems and ongoing risk not ameliorated by the use of any or all of the above strategies, islet cell transplantation with its apparent re-connecting of the counter-regulatory response in its fullest sense (reduction of insulin secretion as blood glucose levels fall) has been shown to be a most effective strategy. The limitations of this technique centre mainly around its very limited availability (until such a time as islet cell culture is an effective strategy), its often only temporary effect (about 50% 3-year success) and the risks associated with immunosuppression required for the procedure.

Chronic cognitive changes and diabetes

In addition to the excess risk of vascular disease occurring in people with diabetes (discussed previously), the epidemiology of cognitive impairment has reliably shown a link between type 2 diabetes and the risk of accelerated cognitive decline. Although the nature of this association was initially unclear, more recent data suggest that there is a significant relationship between cognitive decline and levels of glucose control in diabetes, which may be ameliorated by improved glucose control in line with other diabetes-related complications. Further, there have been independent studies looking at the frequency of Alzheimer's disease in the population which also describe a clear relationship between it and diabetes, so there are a number of different issues in the development of chronic cognitive change in individuals with diabetes, addressed below.

Hypoglycaemia-related chronic cognitive dysfunction

After a hypoglycaemic coma, recovery of neurological function is usually rapid with no discernable cognitive effect after 36 h. However, a single episode of severe hypoglycaemia, if coma is protracted, can (rarely) result in permanent neurological dysfunction and structural abnormality, with lesions described predominantly in the frontal areas and deep grey matter. Such lesions are rarely encountered in day-to-day practice. The more common clinical picture of recurrent variable hypoglycaemia over many years has a more uncertain impact on cognitive function. Most investigators fail to determine any specific detriment of such experience when studying its effect in adults, but occasional reports of predisposition to later life cognitive decline and cortical atrophy have been documented. Perhaps the most complete documentation of such risk was made in 2003 in a group of 74 young adults with type 1 diabetes (all >10 years' duration), in whom a cognitive battery of tests was undertaken, along with an MRI, and analysed according to prior hypoglycaemic experience (total severe hypoglycaemic episodes) and evidence of retinopathy as a marker for hyperglycaemia. In this study hypoglycaemic experience had no detectable deleterious long-term effect on either cognitive function or brain structure, although the group with retinopathy had significant impairments of aspects of cognitive function and small focal white matter lesions in the basal ganglia. Data for hypoglycaemic effects in children are equally reassuring, except for those who develop diabetes very early in life (<5 years old), in whom severe hypoglycaemia at such a young age appears to have a significant (if relatively small) effect on later measures of intelligence.

Ischaemia-related cognitive decline

As described earlier in this chapter, type 2 diabetes is associated with an increased risk of stroke, and although large infarct events clearly have significant impact on an individual's cognition, population studies have additionally described increased cortical atrophy occurring in patients with diabetes and no focal lesions,[48] which are postulated to be either a micro-angiopathic effect of diabetes or multiple small macrovascular disease-mediated infarcts, possibly related to hypertension or the effects of other metabolic derangement occurring in patients with poorly controlled diabetes such as uraemia with 'middle molecule'-mediated cognitive decline. Conclusive data are, however, not yet available because, although studies of cognitive decline with age in diabetes have been undertaken, and neuroimaging studies with large numbers of patients have also been described, there is not yet a large study that has combined both these measurements in the same population. However, MRI studies have also identified white matter hyperintensities (leukoaraiosis), which are felt to represent 'ischaemic demyelination' secondary to occlusion of small penetrating arteries. Further, the frequency of such lesions is associated with the level of glycaemic control over time. More recent and more detailed gadolinium-enhanced MRI investigation of volunteers with diabetes compared with individuals without diabetes has revealed increased blood–brain barrier permeability in patients with diabetes and white matter lesions,[50] suggesting that this may reflect one of the underlying causes of cerebral dysfunction in patients with diabetes, and potentially other conditions similarly affecting the brain, such as hypertension.

In terms of frequency it is likely that such vascular-mediated cerebral changes are the most important cause of the amplified cognitive decline over time seen in patients with diabetes (both type 1 and type 2) compared with the population without diabetes. In this recently opened field of investigation, however, there are other possibilities for the cause of such decline, so that definitive statements about the relative importance of different causes will require further study for clarification.

Diabetes and Alzheimer's disease

As both diabetes and Alzheimer's disease tend to occur in older populations, the association between the two conditions was for many years felt to be purely coincidental. However, recent studies into the association have clearly identified that there is indeed a link that is more powerful than chance alone (although no causality can at this stage be implied). One recent longitudinal study looked at an ageing population of nuns and priests, following them with both cognitive function testing and formal examinations for the development of Alzheimer's disease. Those of the population with diabetes had a 65 per cent increase in the risk of developing Alzheimer's disease (based on international diagnostic guidelines) over 5 years and a 44 per cent increase in the speed of cognitive decline overall. In addition to such clinical data, imaging studies revealed a characteristic early effect on the hippocampus and amygdala in patients with Alzheimer's disease. A recent large population study of MRI in elderly individuals (>500 individuals) with and without diabetes showed more atrophy in the those with diabetes than those without, with the greatest atrophy seen in those with the highest levels of insulin resistance, and occurring independent of any vascular abnormalities.

Although there is not yet any human postmortem study showing the characteristic neuropathological changes of Alzheimer's disease associated with diabetes (which would obviously clinch the case), there is now experimental animal evidence that has found characteristic Alzheimer-type change in animals exposed to hyperglycaemia over time. At this stage, then (although the cause of the link is unclear), one can reliably state that the risk of Alzheimer's disease is indeed elevated in diabetes. Interestingly, work has also been reported looking at the glucose metabolic status of patients with Alzheimer's disease, which would tend to suggest that diabetes is more common in this group than in the comparable age- and sex-matched population with dementia of non-Alzheimer type. This study did involve some postmortem studies and made the link between Alzheimer's disease and type 2 diabetes on the basis of amyloid β protein deposition occurring in the brain in Alzheimer's disease and the pancreas in type 2 diabetes as a possible unifying source of causation.

9.7 Conclusion

It is perhaps to be expected that the brain, as an organ exclusively dependent on the supply of glucose for its continuing functions, and supplied with a rich vascular tree for this purpose, can have its function dramatically influenced in a condition that changes those glucose levels, and exposes individuals to a wide (non-physiological) range of glycaemic experience from episodic hypoglycaemia to chronic hyperglycaemia. All aspects of the complex interplay of modulators (see Figure 7.1), which produces the unique cognitive outcomes of personality, character and intelligence that characterize individuals, can be affected by the consequences of diabetes (either directly or indirectly). Most of such effects have been systematically investigated only in the course of the last decade or so, such that the present state of knowledge is really only scratching the surface of the issues. However, now that some of the more important issues have been brought into the spotlight, and many of the underlying cerebral mechanisms are being elucidated,[57] the next decade should, based on the increasing awareness of the cerebral molecular changes associated with diabetes, start to yield not just new descriptions of problems, but the hope for answers to the issues of defective cognitive and cerebral function that can accompany diabetes.

Case study

A 30-year-old man with type 1 diabetes of 16 years' duration is admitted to hospital with shoulder pain (dislocation) and a minor head injury after a road traffic accident (RTA), in which no other cars were involved as he crashed into a tree. He has no recollection of the accident, but is accompanied by police who were following him at the time of the accident and describe him as driving erratically and initially acting as if drunk when stopped after the accident, although his breathalyser test was negative. On arrival in A&E (30 min after the accident) his blood sugar value is 10.1 mmol/l.

His usual metabolic control is good (HbA1c 7 per cent [53 mmol/mol]) using 'basal-bolus' insulin therapy, and hypoglycaemia has not been raised as an issue previously in clinic; regular routine medical screening has never detected diabetes complications or other medical conditions.

Describe the processes of examination, investigation and treatment that you might offer to determine the implications of this episode to his overall management.

Answer
This man's RTA most likely represents the result of a bout of hypoglycaemia, even though the blood glucose was not measured

at the time and levels on arrival at hospital were not low (a result of post-RTA adrenergic counter-regulation).

The fact that he had no symptoms alerting him to the hypoglycaemia, but had cognitive impairment (erratic driving), strongly suggests that he has impaired awareness of hypoglycaemia, which most commonly accompanies regular episodes of hypoglycaemia occurring in daily life, and which (almost by definition) may elude identification in routine clinical practice unless specifically sought by targeted questions/examination.

In the first place he should be dissuaded from further driving until the nature of this problem is clearer and investigation is undertaken.

- Has he had any episodes of severe hypoglycaemia in the last year?
- Is there evidence of any physical cause for hypoglycaemia? (Hypothyroidism/hypoadrenalism/renal impairment as initial screen)
- Does he undertake regular blood glucose monitoring and, if so, is it at times and a frequency appropriate to the insulin regimen and levels of control that he achieves (expectation four to six tests per day based on national/international guidelines)? If not, he should start and be reviewed rapidly after its inception.
- Is there evidence of any trends in blood glucose control with hypoglycaemia risk from this monitoring (give particular attention to risk periods for each insulin – basal insulin = overnight, fasting and pre-meals, bolus insulin 1–2 hours after meals)?
- Give consideration to collateral history from a partner or family member regarding his awareness of hypoglycaemia (who knows first if he's low – them or him?) and behaviour while low (does he ignore early symptoms routinely?). Give consideration to formal assessment of hypoglycaemia awareness using validated tools (e.g. Clarke Questionnaire/Gold Score).
- If no obvious pattern emerges, give consideration to a period of continuous glucose monitoring, with particular emphasis on the overnight period.
- If investigations reveal either >5 per cent of monitoring in 'hypo' range, or a standard deviation of blood glucose monitoring results greater than 0.4 times the average level, then recurrent hypoglycaemia should be considered as a 'real and present danger' for repeated episodes, prompting therapy strategy change.

Strategies that have been shown to be successful in reduction of hypoglycaemia experience vary according to the pattern of problems experienced by an individual, but include:
- *Structured* education programmes (e.g. DAFNE or similar)
- Basal insulin change (either overall reduction or switch to long-acting analogue from human intermediate)
- Bolus insulin training to better match carbohydrate requirements/ or 'wizard-based' intervention to reduce corrective bolus insulin use
- Regular snacking
- Alarms on blood glucose meter to prompt testing before times of risk

- Use of continuous subcutaneous insulin infusion (CSII) pumps
- Use of 'real-time' or 'patient-centred' continuous glucose monitoring devices (with or without CSII)
- In extreme and recalcitrant circumstances where 'life and limb' are threatened, islet cell transplantation.

Further reading

Arvanitakis Z, Wilson RS, Bienas JL, Evans DA, Bennett DA. Diabetes mellitus and the risk of Alzheimer's disease and decline in cognitive function. *Arch Neurol* 2004;**61**: 661–666.

Belch J, MacCuish A, Campbell I, et al. The prevention of progression of arterial disease and diabetes (POPADAD) trial: factorial randomised placebo controlled trial of aspirin and antioxidants in patients with diabetes and asymptomatic peripheral arterial disease. *BMJ* 2008;**337**:a1840.

Bruno A, Kent TA, Coull BM, Shankar RR, et al. Treatment of Hyperglycemia In Ischemic Stroke (THIS): A randomized pilot trial. *Stroke* 2008;**39**;384–389.

Calvin AD, Aggarwal NR, Murad MH, et al. Aspirin for the primary prevention of cardiovascular events: A systematic review and meta-analysis comparing patients with and without diabetes. *Diabet Care* 2009;**32**:2300–2306.

Cox DJ, Gonder-Frederick LA, Clark W. Driving decrements in type 1 diabetes during moderate hypoglycaemia. *Diabetes* 1993;**42**:239–243.

Cranston I, Lomas J, Maran A, Macdonald I, Amiel SA. Restoration of hypoglycaemia awareness in patients with long-duration insulin-dependent diabetes. *Lancet* 1994;**344**: 283–287.

Cranston IC, Reed LJ, Marsden PK, Amiel SA. Changes in regional brain ^{18}F-fluoro-deoxyglucose uptake at hypoglycaemia in type 1 diabetic men associated with hypoglycaemia unawareness and counter-regulatory failure. *Diabetes* 2001;**50**: 2329–2336.

Cryer PE, Davis SN, Shamoon H. Hypoglycaemia in diabetes. *Diabet Care* 2003;**26**: 1902–1912.

Deary IJ. The effects of hypoglycaemia on cognitive function. In: Frier BM, Fisher BM (eds), *Hypoglycaemia in Diabetes: Clinical and physiological aspects*. London: Edward Arnold, 1993: pp 80–92.

Greenwood CE, Kaplan RJ, Hebblethwaite S, Jenkins DJA. Carbohydrate-Induced memory impairment in adults with type 2 diabetes. *Diabet Care* 2003;**26**: 1961–1966.

The Heart Outcomes Prevention Evaluation (HOPE) Study Investigators. Effects of ramipril on cardiovascular and microvascular outcomes in people with diabetes mellitus: results of HOPE study and MICRO-HOPE substudy. *Lancet* 2000;**355**:253–259.

Intercollegiate Stroke Working Party. *National Clinical Guidelines for Stroke*, 2nd edn. London: Royal College of Physicians, 2004.

Janson J, Laedtke T, Parisi JE, O'Brien P, Petersen RC, Butler PC. Increased risk of type 2 diabetes in Alzheimer disease. *Diabetes* 2004;**53**:474–481.

Klein JP, Waxman SG. The brain in diabetes: molecular changes in neurons and their implications for end-organ damage. *Lancet Neurol* 2003;**ii**:548–554.

Ryan CM, Geckle MO, Orchard TJ. Cognitive efficiency declines over time in adults with type 1 diabetes: effects of micro- and macrovascular complications. *Diabetologia* 2003; **46**:940–948.

CHAPTER 10
Diabetes and Mental Health

David P Osborn[1] and Richard IG Holt[2]

[1]UCL, Mental Health Sciences Unit, UCL, London, UK
[2]Human Development and Health Academic Unit, Faculty of Medicine, University of Southampton, Southampton, UK

 Key points

- People with diabetes are at increased risk of both depressive and anxiety disorders.

- People with mental illness are at increased risk of developing diabetes; this has been observed in common mental disorders such as depression, as well as severe mental illnesses such as schizophrenia and bipolar disorder.

- The aetiology is probably multifactorial, and may include obesity, the effect of chronic stress on biological systems, lifestyle factors such as poor diet and exercise, and social deprivation.

- Depressed people with diabetes have worse outcomes in terms of glycaemic control, quality of life, use of services, sick leave, long-term diabetic complications and increased mortality.

- Antipsychotic medications are often associated with marked weight gain and may predispose to diabetes. The association between diabetes and antipsychotics has been observed more frequently with second-generation agents, but may occur with any agent. Overall, it seems that other factors, such as lifestyle, are more important in the pathogenesis of diabetes than the drugs.

- Social adversity and stigma may prevent people with mental health problems from receiving adequate physical health care and addressing this inequality is an international priority.

Diabetes: Chronic Complications, Third Edition. Edited by Kenneth M. Shaw, Michael H. Cummings.
© 2012 John Wiley & Sons, Ltd. Published 2012 by John Wiley & Sons, Ltd.

Therapeutic key points

- People with diabetes should be screened regularly for depression and anxiety and receive appropriate pharmacological and psychological treatments. These treatments can improve both diabetes and mental health outcomes.

- Antidepressant medications are effective treatments but can induce weight gain, which may worsen control of diabetes; the choice of agent should be tailored to the individual. Psychological treatments can be equally effective in addressing mild-to-moderate forms of depression and are likely to be more effective in improving diabetes outcomes.

- People with severe mental illnesses often receive inadequate physical health care, with lower levels of physical screening and less assertive management.

- Cardiovascular risk management is now emphasized for people with both schizophrenia and bipolar disorder and this should include annual screening and appropriate management of diabetes.

- Weight reduction, smoking and exercise programmes can be successful in people with severe mental illnesses and may be better options than switching or stopping antipsychotic medication.

10.1 Introduction

The interface between poor physical health and poor mental health is well established across many medical disciplines and it is essential that providers of diabetes care are familiar with the way that mental health issues interact with diabetes.

Diabetes confers an increased risk of common mental disorders, including depression and anxiety. These conditions are important not solely because of the distress that they cause, but because they affect diabetes management and lead to worse physical and functional outcomes and even increased mortality rates. Common mental disorders in people with diabetes are associated with poor glycaemic control and increased use of health services.

Diabetes is also more common in people with severe mental illnesses, such as schizophrenia and bipolar affective disorder. This may result from an increased prevalence of diabetes risk factors, such as poor diet, obesity and lack of exercise, but also from the mental illness itself and the medications used to ameliorate the condition.

Interventions for both common and severe mental illnesses can be effective in improving both mental and physical health in diabetes. Screening for mental disorders in people with diabetes is recommended by international guidelines, as is screening for diabetes and other cardiovascular risk factors in individuals with severe mental illnesses. This chapter describes the most important mental health conditions associated with diabetes, outlines some of the theories linking the conditions, as well as describing the interventions that can be employed to improve physical and mental health outcomes when the conditions co-occur.

10.2 Epidemiology and description of clinical conditions

Depression and common mental disorders in diabetes

Depression is a common, disabling condition in the general population. Almost one in five people can expect to experience a depressive disorder at some point in their lifetime. The World Health Organization estimates that depression will be one of the leading global causes of disability by 2020, second only to heart disease. By 2030, depression is expected to top this list.

Depressive disorders are characterized by sustained lowering of mood over a period of at least 2 weeks. Symptoms and signs are traditionally divided into psychological and biological groups. The psychological markers include a predominance of negative thinking or cognitions. This frequently includes hopelessness, worthlessness and unwarranted guilt within the individual. When profound, this hopelessness may extend to produce suicidal ruminations, plans and attempts to end life that are not infrequently fatal. Concentration is often diminished and the individual may report sleep disturbance, classically with early morning wakening, loss of appetite, lowered libido and a lack of enjoyment of the usual pleasurable activities (anhedonia). However, a reverse pattern, with increased appetite and sleep, is also recognized. Energy levels are often decreased and the individual reports a lack of motivation for even the most basic day-to-day tasks.

International classification systems subdivide depressive disorders according to severity, namely mild, moderate and severe in both the *International Classification of Disease*, 10th revision (ICD-10) the *Diagnostic and Statistical Manual of Mental Disorders*, 4th edn (DSM-IV), the two most established systems used in the USA and across the world. These definitions mainly hinge on the number of symptoms present in an individual; however, many clinicians prefer to view depression as a continuum rather than applying these arbitrary categorizations.

Poor physical health is one of the most established risk factors for depression; diagnoses of cardiovascular diseases, cancers, and endocrinological and neurological disorders from across the medical spectrum all predispose to depression.

First recognized by Thomas Willis in the seventeenth century, the association between diabetes and depression has been highlighted in the scientific literature for many years. The early estimates of depression prevalence varied widely in populations with diabetes, probably reflecting the variance in study designs and settings. The early studies were criticized for methodological weaknesses, e.g. recruiting only patients with the most severe diabetes from specialist clinics, using non-standardized instruments to ascertain cases of depression, or failing to explore possible confounding and causal relationships in any association between diabetes and depression. Variables, such as social deprivation, ethnicity and smoking, are all associated with both diabetes and depression and might explain the high rates of depression. Yet they were rarely considered or accounted for during the study design or analysis in many studies.

More recent and robust investigations, involving representative samples of adults with diabetes now indicate that the prevalence of depression is approximately two to three times higher, compared with the general population. Increased rates of depression have been demonstrated in individuals with both type 1 and type 2 diabetes mellitus. A recent systematic review of prevalence studies in type 1 diabetes concluded that the risk of depression was 12 per cent in those with diabetes compared with 3.2 per cent of comparison individuals without diabetes.[1] When the review was limited to the highest quality studies, this prevalence figure dropped to a prevalence of 7.8 per cent in type 1 diabetes. A review of studies including both types 1 and 2 diabetes, including 20 papers, found an average depression prevalence rate of approximately 15 per cent, ranging from 8.5 per cent to 40 per cent in different settings.[2] There is also evidence, at least in type 2 diabetes, that the risk of depression may differ according to gender with women more affected, although the consequences appear to be worse in men with diabetes. The rates of depression are higher in those with diabetes complications and in people receiving insulin therapy.

The relationship between diabetes and depression appears to be bi-directional (Figure 10.1). Although it makes intuitive sense that people with diabetes may develop depressive disorders, it is also true that people with depression are at an increased risk of developing diabetes. The possible pathways for this relationship are discussed under aetiology below.

10.3 Other common mental disorders

Anxiety disorders

Much of the diabetes and mental health literature has focused on depression, but this neglects the fact that anxiety disorders may be as disabling as depression and that depressive and anxiety symptoms frequently co-occur. Many mental health researchers now use the term 'common mental disorders' as an umbrella term to acknowledge this overlap. In diabetes,

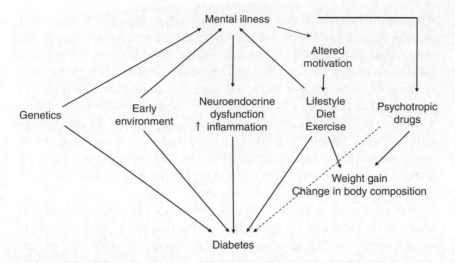

Adapted from Holt et al Diabet Med. 2004;21(6):515-23

Figure 10.1 Possible mechanisms explaining the increased risk of diabetes in people with mental illness. (Adapted from Holt RIG, Peveler RC, Byrne CD. Schizophrenia, the metabolic syndrome and diabetes. *Diabet Med* 2004;**21**:515–523.)

there is evidence that screening and managing anxiety disorders are equally important.

There is a range of anxiety disorders and their description is beyond the scope of this chapter; however, the key symptoms and signs are the presence of overriding psychological worry, either persistent or occurring in discrete episodes. The common features include nervousness, trembling, muscular tension, sweating, light-headedness, palpitations and dizziness. In classification systems such as ICD-10, the clusters of symptoms include: (1) apprehension (feeling on edge, worrying about the future, difficulty concentrating), (2) motor tension (such as headaches, restlessness, trembling) and (3) autonomic overactivity (tachycardia, fast breathing, sweating and dizziness).

A recent UK general population household survey involving 8580 people, including 249 with self-reported diabetes, assessed a variety of mental health outcomes.[3] The strength of this study is not only the recruitment of a population-based sample, but also that it used a structured research interview to determine psychiatric caseness of common mental disorders. This method is far more accurate than using briefer screening questionnaires. The headline finding was that people with diabetes were 1.5 times more likely to have a common mental disorder and this association was particularly strong for mixed anxiety and depression (odds ratio 1.7). The implication is that anxiety symptoms, as well as depressive symptoms, should be identified and managed in people with diabetes. The authors also demonstrated the impact of poor mental health; among those with diabetes, common mental disorders resulted in people being more disabled, less able to control their diabetes and taking more days off work. They also experienced worse outcomes on quality-of-life scales.

Aetiology of depression and common mental disorders in diabetes

The association between diabetes and common mental disorders is far more than a reaction to the stress of living with a chronic condition, although this is an important factor. It is understandable that the frequent monitoring required in diabetes, as well as the need for dietary restrictions and long-term pharmacotherapy, may take its toll in terms of both stress and clinically significant psychiatric disorders. However, there may be a range of other factors that explain the high prevalence of depression and other common mental disorders in adults with diabetes.

Lifestyle factors, smoking and obesity

Obesity, poor diet and physical inactivity are all risk factors for diabetes, but they are also independently associated with depression, as is smoking tobacco. The direction of association may again be bi-directional. Certainly depressed mood or anxiety disorders may lead to lack of exercise, poor dietary choices and in some cases weight gain from over-eating. Moreover there is accumulating evidence that people who are morbidly obese are more likely to be depressed. These common risk factors, for both physical and mental health disorders, may explain the high comorbidity between diabetes and poor mental health, but the timing probably varies from individual to individual. For some, the physical risk factors may predate the onset of both diabetes and depression, whereas for others, the depression might worsen the physical risk factors (e.g. impacting on diet and exercise) which in turn might lead to new-onset diabetes.

Biological mechanisms and chronic stress

The impact of chronic poor mental health on human biological systems remains an area of active research. There is a wealth of evidence that the normal diurnal variation in cortisol concentration is disrupted in people with depression. This chronic dysfunction of the hypothalamic–pituitary–adrenal axis may alter body composition and increase insulin resistance in people with common mental disorders, leading to subsequent diabetes. This provides one mechanism to explain why longitudinal studies have demonstrated that clinical depression is a risk factor for developing diabetes. A recent review retrieved a limited number of longitudinal studies, but concluded that the risk of developing diabetes in people with depression was as high as 37 per cent.[4]

Another potential mechanism is the development of chronic inflammation; cytokines and other inflammatory markers, such as increased C-reactive protein, tumour necrosis factor (TNF)-α and proinflammatory cytokines, are increased in diabetes and the metabolic syndrome, and have been implicated in causing sickness behaviour and depression. Hyperglycaemia may also adversely affect brain function directly.

However, as yet, clinical studies have not been large enough or long enough to disentangle these temporal relationships and the biological mechanisms that may link chronic stress and diabetes.

Genetic and intrauterine factors

There has been some support for the theory that diabetes and common mental disorders may share common genetic or early life risk factors that predispose the individual to both conditions. The field is in its early stages, but there are reports to suggest that common genetic polymorphisms may influence the risk of both diabetes and certain psychiatric disorders, with overlapping chromosomal loci reported in some studies. Less compelling evidence includes the findings of increased rates of diabetes in the relatives of people with mental disorders. Of course this may simply reflect the well-recognized fact that relatives share similar clusters of environmental risk factors including diet and exercise.

Similarly, there are hypotheses that adverse intrauterine conditions may give rise to a common vulnerability to both diabetes and mental health problems. Putative factors include inadequate embryonic nutrition and subsequent low birthweight. Both have been shown to be associated with impaired glucose regulation in adulthood. There is certainly evidence that underweight babies are more prone to affective disorders in their adult life. Once again, the exact relationship between these variables is difficult to tease out, given the need for well-designed, lengthy studies, with multiple follow-up points and sufficient sample size.

Social and psychological factors

Health inequalities, between the richest and poorest sections of society, are well established, both within geographical regions and between regions. The poor mental and physical health of disadvantaged sections of society continues despite national and international campaigns to narrow the gap. People with lower incomes, who do not own their homes, who are unemployed and who have spent less time in education, are at increased risk of both diabetes and depression as well as a host of other poor health outcomes. Although social deprivation explains some of the association between poor physical and mental health, studies that have controlled for these variables usually find that poor mental health and physical health remain associated, irrespective of social deprivation. Therefore social adversity is not the whole story in the association between diabetes and psychiatric disorders.

Impact of depression and common mental disorders in diabetes

Affective and anxiety disorders require treatment in their own right, to minimize the distress that they cause, and the impact on functional and social outcomes including quality of life. Untreated, they also confer a range of negative outcomes in people with comorbid physical conditions. When patients with medical depression are compared with non-depressed patients, the former have a higher degree of physical symptoms and signs and worse adherence to their treatment regimens, including both pharmacological interventions and lifestyle modification programmes.

The impact of poor mental health in diabetes is particularly concerning. Those who have comorbid common mental disorders are likely to have worse glycaemic control than those with good mental health. They seem to be less able or willing to undertake self-monitoring of blood glucose and manage their hypoglycaemic medication, missing more doses and making greater use of emergency and non-urgent health services related to their diabetes. Longitudinal studies have also demonstrated that depression increases the risk of both microvascular and macrovascular complications of diabetes. Mortality is also increased in those with depression, even if this is relatively mild. A US study, involving 359 participants with diabetes, divided the participants into high, medium and low severity of depression, using a validated depression symptom checklist.[5] Participants were assessed for outcomes including glycaemic control, using HbA1c, their knowledge of diabetes, interruptions in oral hypoglycaemic agents and their adherence to dietary recommendations. Those with the highest depression severity fared worse on all these outcomes, including both mental and physical functioning. They also had higher health-care costs associated with greater health-care utilization over 6 months.

The impact of depression may be of particular concern in those with established diabetic complications. Ismail et al.[6] explored the impact of depression in people with diabetes who presented with their first foot ulcer. They recruited 253 people with an ulcer and found that a third of the sample had a clinically significant depressive disorder using an established psychiatric research instrument. They performed survival analysis over the follow-up period of 18 months and showed that mortality rates were raised threefold in those with major or minor depression, compared

with non-depressed participants. The presumed mechanism for poor physical outcomes in depressed people with diabetes is glycaemic control, but
there were no differences in HbA1c in this cohort study. The authors
suggest a range of possible causal mechanisms, including various biological
pathways such as decreased autonomic tone, low heart rate variability,
impaired platelet function and disturbance of the hypothalamic–pituitary–
adrenal axis. Once again, the lack of large cohort studies of adequate
duration prevents us from drawing firm conclusions about these mechanisms; however, it seems clear that those with diabetic complications and
comorbid depression require more intensive interventions, in terms of
screening for depression and active management of both mental and
physical health conditions.

These conclusions have been reinforced by a systematic review and
meta-analysis of 31 studies, published in 2010, regarding the health-care
costs of comorbid mental disorders in people with diabetes.[7] Almost all
health-care costs, including inpatient, outpatient and emergency visits, as
well as medication costs, were increased in people with comorbid mental
health conditions, although the effect sizes were described as small to
moderate. Unsurprisingly, the costs of mental health care were also
increased in those with co-occurring diabetes and mental disorders.

The precise reasons for increased costs may be manifold. One key
hypothesis is that those with more severe physical conditions and worse
diabetic control may be more prone to depression and other mental disorders. However, studies that have controlled for physical illness severity
show that poor mental health is an independent predictor of higher
health-care costs.

10.4 Management of common mental disorders

Identification

As rates of depression and other common mental disorders are so high
in people with diabetes, guidelines recommend routine screening for the
conditions as part of diabetic care. Examples include the UK National
Institute for Health and Clinical Excellence (NICE), which states that
health-care professionals must be aware of the importance of anxiety
and depression, and have the skills to both identify and then manage
or refer people appropriately to specialist services. This is particularly
important if patients are having difficulties managing their diabetes, and
this is impacting significantly on the patient's quality of life or physical
wellbeing.

There are several brief screening questionnaires that can be used to
identify probable psychiatric disorder in people with diabetes. It is

---

Box 10.1 Screening questionnaires for depression in people with diabetes

Most well validated for people with diabetes
Beck Depression Inventory (BDI)
Center for Epidemiologic Studies Depression Scale (CES-D)
Patient Health Questionnaire (PHQ)
Hospital Anxiety and Depression Scale (HADS)
Problem Areas in Diabetes (PAID) scale

Less well validated for people with diabetes
Zung Self-rating Depression Scale (Zung-SDS)
Short Form (SF) Medical Outcomes Survey

Well validated for the general population but not for people with diabetes
Hamilton Rating Scale for Depression (HRSD)
Geriatric Depression Scale (GDS)
WHO Well-being Index (WHO-5/WHO-10)
General Wellbeing Questionnaire (WBQ)
Montgomery–Åsberg Depression Rating Scale (MADRS)
Symptom Check List (SCL)
General Health Questionnaire (GHQ)
Diagnostic and Statistical Manual of Mental Disorders (DSM)
European Quality of Life-5 Dimensions (EQ-5D)

---

recommended that all patients are screened annually, and in the UK general practitioners are remunerated for providing such screening.

Examples of screening questionnaires include the Hospital Anxiety and Depression Scale (HADS).[8] This instrument was developed for use in patients with physical disorders and, in contrast to that suggested by the name, has also been validated in patients with physical conditions in community settings. It does not over-emphasize the somatic or biological symptoms of depression, such as low appetite or weight loss, which co-occur in many physical illnesses. Inclusion of these symptoms in other questionnaires can give rise to elevated prevalence rates from false positives. An alternative to the HADS is the Patient Health Questionnaire (PHQ-9),[9] widely used in UK primary care settings. Box 10.1 summarizes the screening questionnaires for depression in people with diabetes.

Even more simple is the two-question screen for depression:
1. During the past month have you often been bothered by feeling down, depressed or hopeless?
2. During the past month have you often been bothered by little interest or pleasure in doing things?

If the answer to either is 'yes' the patient should be asked if he or she want helps with this problem. If the answer to this supplementary question is also 'yes', then it is reasonable to make a formal assessment of depression and offer treatment if appropriate.

Interventions

The usual treatments for common mental disorders include pharmacological interventions for moderate-to-severe disorders, and psychological and psychosocial interventions for disorders of all severities.

Pharmacological interventions

In general, most antidepressant medications increase synaptic levels of central nervous system (CNS) monoamines, by either inhibiting their breakdown or preventing their reuptake. The standard antidepressants of the mid-twentieth century were tricyclic antidepressants such as amitriptyline and nortriptyline. Their use was gradually overtaken in the 1980s and 1990s by the serotonin-specific reuptake inhibitors (SSRIs), which are possibly better tolerated and certainly safer in overdose. Examples include sertaline, fluoxetine and citalopram. A new wave of antidepressant medications followed including serotonin–noradrenaline reuptake inhibitors (SNRIs), such as venlafaxine and the newer compound mirtazepine, a noradrenaline and serotonin-specific antidepressant (NaSSA). Box 10.2 lists some of the most common antidepressant agents by class.

Most guidelines suggest that there is little to differentiate the efficacy of different antidepressants in terms of depression outcomes, so the choice of agent is often made by consideration of the side-effect profile and patient preference. However, they should always be prescribed in adequate doses. The tricyclic antidepressants are less favoured when cardiac conditions are present because of their cardiotoxicity, when sedation would be a problem, or when patients are at increased risk of suicide. SSRIs are more prone to gastrointestinal side effects and there are concerns about discontinuation syndromes if they are stopped abruptly. Mirtazapine can predispose to weight gain and therefore is less suitable for patients with diabetes where excess cardiovascular risk is already a concern. However, weight gain can also be a problem with the tricyclic antidepressants.

Usual treatment guidelines state that antidepressant agents may be required for 4–6 weeks before a response is observed. If a patient remits, treatment should be maintained for 6–12 months to minimize the risk of relapse. In patients with recurrent depressive disorders, treatment is often required for 2 years or more. If a patient has not responded to one antidepressant, then switching between agents, either within class or to another class, is recommended. Non-responsive cases and those with marked risk of suicidal behaviour require prompt referral to specialist mental health services.

Antidepressants and diabetes outcomes

There is good evidence that treating common mental disorders with pharmacological agents can improve psychiatric outcomes, but evidence is

---

Box 10.2 Types of antidepressants

SSRIs are recommended as first-line treatment for people with diabetes

Selective serotonin reuptake inhibitors (SSRIs)
Citalopram
Escitalopram
Fluoxetine
Paroxetine
Sertraline

Serotonin–noradrenaline reuptake inhibitors (SNRIs)
Duloxetine
Venlafaxine

Noradrenaline- and serotonin-specific antidepressants (NaSSAs)
Mirtazapine

Noradrenaline reuptake inhibitors (NARI)
Reboxetine

Noradrenaline–dopamine reuptake inhibitors (NDRIs)
Bupropion

Noradrenaline–dopamine disinhibitors (NDDIs)
Agomelatine

Tricyclic antidepressants (TCAs)
Amitriptyline
Clomipramine
Clomipramine
Doxepin
Dosulepin
Imipramine
Trimipramine
Nortriptyline

Monoamine oxidase inhibitor (MAOIs)
Isocarboxazid
Moclobemide (reversible)
Phenelzine
Tranylcypromine

---

emerging that physical outcomes, including glycaemic control, may also improve, although the data are more conflicting. There are positive studies involving both SSRIs and tricyclic antidepressants, but a recent systematic review has suggested that sertaline may be the antidepressant medication most beneficial for improving glycaemic control.[10] When antidepressants are used in diabetes, interactions between drugs should be considered, e.g. agents such as fluoxetine inhibit enzymes involved in the breakdown of oral hypoglycaemic agents, potentially resulting in hypoglycaemia.

Psychological interventions

There is ample evidence that brief psychological therapies can be beneficial for people with depression and other common mental disorders. The most common interventions include cognitive–behavioural therapy (CBT), interpersonal therapy (IPT), motivational interviewing, counselling and psychodynamic therapy. CBT includes methods for identifying and challenging maladaptive thought patterns or cognitive styles in people with depression. The patient learns to debate these unhelpful thoughts, which otherwise serve to maintain the depression, as well as addressing behavioural issues that can otherwise prevent recovery.

Psychological interventions in diabetes

A systematic review of 25 randomized controlled trials (RCTs) of psychological therapies involving patients with diabetes was published in *The Lancet* in 2004.[11] The review carefully assessed the quality of the trials including issues such as the use of a suitable control group, masking of the researchers to treatment allocation and the validity of the outcome measures.

The results of the meta-analysis revealed that both psychological distress and mean HbA1c were lower when patients received active psychological interventions, compared with the control groups. The interventions, however, did not improve the control of bodyweight, or self-monitored blood glucose concentration. Most of the trials included in the review involved a form of CBT (usually between 6 and 12 sessions); the next most common intervention was motivational interviewing. The latter technique was originally developed as an aid to address unhealthy lifestyles and might be usefully employed to help with diabetes self-care, including diet, exercise, self-monitoring and adherence to treatments. The authors commented that there was a disappointing lack of trials exploring specific therapies for people with diabetes.

There have, however, been some attempts to evaluate specific models of care for people with diabetes and poor mental health, but results have been mixed, with more promising results emerging recently. One example was the pathways study, published in 2004.[12] This RCT involved over 300 patients with diabetes and depression and compared a form of intensive case management with treatment as usual. It demonstrated better depression outcomes, but no accompanying improvement in diabetic control. By contrast, a recent meta-analysis of 15 trials showed that psychotherapy produces best results (mentally and physically) when it is combined with self-management education and therefore this should be first-line treatment for depression in types 1 and 2 diabetes.[8] The same review also demonstrated that models of collaborative care are successful for patients with type 2 diabetes and depression in primary care settings.

It is noteworthy that exercise is effective in improving mild depression and should be encouraged for its physical and mental health benefits.

In conclusion, there is compelling evidence that physical and mental health can be improved by both pharmacological and psychological interventions, often combined with self-management and collaborative care across the primary–secondary care interface.

10.5 Severe mental illnesses

Illnesses, such as schizophrenia and bipolar affective disorder, are often classified as severe mental illnesses. The term has attracted criticism because it may imply that other psychiatric disorders are not severe. Indeed many depressive disorders and eating disorders may be equally severe and have fatal outcomes. However, the term encapsulates two disorders that often share chronic, relapsing–remitting courses and increase the risk of cardiovascular disease and diabetes.

Schizophrenia
Schizophrenia has a lifetime prevalence of 0.5–1 per cent in the general population with an onset usually occurring in the late teens or twenties. Although some patients have a single episode and recover completely, many others will have future relapses of the condition. A smaller percentage never recovers, has markedly diminished levels of functioning and may require long-term care.

The illness is characterized by the presence of 'positive symptoms' such as delusions and hallucinations, and several subtypes are described, e.g. paranoid, simple and hebephrenic, according to the predominance of different symptoms. The symptoms must be present for at least 1 month in ICD-10 and for 6 months in DSM-IV. In the more chronic forms of the disorder, patients may develop 'negative symptoms'. These include lack of motivation and drive, poverty of thought and speech (that is a decreased quantity), poor self-care and other forms of self-neglect. Many people with schizophrenia live fulfilling lives in the community, but, similar to many other mental health disorders, the condition is associated with a marked stigma and this often prevents people from accessing work and other opportunities in the wider community, resulting in social exclusion. Depressive symptoms are common and suicide is a major concern in people with schizophrenia; the risk is markedly elevated throughout the life course, compared with the general population.

Some people with schizophrenia lack insight into their condition, particularly when the illness is in the acute phase or when a relapse occurs. At this point, some people require involuntary treatment in hospital but this can often be avoided if a relapse is treated early enough. Community mental health teams, emergency home treatment (or crisis) teams and primary care can all work together as an alternative to hospital admission.

Bipolar affective disorder

Bipolar disease is a mood disorder, previously known as manic depression, with a prevalence of 0.5–1 per cent. Once again, it is often a chronic, relapsing–remitting condition, with onset in early adulthood and an equal sex distribution. The diagnosis is only made when someone has suffered more than one episode of prolonged abnormal mood, including periods of mania (or its less severe form, hypomania) and depression.

When a patient is manic, the mood is elated and this is accompanied by increased speed of thoughts and speech, grandiose thinking (an inflated sense of personal abilities and status) and, if the patient has a manic psychosis, delusions and/or hallucinations are present. The patient sleeps less, may be agitated and energized, may overspend or indulge in sexual activity that is out of character. The risks include incurring financial debts, sexually risky behaviour, vulnerability to exploitation, damage to personal and work relationships, frustration with others and occasionally violence. Once again, if insight is lost, the patient may require involuntary hospital care to ensure his or her safety. The difference between mania and hypomania is a matter of degree. In hypomania, the individual may be able to maintain their occupational and social functioning to some level.

As well as manic episodes, people with bipolar affective disorder are prone to severe episodes of depression. These episodes may be equally debilitating but are similar in nature to the description of depression above.

10.6 Severe mental illnesses and diabetes

The association between schizophrenia and diabetes has been described for more than a century. Following these early reports, a number of case series described people with schizophrenia who had impaired glucose tolerance and frank diabetes early in the twentieth century and before the advent of antipsychotic medication. The last decade, however, has seen far greater interest in the relationship and a more intense research endeavour to determine the reasons underlying the association and to evaluate methods to address the conditions when they co-occur.

Despite this, high-quality epidemiological studies are still lacking, although this situation has improved more recently. A recent systematic review retrieved all studies of diabetes that also included a comparison group. The relative risk of diabetes appeared to be increased twofold in people with severe mental illnesses including bipolar disorder.[13]

The association between severe mental illnesses and diabetes is important in its own right but also in the context of cardiovascular disease. People with severe mental illnesses are more likely to die prematurely from cardiovascular disease than from suicide. The rate of cardiovascular deaths is increased approximately threefold in people with severe mental illnesses aged under 50 years and twofold in those aged between 50 and 70 years compared with the general population. This association remains even after controlling for smoking and social deprivation.[14]

Aetiology

There may be many explanations for the increased rates of diabetes in people with severe mental illnesses (see Figure 10.1). Some are similar to those highlighted for the common mental disorders, including the biological impact of chronic stress, social adversity and increased diabetes lifestyle risk factors. Diet and exercise levels are frequently suboptimal in severe mental illness. People with schizophrenia eat diets with less fibre, less fruit and vegetables and more fat than healthy people, and this is seen at the onset of the illness and later in the course of the conditions.[15] They are far less likely to take even moderate levels of exercise, and these associations remain even after controlling for the potential confounding effects of social deprivation.

Although severe mental illnesses affect people from all backgrounds, there is often an impact on social functioning and accompanying social deprivation. Less than 20 per cent of people with schizophrenia are in competitive employment and more people with severe mental illnesses live in deprived areas. The health inequalities associated with poverty may therefore underpin the elevated risk of diabetes in this group.

Biological links between diabetes and severe mental illnesses

Living with a chronic severe mental illness is obviously stressful; long-term symptoms such as paranoia, auditory hallucinations and depression, as well as repeated hospitalization, lead to prolonged autonomic over-activity and anxiety. It is hypothesized that this stress may affect the hypothalamic–pituitary–adrenal axis with a subsequent change in body composition and increase in insulin resistance in people with severe mental illnesses, a model similar to that described for common mental disorders. There has also been interest in possible common genetic markers for both diabetes and schizophrenia, a common vulnerability, although the research is in its infancy and by no means conclusive. It seems likely that environmental factors, including diet, exercise, subsequent obesity and possibly antipsychotic medications, are likely to play the greater role in the association between diabetes and severe mental illnesses.

Unlike depression, the association between severe mental illness and diabetes appears to be unidirectional. There is no evidence that diabetes leads to schizophrenia or bipolar disorder in the way that physical illnesses such as diabetes can lead to increased rates of depression and anxiety.

Diabetes and antipsychotic medication

Antipsychotic medications are a key element in the treatment of severe mental illnesses. This is true for both schizophrenia and increasingly bipolar affective disorder, as well as the other less common psychoses. They are used in the acute phases of the illnesses for symptom control and also for maintenance treatment between episodes to decrease the likelihood of relapse. Although psychological therapies are effective in these conditions, they are not recommended as alternatives to medication in evidence-based treatment guidelines. The requirement for long-term medication, over many years, brings the risk of long-term side effects and there is accumulating evidence that people treated with antipsychotics are at increased risk of developing impaired glucose tolerance and diabetes.

There has been controversy about the relative risk of diabetes with different antipsychotics and also the degree to which the illnesses and the medication contribute to the elevated rates of diabetes in people with severe mental illnesses compared with traditional diabetes risk factors.

Antipsychotics are grouped into two main categories: (1) first-generation antipsychotics (FGAs) or 'typical' or 'conventional' antipsychotics, and (2) second-generation antipsychotics (SGAs) or 'atypical' antipsychotics. The FGAs were developed in the mid-twentieth century and include haloperidol, chlorpromazine and trifluoperazine. It is presumed that their therapeutic benefit is derived from the blockade of central dopamine receptors. This action also produces their most troublesome side effects, namely movement disorders which include parkinsonism and other extrapyramidal side effects (EPSs), as well as hyperprolactinaemia and its associated sexual dysfunction. The SGAs were introduced in the mid-1990s and include olanzapine, risperidone, quetiapine and clozapine. They are termed 'atypical' because they do not solely act to block dopamine receptors and are less prone to invoke EPSs. This lack of neurological side effects was seen as a major breakthrough and many treatment guidelines began to recommend that SGAs be routinely used as first-line treatment in schizophrenia. By 2010, the number of prescriptions for SGAs far outweighed those for FGAs in UK primary care. Table 10.1 lists the most common first- and second-generation antipsychotic medications.

However, SGAs are generally associated with more weight gain and possibly other metabolic complications, such as dyslipidaemia, than the

Table 10.1 Examples of first- and second-generation antipsychotics

First-generation antipsychotics	Second-generation antipsychotics
Butyrophenones	Clozapine
Haloperidol	Olanzapine
Benperidol	Risperidone
	Quetiapine
Phenothiazines	Ziprasidone
Chlorpromazine	Amisulpride
Fluphenazine	Paliperidone
Perphenazine	Zotepine
Prochlorperazine	Sertindole
Thioridazine	Aripiprazole
Trifluoperazine	
Pimozide	
Thioxanthenes	
Clopentixol	
Flupentixol	
Zuclopentixol	

FGAs. There is a hierarchy of risk of weight gain, with olanzapine and clozapine being most problematic. In most countries the use of clozapine is reserved for people with treatment-resistant conditions because it also carries a risk of agranulocytosis, so regular blood monitoring is required to identify falls in white cell counts. Olanzapine is one of the most widely prescribed antipsychotics worldwide and is used to treat schizophrenia and mania in both the acute and maintenance phases of the conditions.

Weight gain is certainly not restricted to these two antipsychotics and may be observed with most agents. The mechanism is uncertain but primarily appears to be caused by an increase in appetite. Patients may gain several kilograms within the first few weeks of treatment and the weight gain may continue for more than a year, albeit at a slower rate.

The weight gain has led to concerns about the effect that SGAs may have on diabetes risk. This issue has not been fully resolved because of the lack of high-quality data; in the absence of adequately powered RCTs, other forms are evidence become important. There have been a number of case reports of individuals developing diabetes on treatment that has gone into remission after treatment cessation. A large number of pharma-coepidemiological studies have been published addressing this issue but many are of poor quality and fail to take account of important confounders. Nevertheless two themes emerge: first, treatment with any antipsychotic is associated with an increased risk of diabetes compared with no treatment and, second, as shown in a recent systematic review comparing

FGAs and SGAs, treatment with an SGA was associated with a small but significantly higher risk of diabetes than treatment with an FGA.[16] Comparisons between different SGAs have produced less consistent findings and furthermore most RCTs have failed to find a significant difference in rates of incident diabetes between people receiving different antipsychotics or indeed between treatment and placebo.

Although further evidence about the relative harm of different antipsychotic agents should emerge as higher-quality longitudinal studies are published over the coming years, currently it appears that the magnitude of any association between SGAs and diabetes is much smaller than the risk of diabetes associated with severe mental illnesses itself and the other common diabetes risk factors.[17]

In bipolar affective disorder, many patients are prescribed combinations of both antipsychotic medications and mood-stabilizing medications. Lithium and sodium valproate are among the most common of these mood stabilizers and they are often prescribed persistently over many years to prevent relapse. Both agents are associated with a potential for weight gain and therefore an additional possible pathway to diabetes.

10.7 Management

The key principle of diabetes care for people with severe mental illness is that they should receive physical health care that is *at least* to the same standard as for people without mental health problems.

Stigma has often been cited as a reason for poor physical health in people with mental health problems. A report from the Disability Rights Commission in 2006[18] coined the term 'diagnostic overshadowing'. Many people who use mental health services state that they receive inferior physical health care on account of their mental illness. They describe health professionals focusing solely on their mental disorder and failing to attend to descriptions of their physical health needs. In other words, the mental health diagnosis overshadows the need for adequate physical investigations and treatments. This might lead to decreased screening rates for diabetes and indeed to inferior diabetes care even after a diagnosis has been established.

It is known that people with severe mental illness are less likely to be examined for eye or foot diabetic complications, despite more clinic visits to their GP, and are less likely to be screened for HbA1c or cholesterol. People with severe mental illness receive less education or cardioprotective medication. One exception to this sad indictment was a UK study in which care was found to be equivalent to the general population, possibly as a result of GP reimbursement.

Table 10.2 Recommendations for screening of people receiving antipsychotic medication

Risk factor	How	When
Obesity	Weight and BMI Waist circumference may be helpful	Every visit, at least weekly when antipsychotics are initiated
Blood pressure	Automated or manual sphygmomanometer	Before treatment initiation, 2–3 months later and then annually
Diabetes	Fasting or random glucose or HbA1c	Before treatment initiation, 2–3 months later and then annually
Cholesterol and triglycerides	Fasting lipid profile	Before treatment initiation, 2–3 months later and then annually
Smoking status	History	Every visit
Family history of diabetes or CVD	History	At first assessment and then annually
Personal history of diabetes or CVD	History	At first assessment and as necessary

BMI, body mass index; CVD, cardiovascular disease; HbA1c, glycated haemoglobin.

There is also an imperative to screen for diabetes in people taking antipsychotic medication. Given the debate about the relative diabetogenic risk of different agents, it is recommended that all people prescribed antipsychotics have a glucose (fasting or random) or HbA1c checked at baseline before treatment commences, 3 months later and then annually. Table 10.2 summarizes the recommendations for screening in people prescribed antipsychotic medication.

Setting of care

Most diabetic screening and management for people with severe mental illnesses should be provided in primary care, not least because people with schizophrenia tend to attend their general practice more frequently than the general population. There is general agreement among mental health and primary care workers that this constitutes the best model, and many mental health practitioners lack confidence with some aspects of physical health care. Primary care should ensure that results of physical investigations and management are communicated to secondary care mental health services. However, there is a considerable minority of people with severe mental illness who do not see their GP, and mental health teams have an obligation to ensure that these people are screened for diabetes (and other physical conditions) and referred for specialist intervention if necessary.

Some community and inpatient mental health teams receive specialist input from GPs or physical health care nurses and this is an optimal model, although clearly more expensive in an era when mental health services are under increasing pressure to decrease costs. However, equitable physical health care cannot be viewed as a dispensable element of modern mental health care.

10.8 Severe mental illnesses and other cardiovascular risk factors

The increased prevalence of cardiovascular disease in people with severe mental illness is explained to a large degree by an increased prevalence of traditional cardiovascular risk factors. Increased rates of diabetes and obesity in people with severe mental illnesses are accompanied by an increased prevalence of dyslipidaemia and hypertension; low high-density lipoprotein (HDL)-cholesterol and hypertriglyceridaemia are common, affecting 25–69 per cent whereas several reports also suggest that hypertension is more common in those with severe mental illness. Smoking is a particular concern; 50–80 per cent of people with schizophrenia smoke. They tend to smoke more cigarettes and inhale more deeply. All these risk factors may interact to elevate the risk of cardiovascular complications.

In the UK, national treatment guidelines have been published by the NICE, for both bipolar disorder and schizophrenia. These guidelines recognize the increased rates of cardiovascular risk factors and recommend that people with severe mental illness should have an annual screen for these risk factors, usually in primary care. Once these risk factors have been measured, a cardiovascular risk score should be calculated, although there are concerns that the usual risk scores may underestimate their risk.

People with illnesses such as schizophrenia are equally likely to attend for cardiovascular screening as the UK general population.[19] However, they may be far less likely to receive interventions in real-life clinical practice, e.g. evidence from primary care suggests that they are less likely to receive statin prescriptions.

Interventions for diabetes and cardiovascular risk in people with severe mental illness
There are very few trials of interventions to address the risk factors for diabetes, or diabetes itself, in people with severe mental illness. Most studies are non-randomized, small, feasibility trials. Therefore, although there are systematic reviews in this field, including reviews of weight reduction and exercise programmes, they are currently inconclusive.

The most important principle is that people with schizophrenia should be offered access to exactly the same lifestyle management and pharmacological protocols as people without mental health problems. Some studies suggest that people with schizophrenia are less aware of the importance of diet and exercise as cardiovascular risk factors. It may be worthwhile spending extra time educating people about healthy lifestyles, although education alone is unlikely to have an impact unless backed up with other behavioural techniques to address issues such as smoking, diet and exercise. The small amount of evidence available indicates that people with schizophrenia can be successful in smoking cessation, and that widespread pessimism among many professionals is unfounded.

As weight gain is a frequent side effect of antipsychotic medication, diet and exercise advice should be discussed at the initiation of treatment and should be revisited at regular intervals thereafter. This requires some sensitivity. Antipsychotic medication is very effective in treating and preventing psychotic symptoms, which themselves carry major risks to the individual. The discussion of side effects needs to recognize the benefits of antipsychotics as well as the potential side effects. Although it would be ideal to avoid antipsychotic treatments that induce weight, options are limited and all agents have their own side-effect profiles such as agitation or parkinsonian symptoms. Poor adherence to antipsychotics is one of the most common reasons for relapses of severe mental illnesses and so the discussion of weight gain and possible metabolic sequelae must be honest, yet balanced. Overall treatment with antipsychotics is associated with a lower mortality rate, including deaths from cardiovascular disease.

When an individual with severe mental illness develops diabetes, decisions about antipsychotic treatment may be more challenging. If the mental disorder has been highly problematic, with repeated hospitalizations, there is good justification to persevere with an antipsychotic that has proved helpful, even if it might affect the diabetes and induce weight gain. If an individual has been stable for many years, in terms of his or her mental state, there may be an argument for considering switching antipsychotic agent, lowering the dose or even having a trial period without antipsychotics. However, this is not straightforward; when the antipsychotic has been prescribed long term, it is probably less likely that it is implicated in new-onset diabetes. As such no single guideline is suitable for all patients and the decision about ongoing medication should be collaborative between clinician and patient. It must involve all relevant professionals, especially those in primary care, and should always include the best evidence-based interventions for the diabetes. It is essential that these decisions be weighed carefully to avoid knee-jerk changes in treatment that may adversely affect either physical or mental health outcomes.

10.9 Conclusion

The association between poor mental health and diabetes is now well established. There are a variety of possible explanations, including social adversity, unhealthy lifestyles, obesity and the impact of chronic stress on the biological mechanisms that underpin the association. Antidepressants and antipsychotic medications, particularly SGAs, induce weight gain. Past and present effectiveness of medications must be considered before stopping or switching medications, but in those who are already obese, the agents least likely to induce weight gain should be chosen.

The stigma of mental illnesses is an equally important problem. This can prevent individuals from seeking help. If they do consult clinicians, people with mental illness often receive inferior care either because their mental health issues take prominence or because the professional assumes that they will not adhere to interventions.

There is good evidence that treating depression and anxiety can lead to improvements in diabetes outcomes and this requires systematic screening for the conditions and then assertive management with the well-established treatments.

We know less about effective interventions for individuals with diabetes and severe mental illnesses. However, we do know that they are equally likely to attend screening and that the same lifestyle and pharmacological interventions can be applied successfully. It may require increased commitment on the part of the individual and interagency working to reduce the current inequalities in physical health care that are experienced by people with schizophrenia and bipolar disorder.

Case studies

Case 1
John is a 62-year-old married man who has had type 2 diabetes for 18 years, which until recently was treated by diet and oral hypoglycaemic medication. He started insulin therapy several months ago because of poor glycaemic control. He has a BMI of $33 \, kg/m^2$. During his most recent consultation, his mood was noticeably low. On direct questioning, he gave a history of significant depressive symptoms lasting for several months, dating back to the initiation of insulin. He had low self-esteem, which was made worse by feelings of inadequacy brought on by his erectile dysfunction. His father also had diabetes and John remembers his father having a below-knee amputation shortly after starting insulin. Management consisted of antidepressant medication, augmented with cognitive–behavioural therapy. His psychologist explored the fears that John had around the use of insulin. John was also treated

with sildenafil and he was able to resume sexual intercourse with his wife.

Case 2

Kate is a 47-year-old woman with a 20-year history of paranoid schizophrenia. She experiences paranoid delusions that the police and mental health professionals want to kill her and auditory hallucinations that make derogatory statements about her. She has attempted to kill herself by overdose on five occasions. She has been treated with the antipsychotic clozapine for the last 18 months, but has gained 10 kg in weight and now has a body mass index (BMI) of 31.2 kg/m². She was diagnosed with type 2 diabetes 6 months ago and she is a life-long smoker. Her psychiatric symptoms are much improved on clozapine and both she and the mental health team are keen that she remains on this antipsychotic. Her diabetes is managed with oral hypoglycaemic medication (metformin 850 mg twice daily) and she regularly attends her GP. Her glycaemic control is now good (glycated haemoglobin [HbA1c] 6.9 per cent [52 mmol/mol]) and she is attending a weight management course and received a free gym referral via the local authority. The GP and her mental health nurse are in regular contact to encourage her in her lifestyle management and she has also been referred to a smoking general cessation clinic.

References

1. Barnard KD, Skinner TC, Peveler R. The prevalence of co-morbid depression in adults with type 1 diabetes: systematic literature review. *Diabet Med* 2006;**23**: 445–448.
2. Anderson RJ, Freedland KE, Clouse RE, Lustman PJ. The prevalence of comorbid depression in adults with diabetes: a meta-analysis. *Diabet Care* 2001;**24**: 1069–1078.
3. Das-Munshi J, Stewart R, Ismail K, Bebbington PE, Jenkins R, Prince MJ. Diabetes, common mental disorders, and disability: findings from the UK National Psychiatric Morbidity Survey. *Psychosom Med* 2007;**69**:543–550.
4. Knol M, Twisk J, Beekman A, et al. Depression as a risk factor for the onset of type 2 diabetes mellitus. A meta-analysis. *Diabetologia* 2006;**49**:837–845.
5. Ciechanowski P, Katon WJ, Russo JE. Depression and diabetes: Impact of depressive symptoms on adherence, function and costs. *Arch Intern Med* 2000;**160**: 3278–3285.
6. Ismail K, Winkley K, Rabe-Hesketh S. Systematic review and metaanalysis of randomised controlled trials of psychological interventions behavioural treatment programme in the UK. *Acta Psychiatr Scand* 2007;**115**:286–294.
7. Hutter N, Schnurr A, Baumeister H. Healthcare costs in patients with diabetes mellitus and comorbid mental disorders–a systematic review *Diabetologia* 2010;**53**: 2470–2479.
8. Zigmond AS, Snaith RP. Hospital anxiety and depression scale. *Acta Psychiatr Scand* 1983;**67**:361–370.

9. Kroenke K, Spitzer RL, Williams JB; The PHQ-9: validity of a brief depression severity measure. *J Gen Intern Med* 2001;**16**:606–613.

10. van der Feltz-Cornelis CM, Nuyen J, Stoop C, et al. Effect of interventions for major depressive disorder and significant depressive symptoms in patients with diabetes mellitus: a systematic review and meta-analysis. *Gen Hosp Psychiatry* 2010;**32**: 380–395.

11. Ismail, K, Winkley, K & Rabe-Hesketh, S. Systematic review and meta-analysis of randomised controlled trials of psychological interventions to improve glycaemic control in people with type 2 diabetes. *Lancet* 2004;**363**:1589–1597.

12. Katon WJ, Von Korff M, Lin EHB, et al. The Pathways Study: a randomized trial of collaborative care in patients with diabetes and depression. *Arch Gen Psychiatry* 2004;**61**:1042–1049.

13. Osborn DPJ Wright CA, Levy G, King MB, Deo R, Nazareth I. Relative risk of diabetes, dyslipidaemia, hypertension and the metabolic syndrome in people with severe mental illnesses. Systematic review and metaanalysis. *BMC Psychiatry* 2008;**8**:843.

14. Osborn DPJ, Levy G, Nazareth I, Petersen I, Islam A, King M. Relative risk of cardiovascular and cancer mortality in people with severe mental illness from the United Kingdom's General Practice Research Database. *Arch Gen Psychiatry* 2007;**64**: 242–249.

15. Osborn DPJ, King MB, Nazareth I. Physical activity, dietary habits and coronary heart disease risk factor knowledge amongst people with severe mental illness. A cross sectional comparative study in primary care. *Soc Psychiatry Psychiatr Epidemiol* 2007;**42**:787–793.

16. Smith M, Hopkins D, Peveler RC, Holt RIG, Woodward M, Ismail K. First- v. second-generation antipsychotics and risk for diabetes in schizophrenia: systematic review and meta-analysis. *Br J Psychiatry* 2008;**192**:406–411.

17. Holt RI, Peveler RC. Antipsychotic drugs and diabetes: an application of the Austin Bradford Hill criteria. *Diabetologia* 2006;**49**:1467–1476.

18. Disability Rights Commission. Equal *Treatment: Closing the gap. A formal investigation into physical Health inequalities experienced by people with learning difficulties and mental health problems*. London: Disability Rights Commission, 2006. Available at: www.drc-gb.org

19. Osborn DPJ, King MB, Nazareth I. Participation in cardiovascular risk screening by people with schizophrenia or similar mental illnesses. A cross sectional study in general practice. *BMJ* 2003;**326**:1122–1123.

CHAPTER 11

Musculoskeletal Complications of Diabetes Mellitus

Stratos Christianakis, Minh Chau Nguyen and Richard S Panush

Division of Rheumatology, Department of Medicine, Keck School of Medicine, University of Southern California, Los Angeles, California, USA

 Key points and key therapeutic points

- Think about musculoskeletal/rheumatological syndromes associated with diabetes. Ask about them. Be alert to them. They are common.

- Use clinical skills, or invite appropriate consultative expertise, to establish these diagnoses. 'In clinical rheumatology science does not often substitute for art nor sophisticated technology for diagnostic acumen'.[1]

- Although not as 'dramatic' as perhaps other aspects of management of diabetes and its complications, attention to musculoskeletal/rheumatological syndromes will offer patients important opportunities for improvement in symptoms and quality of life and reduction of attendant morbidity.

- The fundamental principles of managing the musculoskeletal/rheumatological complications associated with diabetes emphasize their recognition followed by supportive care, symptomatic relief and optimizing glycaemic control.

- The carpal tunnel and flexor tenosynovitis ('trigger finger') syndromes accompanying diabetes are illustrative examples of this. They should be relatively easy to identify, can usually be managed satisfactorily medically, only rarely need surgical intervention and are reminders to strive for good control of the underlying diabetes.

11.1 Introduction

Musculoskeletal (MS)/rheumatological symptoms are common in patients with diabetes mellitus, particularly as they live longer. Although these may not be considered as dramatic or important as those reflecting vascular disease, they are prevalent, painful, debilitating and impair functional ability and quality of life. If patients with diabetes are to receive optimal care, it is important that they be recognized and managed. We review the salient features of MS manifestations of diabetes mellitus as soft tissue-related, articular and systemic conditions (Box 11.1).

Diabetes: Chronic Complications, Third Edition. Edited by Kenneth M. Shaw, Michael H. Cummings.
© 2012 John Wiley & Sons, Ltd. Published 2012 by John Wiley & Sons, Ltd.

Box 11.1 Classification of musculoskeletal manifestation of diabetes

Soft tissue related
- Adhesive capsulitis
- Diabetic cheiroarthropathy
- Flexor tenosynovitis
- Dupuytren's contracture(s)
- Carpal tunnel syndrome

Articular
- Crystal-induced arthropathies: calcium pyrophosphate dehydrate crystal deposition disease, monosodium urate (grout), basic calcium pyrophosphate
- Osteoarthritis
- Charcot (neuropathic) joints

Systemic
- Diffuse idiopathic skeletal hyperostosis (DISH)
- Musculoskeletal infections
- Diabetic muscle infarction
- Diabetic amylopathy

Soft tissue-related conditions are related often to limited joint mobility, whether it be the stiff skin and joint contractures of diabetic cheiroarthropathy and Dupuytren's contractures, or the 'frozen shoulder' of adhesive capsulitis. Articular conditions are generally characterized by osteoarthritis (primary or a consequence of impaired proprioception [neuropathic arthritis]) or metabolic perturbations (calcium pyrophosphate crystal deposition disease [CPPDD] and gout). Systemic manifestations include neuropathies, myopathies, osteopenia, hyperostosis and amyloidosis.

11.2 Pathophysiology

The pathophysiology of MS/rheumatic complications in diabetes is quite variable across these heterogeneous syndromes. Although it remains mostly speculative, certain observations merit comment. Cheiroarthropathy and limited joint mobility are unique to people with diabetes and presumably reflect pathways important in the underlying disease. Other MS manifestations, such as trigger finger and adhesive capsulitis, occur in the general population but are more common in people with diabetes; why this occurs is not known. Atherosclerosis and neuropathy are indeed associated with uncontrolled diabetes, which place patients with diabetes at increased risk of certain MS complications such as avascular necrosis, osteomyelitis, and the development of Charcot (neuropathic) joints.

Poor glycaemic control in patients with diabetes may affect quality and quantity of connective (soft) tissue. Sustained hyperglycaemia results in non-enzymatic glycation of proteins, including connective tissue proteins. Although this reaction is spontaneous, it depends on both the duration and degree of hyperglycaemia and the permeability of connective tissue proteins to glucose. Once collagen and connective tissue proteins become glycated, they may undergo further reactions that produce advanced glycation end-products (AGEs).[2] These abnormal connective tissue proteins have impaired structure and function and may contribute to stiffening of musculoskeletal tissue. This could be due to formation of protein cross-links and alterations in enzymatic activity; ligand binding and connective tissue half-life may also be influenced.[3] Moreover the AGEs (including glycosylated collagen) are antigenic and have been shown to induce an antibody-mediated reaction in connective tissue. AGEs are also capable of forming immune complexes that may be linked to atherosclerosis.[4]

In addition receptors for advanced glycation end-products (RAGEs) have been found on the cell surface of fibroblasts, smooth muscle cells, macrophages, endothelial cells and astrocytes. RAGEs can be stimulated by AGEs as well as some proinflammatory cytokines. Activation of these receptors is thought to cause oxidative stress as well as initiate proinflammatory signalling pathways that involve the production of cytokines, including interleukin-1 (IL-1), IL-6 and tumour necrosis factor (TNF). This environment can lead to tissue damage. AGEs and RAGEs have potential but still ill-defined roles in the pathophysiology of diabetic complications.

Finally, obesity is strongly associated with type 2 diabetes. For reasons that are not, obesity seems to be associated with enhanced basal inflammatory tone. Obese patients have excessive accumulation of adipose tissue, both subcutaneously and in skeletal muscle. Adipocytes had been thought to simply be a repository for storage of energy; however, they may play a larger role in the pathogenesis of a proinflammatory environment through the release of adipokines and the production of free fatty acids. Intramyocellular accumulation of lipids affects kinase signalling pathways, which confounds the response of skeletal muscle to insulin.[5] Thus, although there is clearly no unifying explanation for the MS manifestations of diabetes mellitus some understandings and speculation are possible.

11.3 Soft-tissue syndromes in patients with diabetes

Adhesive capsulitis (frozen shoulder)

Adhesive capsulitis describes stiffening of the glenohumeral joint. This condition is not unique to patients with diabetes although it is more common in the diabetic population; its incidence has been reported to be as high as 30 per cent. It occurs at a younger age in people with diabetes, can last longer and be more recalcitrant to therapy.[6] Adhesive capsulitis is poorly understood and probably best conceived as a syndrome reflecting primary, idiopathic problems or as a secondary complication from other shoulder diseases, and may evolve to the non-specific 'frozen shoulder' malady.

Adhesive capsulitis is associated with significant loss of active and passive range of motion, cause severe pain and thus can adversely affect quality of life. Patients typically develop gradual stiffness and pain over several months; pain is frequently nocturnal and patients are unable to lie on the involved shoulder. External rotation and abduction are usually limited. People with diabetes tend toward bilateral involvement.[7] Risk factors for the development of adhesive capsulitis in people with diabetes include disease duration and age.[6] In the evaluation of an adhesive capsulitis, plain radiographs should be obtained to exclude other causes of shoulder pain. The condition has been described as having three distinct phases: painful, adhesive and resolution phases. The problem is typically self-limited but can last months and, in people with diabetes, adhesive capsulitis can be more refractory to management. Conservative management includes pain control and physical therapy as tolerated. The benefit of subacromial or intra-articular shoulder injections remains controversial. In refractory cases, manipulation under anaesthesia has been considered.[6]

Limited joint mobility (diabetic cheiroarthropathy)

Limited joint mobility (LJM) or diabetic cheiroarthropathy uniquely involves the small joints of the hands of people with diabetes. The cause of LJM is unclear; it is probably multifactorial, with some possible underlying mechanisms including increased non-enzymatic glycosylation of collagen protein due to chronic hyperglycaemia, alterations in collagen cross-linking, leading to resistance to collagenase degradation, and altered collagen synthesis.[7,8] The end-result is increased collagen deposition in people with diabetes and this syndrome. Interestingly this appears to happen in periarticular collagen rather than articular collagen. Excess collagen deposition causes the skin on the dorsal aspect of the hand to become thickened, tight and waxy. Patients often complain of stiffness, loss of dexterity and weakness. Pain is variable and may be accompanied by paraesthesias. Flexion deformities also develop over the metacarpophalangeal and interphalangeal joints, manifested by the 'prayer sign' – an inability to fully approximate the palms together with the wrist in full flexion (Plate 11.1).[9] The condition is typically bilateral and, if contractures develop, they most often occur in the fifth digit.

LJM occurs most commonly in patients with type 1 diabetes, with an incidence approaching 50 per cent.[7] It is frequently encountered together with Dupuytren's contracture(s). Perhaps more important than the skin tightening and physical symptoms associated with LJM are the other associations noted in people with diabetes who have cheiroarthropathy – increased incidence of microvascular disease (proliferative retinopathy, nephropathy and neuropathy).[8] Indeed LJM may reflect microvascular disease, resulting in the increased formation of damaging oxygen free radicals.[8] As all these complications are thought to relate to poor diabetic control, management of LJM includes strict blood sugar control in addition to a programme of hand therapy. Corticosteroid injections have not played a major role in the management of LJM.

Trigger finger (flexor tenosynovitis)

Although not unique to people with diabetes, flexor tenosynovitis or trigger finger is a frequent diabetic complication of the hands. The estimated incidence is as high as 11 per cent in people with diabetes compared with less than 1 per cent in those who do not have diabetes.[7] It seems to be associated with the duration of diabetes and is thought to have the same pathogenesis as diabetic cheiroarthropathy.[7]

Flexor tenosynovitis is a fibrous tissue proliferation in the tendon sheath that leads to limitation of the normal movement of the tendon. For uncertain reasons, possibly due to repetitive use, the flexor tendon becomes irritated as it slides through the tendon sheath. Recurrent irritation causes the tendon to thicken and nodules may form, making its passage through the tendon sheath more difficult. Patients often complain of a catching sensation or 'locking' phenomenon when the affected finger is flexed. This may be associated with severe pain, especially when the finger is extended. Physical examination reveals a palpable nodule that is typically in the area overlying the metacarpophalangeal joint at the distal palmar crease. There is also thickening along the affected flexor tendon sheath on the palmer aspect of the finger. Frequently 'locking' or 'triggering' can be duplicated by passive or active flexion of the finger. With movement of the finger, the nodule can also be felt to move. Initial treatment usually involves instillation of corticosteroid injection into the tendon sheath. Alternatively topical anti-inflammatory medications, oral anti-inflammatory drugs and physical therapy with appropriate modalities may be beneficial. It is rare to refer such patients for surgical intervention.

Dupuytren's contracture

Dupuytren's contracture is a fibrotic disorder of the aponeurosis.[7,8] The palmar fascia of the hand insidiously and asymptomatically becomes thickened (Plate 11.2). Eventually patients experience joint stiffness and limited extension of the digits. As scarring of the palmar fascia progresses, nodules form and there are contractures of the digits at the metacarpophalangeal joints. Function and dexterity of the hand and fingers are lost. The underlying mechanism of Dupuytren's contracture is unclear, but the condition is associated with proliferation and disorder of fibroblasts, which presumably leads the clinical abnormalities. Dupuytren's contracture occurs more commonly in the diabetic population (up to 60%) and frequently involves the middle and ring fingers.

Dupuytren's contractures in people with diabetes tend to be less severe than in other populations. Risk factors for its development include duration of diabetes and age. Treatment involves strict glycaemic control, symptomatic therapies and a hand therapy programme; in sever refractory instances, surgical release can be performed.

Carpal tunnel syndrome

Carpal tunnel syndrome (CTS) is a painful neuropathic condition in which the median nerve becomes entrapped by the carpal ligament, and other structures in the carpal tunnel, as it passes through the wrist. The same mechanisms that cause LJM are postulated to cause CTS. Unlike LJM, CTS is related to disease duration, but not glycaemic control. Patients typically complain of pain and/or paraesthesias in the median nerve distribution of the hand. In rare circumstances, symptoms can radiate to the forearm. The pain and paraesthesias tend to be worse at night and can often wake patients from sleep when the nerve is inadvertently compressed. In more severe cases, patients complain of weakness or clumsiness when using the hands (such as frequently dropping objects, loss of hand dexterity, and difficulty buttoning clothes or turning keys or doorknobs).

Clinical signs may include weakness of thumb abduction and opposition and atrophy of the thenar eminence. Repetitive activities that involve flexing or extending the wrist (such as typing, driving or holding objects (book or telephone)) for prolonged periods can trigger symptoms. Physical examination will often reveal Tinel's and/or Phalen's signs. In severe instances, atrophy and weakness of the thenar muscles are observed. The diagnosis is usually established clinically; nerve conduction studies may be confirmatory or considered when findings are equivocal. The incidence of CTS in people with diabetes has been reported to be as high as 25 per cent, and it seems to be more common in women.[8] Treatment is initially conservative and involves anti-inflammatory agents, splinting and avoidance of provocative activities. Corticosteroids can be injected into the carpal tunnel; surgical intervention should be infrequent, and certainly not the initial therapy.

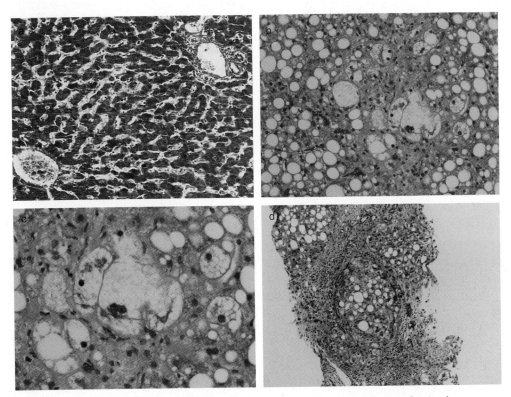

Plate 3.1 Non-alcoholic steatohepatitis histology. (a) Normal liver parenchyma; (b) simple macrovesicular steatosis; (c) a 'balloon' cell and (d) cirrhosis: a regenerative nodule of hepatocytes encapsulated by fibrous septa extending from portal tracts. (Courtesy of Dr Cynthia Guy, Duke University, Durham, NC, USA.)

Diabetes: Chronic Complications, Third Edition. Edited by Kenneth M. Shaw,
Michael H. Cummings.
© 2012 John Wiley & Sons, Ltd. Published 2012 by John Wiley & Sons, Ltd.

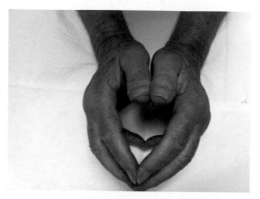

Plate 11.1 Illustration of the 'prayer' sign in the cheiroarthropathy of diabetes.

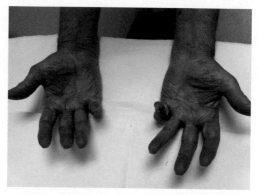

Plate 11.2 Dupuytren's contracture(s) in a patient with diabetes.

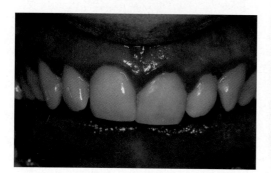

Plate 12.1 Gingivitis: 19-year-old patient with diabetes and gingivitis affecting the upper anterior dentition. Note that the gingival inflammation occupies the marginal 2–3 mm of the gingiva and follows the contour of the teeth. The interdental papillae (triangular areas of gingiva between the teeth) are swollen and inflamed.

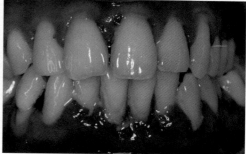

Plate 12.2 Periodontitis (clinical appearance): 22-year-old patient with diabetes and advanced periodontitis affecting the entire dentition. The lower anterior teeth in particular show many features of periodontitis: abnormal gingival anatomy due to tissue destruction, gingival recession, gingival swelling and inflammation, spontaneous bleeding and abundant plaque deposits.

11.4 Articular manifestations

Crystalline arthropathies

Crystalline-induced arthropathies are common in patients with diabetes. Hyperuricaemia often precedes the development of diabetes and may have a pathological role in the metabolic syndrome. Calcium pyrophosphate dehydrate deposition disease (CPPDDD) and diabetes have been associated in such conditions as haemochromatosis and acromegaly, where perturbations of insulin and/or insulin-like growth factor may be relevant.[10] In addition, syndromes associated with basic calcium phosphate (BCP) crystals, such as calcific tendonitis, are clearly associated with diabetes.[11] Similar calcific processes certainly occur in blood vessels of patients with diabetes as well as in spinal ligaments in diffuse idiopathic skeletal hyperostosis (DISH). Metabolic changes, consequent on chronic high glucose and insulin levels, may produce important changes in connective tissues that might predispose to pathological calcification. Soft-tissue calcifications and periarthritis seen in shoulder radiographs in people with diabetes are more likely to be symptomatic than in those without diabetes.

Osteoarthritis

Although it is not that diabetes predisposes generally to osteoarthritis, certain associations merit brief exposition. Obesity is a common risk factor for both osteoarthritis and diabetes although epidemiological studies teasing out relative risk contributions are difficult to interpret.[11] The high independent prevalence of diabetes and osteoporosis alone is enough to explain the overlap of disease states as being by chance. C-reactive protein (a quantitative marker of the acute phase response linked to atherosclerosis, obesity and diabetes) correlated with the development of osteoarthritis of the knee.[12] Also interesting is a possible association of diabetes and risk of developing hand osteoarthritis, which is obviously not influenced directly by weight strain. Significantly higher prevalence of hand osteoarthritis was noted in the subset of patients with a combination of overweight status, diabetes and hypertension. Further, this increased disease burden was noted in a relatively younger patient population.[13] Peripheral neuropathy, a common complication of diabetes, may also adversely affect joints and increase the risk of advanced, aggressive forms of osteoarthritis due to proprioceptive derangement (see next).[14]

Charcot arthropathy

Charcot arthropathy, a form of neuropathic arthropathy, is a serious complication of diabetes. It is characterized by fracture, joint derangement and subluxation of the affected joint in the presence of a significant sensory deficit. The end-result of this arthropathy is often obliteration of the joint space altogether. Charcot arthropathy typically affects the foot (less so the knee) in patients with diabetes and peripheral neuropathy. It can often mimic other joint conditions and invariably develops into a chronic arthritis with severe deformity and limitation of motion. Late stages are often complicated by refractory skin ulcers and may culminate in amputation.

Onset of arthropathy can also be difficult to ascertain, because swelling or warmth of the affected joint may be insidious or sudden. Invariably, patients with long history of poorly controlled diabetes are at higher risk, and most patients have unilateral disease. As a result of the implications of poor proprioception and impaired pain sensation, the arthropathy usually declares itself clinically after the major structural derangements have taken place.

Treatment options for Charcot arthropathy are limited. Non-weight bearing and immobilization of the affected limb are necessary. Intravenous and oral bisphosphonates, as well as intranasal calcitonin, have been recently tried for symptomatic care. Surgical interventions such as arthroplasty and fusion are deferred due to the impairment of proprioception, fear of asymmetrical wear, loosening and ultimately risk of infection in people with diabetes.

11.5 Systemic musculoskeletal conditions

Hyperostosis

Diffuse idiopathic skeletal hyperostosis is characterized by calcification and ossification of soft tissues, mainly ligaments and entheses.[15] The hallmark of DISH is asymmetrical hyperostosis jutting from the axial spine (Figure 11.1); however, these hyperostoses occur at peripheral entheses as well, distinguishing it from osteoarthritis. Although the aetiology of DISH is unknown, several metabolic factors may be associated with this condition, including diabetes, diabetic family history and obesity.[11,16] Prevalence of DISH in people with diabetes has been shown in one recent study to be 12.1 per cent, although not statistically different from the control group.[17] Patients' complaints range from being asymptomatic to suffering from significant pain at affected areas. Treatment is symptomatic and supportive.

Diabetic osteopenia

Osteoporosis in people with diabetes is of considerable concern. All people with diabetes have adynamic bone disease. Factors contributing to this are multiple, probably differ for types 1 and 2 disease, and may involve insulin and insulin-like growth factor I (IGF-I) pathways, accumulation of

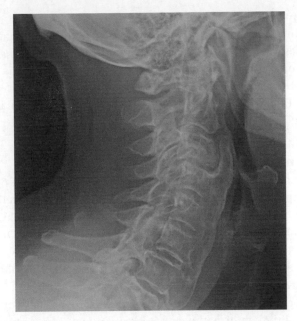

Figure 11.1 Diffuse idiopathic skeletal hyperostosis.

advanced glycation end-products and calcium metabolism. Age of onset of diabetes (i.e. in adolescence) may be important, because this affects peak bone mass. Some have found type 2 diabetes to be associated with increased bone mineral density (BMD). Bone fragility may contribute to fracture risk independent of BMD, and BMD may not reflect fracture risk in some individuals. Bone metabolism is also influenced by the late complications of diabetes (e.g. renal failure). The risk of fracture reflects other confounders – falling secondary to visual impairment, cerebrovascular disease or neuromuscular/MS disease. Localized bone loss related to diabetic neuropathy may increase the risk of fracture at the foot and ankle.[18]

Specific therapies too (e.g. thiazolidinediones) may influence fracture rates.[19]

Musculoskeletal infections

Osteomyelitis is a common MS morbidity in diabetes. It is usually located in the toes, metatarsal heads, calcaneus and malleoli of patients with diabetes. It is often associated with poor proprioception and uneven weight bearing. *Staphylococcus aureus* and streptococci are the most common organisms in soft-tissue infections. Cellulitis or pyomyositis can develop, with resultant infections of underlying tendons and bones, and/or septic arthritis. Diabetes is an important risk factor for pyogenic arthritis of the knee, hip or shoulder joints. Septic arthritis should be considered for any joint effusion in a person with diabetes, with careful and appropriate evaluation and examination of synovial fluid mandatory. Bone scanning has been for suspected bone and soft-tissue infections, but false-positive scans have limited the use of this method. Magnetic resonance imaging (MRI) appears to be quite sensitive and specific for diagnosing osteomyelitis and pyomyositis, and should be widely used in imaging diabetic foot problems.[7]

Diabetic muscle infarction

Diabetic muscle infarction is a rare complication of long-standing diabetes. Classic symptoms include abrupt onset of pain and local swelling of the lower extremity. The painful lesion usually persists for weeks, and may then spontaneously resolve over several weeks to months. Of note, half the patients have recurrent episodes. A muscle commonly affected is quadriceps, but calf muscles may be involved as well. This phenomenon is unrelated to atheroembolism or occlusion of major arteries. This is considered to be one of many of the micro- and macrovascular complications of diabetes, although its pathogenesis is not known. Muscle biopsy can be helpful in establishing the diagnosis, but histological findings are not specific. Features include large areas of muscle necrosis and oedema, regenerating muscle fibres, lymphocytic interstitial infiltration, and occlusion of arterioles and capillaries by fibrin.[20]

Other diagnostic possibilities – pyomyositis, gangrene, fasciitis, thrombosis and malignancy – must be thoughtfully considered. Clinicians should be alert to the diagnosis of diabetic muscle infarction in patients with established microangiopathy who present with an isolated painful muscle. T_2-weighted MRI is valuable for confirming the diagnosis.[21] MRI shows oedema in the affected muscles. Addition of gadolinium helps differentiate acute inflammation and infarction, but must be used judiciously in people with diabetes and impaired kidney function due to the risk of nephrogenic systemic fibrosis.

Treatment of diabetic muscle infarction includes restriction of the use of the affected muscle and administration of analgesics. Most patients experience spontaneous resolution, although recurrences are common. Those with recurrence or bilateral occurrences tend to have significant vascular complications of diabetes and therefore a poorer prognosis.

Diabetic amyotrophy

Diabetic amyotrophy is a disabling illness that is distinct from muscle infarction and diabetic neuropathy. It is characterized by acute or subacute asymmetrical muscle weakness and wasting, and by diffuse, proximal, lower limb muscle pain and asymmetrical loss of tendon jerks. The shoulder girdle may be affected, but less commonly. It typically occurs in older men with type 2 diabetes, and is often associated with weight loss, sometimes as much as 40 per cent of premorbid body mass. Cause and incidence of diabetic amyotrophy are uncertain. It is a diagnosis of exclusion; other explanations for weight loss and neurological signs and symptoms must be evaluated. Management focuses on glycaemic control and symptomatic/supportive therapy. Most patients improve, although this may be gradual and incomplete. Some studies suggested a putative role for immune-mediated inflammatory microvasculitis causing ischaemic damage of the nerves.[22] If so immunotherapies might be considered; no trials have been shown to support this hypothesis.

11.6 Concluding comments

Musculoskeletal/rheumatological complications add to the morbidity, and occasionally mortality, of patients with diabetes. Many of these are common and all are readily recognizable if considered. Most are manageable. Indeed several reflect pathophysiological factors inherent to the underlying diabetes. Attention to these will improve the lives of affected patients.

Case studies

Discussions about the case studies will be found in the chapter on multiple choice questions, under the section for Chapter 11.

Case study 1
A 56-year-old man, with 21 years of poorly controlled diabetes mellitus, was seen in the office complaining of 'arthritis'. He had 3 years of worsening joint pain, mainly in the wrists, fingers and left shoulder. He did not relate significant swelling of the hands or any warmth or redness. He reported 10 minutes of morning stiffness relieved with non-prescription non-steroidal anti-inflammatory drug (NSAID) use. On physical examination there was bilateral wrist as well as second and third metacarpophalangeal synovial thickening. He had bilateral fifth digit Dupuytren's contractures. Laboratory data showed serum glutamic–oxaloacetic transaminase 285 U/l, serum glutamic–pyruvic transaminase 350 U/l, haemoglobin 11.2 g%, uric acid 8.2 mg%, normal erythrocyte sedimentation rate and C-reactive protein levels, no antibodies to centromere or SCL-70 antigens or to cyclic citrullinated protein, negative test for rheumatoid factors, and ferritin level 2500 ng/ml. Radiographs of hands are shown in Figure 11.2.

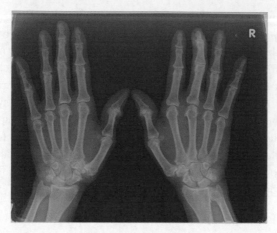

Figure 11.2 Hand films, case study 1. See main text for discussion.

Case study 2

A 58-year-old woman has been cared for by her primary care physician for type 2 diabetes that has not been ideally controlled. Her most recent HbA1c was 8.9 per cent. She worked as a baker and admitted that she was not compliant with her diet. She also consumed a glass of wine three times weekly. She was on maximum doses of oral diabetic medications, and her physician wished to start her on insulin. For the last 6 months, she complained of numbness in her toes. She has had numbness in her right hand for 2 months. She noted occasional difficulty grasping and gripping objects at home and at work. Physical examination was notable for loss of vibratory and pin-prick sensation; the grip strength in her right hand was diminished. There was no atrophy and Phalen's test was equivocal. Nerve conduction study showed slowing of sensory conduction across the wrist.

Case study 3

A 24-year-old graduate student with type 1 diabetes presented for urgent care for left shoulder pain. He used an insulin pump, and his sugar was well controlled. Shoulder pain began 2 months ago. He initially attributed the pain to naps on the couch in the student lounge. Sometimes he would awaken with neck soreness and pain radiating to the shoulder. It never spread down his arm. His shoulder ached, and he could no longer play basketball with his friends. There was no identifiable traumatic episode. Physical examination found normal range of motion of his neck and no tenderness or pain in the right arm. His left shoulder had severely limited range of motion with pain in all planes. He could abduct and flex to only 90°. There was normal sensation, and his distal muscle strength was not diminished. Deep tendon reflexes were normal. Radiographs of his left shoulder showed normal bone alignment, no fractures, and no abnormalities in the soft tissue.

References

1. Carias K, Panush RS. Acute arthritis. *Bull Rheum Dis* 1994;**43**(7):1–4.
2. Ahmed N. Advanced glycation endproducts – role in pathology of diabetic complications. *Diabet Res Clin Pract* 2005;**67**:3–21.
3. Rosenbloom AL, Silverstein JH. Connective tissue and joint disease in diabetes mellitus. *Endocrinol Metab Clin North Am* 1996;**25**:473–483.
4. Turk Z, Ljubic S, Turk N, Benko B. Detection of autoantibodies against advanced glycation endproducts and AGE immune complexes in serum of patients with diabetes mellitus. *Clin Chim Acta* 2002;**303**:105–115.
5. Nawrocki AR and Scherer PE. The delicate balance between fat and muscle: adipokines in metabolic disease and musculoskeletal inflammation. *Curr Opin Pharmacol* 2004;**4**:281–289.
6. Balci N, Balci MK, Tüzüner S. Shoulder adhesive capsulitis and shoulder range of motion in type II diabetes mellitus: association with diabetic complications. *J Diabet Complications* 1999;**13**:135–140.
7. Arkkila P, Gautier J. Musculoskeletal disorders in diabetes mellitus: an update. *Best Pract Res Clin Rheumatol* 2003;**17**:945–970.
8. Smith L, Burnet S, McNeil J. Musculoskeletal manifestations of diabetes mellitus. *Br J Sports Med* 2003;**37**:30–35.
9. Papanas N, Maltezos E. The diabetic hand: a forgotten complication? *J Diabet Complications* 2010;**24**:154–162.
10. Mavrikakis M, Drimis S, Kontoyannis D, et al. Calcific shoulder periarthritis (tendinitis) in adult onset diabetes mellitus: a controlled study. *Ann Rheum Dis* 1989;**48**: 211–214.
11. Burner TW, Rosenthal AK. Diabetes and rheumatic diseases. *Curr Opin Rheumatol* 2009;**21**:50–54.
12. Sowers M, Jannausch M, Stein E, Jamadar D, Hochberg M, Lachance L. C-reactive protein as a biomarker of emergent osteoarthritis. *Osteoarthr Cartilage* 2002;**10**: 595–601.
13. Dahaghin S, Bierma-Zeinstra S, Koes B, et al. Do metabolic factors add to the effect of overweight on hand osteoarthritis? The Rotterdam Study. *Ann Rheum Dis* 2007;**66**:916–920.
14. Shakoor M, Agrawal A, Block J. Reduced lower extremity vibratory perception in osteoarthritis of the knee. *Arthr Rheum* 2008;**59**:117–121.
15. Resnick D, Niwayama G. Radiographic and pathologic features of spinal involvement in diffuse idiopathic skeletal hyperostosis (DISH). *Radiology* 1976;**119**:559.
16. Mader R, Lavi I. Diabetes mellitus and hypertension as risk factors for early diffuse idiopathic skeletal hyperostosis (DISH). *Osteoarthr Cartilage* 2009;**17**:825–828.
17. Sencan D, Elden H, Nacitarhan V, Sencan E, Kaptanoglu E. The prevalence of diffuse idiopathic skeletal hyperostosis in patients with diabetes mellitus. *Rheumatol Int* 2005;**25**:518–521.
18. Hordon LD. Bone disease in diabetes mellitus. *UpToDate* 2010;19.2.
19 Yaturo, S. Diabetes and skeletal health. *J Diabet* 2009;**1**:246–254.
20. Rocca PV, Alloway JA, Nashel DJ. Diabetic muscular infarction. *Semin Arthr Rheum* 1993;**22**:280–287.
21. Chow KM, Szeto CC, Griffith JF, Wong TY, Li PK. Unusual muscle pain in two patients with diabetic renal failure. *Hong Kong Med J* 2002;**8**:368–371.
22. Chan YC, Lo YL, Chan ES. Immunotherapy for diabetic amyotrophy. *Cochrane Database Syst Rev* 2009;(3):CD006521.

CHAPTER 12

Diabetes and Oral Health

Philip M Preshaw
School of Dental Sciences and Institute of Cellular Medicine, Newcastle University, UK

 Key points

- Oral complications commonly associated with diabetes include periodontal disease, xerostomia, dental caries and candidiasis.

- The risk for periodontitis is increased approximately threefold in patients with diabetes compared with those without.

- The inflammation associated with periodontitis can have a negative impact on glycaemic control.

- Dry mouth can be a major problem in diabetes and greatly increases the risk for dental caries and candidiasis.

- Liaison with the dental health-care team is essential for providing patient-centred care for people with diabetes.

 Therapeutic key points

- All patients with diabetes should be questioned about their oral health and access to dental care.

- Assessment of oral health status by visual inspection of the oral cavity should form part of routine diabetes management.

- Patients with diabetes should be informed about their increased risk for oral complications and appropriate referrals made to the dental health-care team.

- Treatment of periodontitis can lead to improvements in glycaemic control, with estimated mean HbA1c reductions of approximately 0.4 per cent.

- Patients with diabetes who smoke should be strongly counselled to quit smoking because it is a major risk factor for oral diseases.

- Fluoride therapy, antiseptic mouth rinses and artificial salivas are indicated in the management of patients with xerostomia.

- Candidiasis is a common problem in patients with diabetes, requiring joint management with the dental team.

Diabetes: Chronic Complications, Third Edition. Edited by Kenneth M. Shaw, Michael H. Cummings.
© 2012 John Wiley & Sons, Ltd. Published 2012 by John Wiley & Sons, Ltd.

12.1 Introduction

Just as the eyes are the window to the soul, the mouth is the window to the rest of the body – that is to say, medical practitioners would benefit from regularly looking into their patients' mouths because many systemic conditions have oral manifestations that may be the first signs of disease. Pharmaceuticals routinely prescribed for management of systemic diseases may have an adverse effect on the health or functioning of the mouth. Oral conditions (specifically periodontal diseases) may increase the risk for a variety of chronic diseases such as diabetes, and possibly also cardiovascular disease and adverse pregnancy outcomes. Oral health has a significant impact on quality of life, and therefore asking patients about their oral health and access to oral health care, together with briefly assessing oral status, should form part of the routine assessment of diabetes patients. For many years, medical practitioners have tended to focus primarily on the rest of the body and ignored the mouth. At the same time, dental practitioners have tended to view the mouth in isolation from the rest of the body. There is now increased awareness that good general health is not possible without good oral health, and this observation should lead to more integrated management of patients by medical and dental healthcare teams. People with diabetes are at increased risk for various oral conditions, particularly periodontal diseases, but also xerostomia, dental caries, dental abscesses and candidiasis.

12.2 Epidemiology of periodontal diseases

Periodontal diseases are highly prevalent, and collectively are the most common diseases known to humans. Classification systems for periodontal diseases are complex and take into account the clinical presentation, rate of disease progression, age at diagnosis, and systemic and local factors that may increase risk. In very broad terms, periodontal diseases can be divided into gingivitis and periodontitis.

Gingivitis

Gingivitis is extremely prevalent, affecting (at least to some degree) the great majority of the UK population. The most common form, *chronic gingivitis*, is plaque-induced inflammation of the gingiva (the gum, specifically that part of the gum that is visible in the oral cavity and wraps, collar like, around the tooth). The condition is usually painless and characterized by gingival erythema and oedema, and increased tendency to bleed (bleeding may be on brushing, flossing or eating, or may occur spontaneously). Gingivitis is entirely reversible after professional cleaning (by a dentist or dental hygienist) together with improved self-performed oral hygiene by the patient. The 1998 UK Adult Dental Health Survey revealed that 72 per cent of dentate adults had visible plaque on their teeth, with on average third of all teeth affected.[1] Similarly, 73 per cent of adults had visible calculus (mineralized plaque deposits), indicating the long-term presence of plaque in the mouths of most UK adults.

Periodontitis

Periodontitis is a much more serious condition, characterized by break-down of the attachment between the gingiva and the tooth, creating a *periodontal pocket*, or space, between the gingiva and the tooth. In contrast to gingivitis, periodontitis affects all the supporting structures of the teeth, including the gingiva, periodontal ligament and alveolar bone (that part of the jaws supporting the teeth). Pocketing is not usually evident on visual inspection, so careful dental examination using a probe to measure the depth of the pockets is an essential part of assessment, routinely performed by dentists and dental hygienists. The condition is slowly progressing, but the tissue damage that occurs is largely irreversible. The pockets deepen as a result of destruction of fibres of the periodontal ligament (referred to as 'loss of attachment') and resorption of alveolar bone, leading to increased tooth mobility and, ultimately, tooth loss. The most common form is *chronic periodontitis* (often referred to simply as 'periodontitis' or 'periodontal disease').

Signs and symptoms include gingival erythema and oedema, gingival bleeding, gingival recession (making patients appear 'long in the tooth'), tooth mobility, drifting of teeth, widening of spaces between teeth, sensitivity (as a result of gingival recession exposing the sensitive tooth root), suppuration from periodontal pockets and tooth loss. Pain (other than tooth sensitivity) is not normally a feature. According to the 1998 UK Adult Dental Health Survey, 43 per cent of UK adults had moderate periodontitis (loss of attachment ≥4 mm) and 8 per cent had severe periodontitis (loss of attachment ≥6 mm).[1] Epidemiological studies conducted in different populations around the world indicate that approximately 10–15 per cent of adults are likely to have severe periodontitis, i.e. periodontitis that is advanced enough to threaten tooth loss. This reflects the extremely high prevalence of this common, and largely hidden, chronic inflammatory disease. Furthermore, periodontitis has negative and profound impacts on many aspects of daily living, affecting confidence, social interactions and food choices.[2] This can be important in diabetes management because it can be more difficult to eat a healthy diet rich in fresh fruit and vegetables if there are many mobile teeth.

Diabetes increases the risk for periodontitis approximately threefold when compared with individuals who do not have diabetes.[3] The level of glycaemic control is a major factor in determining increased risk. In the US National Health and Nutrition Examination (NHANES) III survey, adults with HbA1c >9 per cent had a significantly higher prevalence of severe periodontitis than those without diabetes (odds ratio = 2.90; 95% confidence interval [CI]: 1.40, 6.03) after controlling for age, ethnicity, education, gender and smoking.[4] Most research has focused on the links between type 2 diabetes and periodontal disease, probably because both conditions have tended to develop in patients in their 40s and 50s. However, type 1 diabetes also increases the risk for periodontitis and all patients with diabetes (including children and young adults) should be considered to be at increased risk for periodontal disease. It is important to note that a *two-way relationship* has been observed between diabetes and periodontal disease: not only is risk for periodontitis increased in patients with diabetes, but the prevalence of diabetes in patients with periodontitis is approximately double that seen in non-periodontitis patients (12.5% vs 6.3% in the NHANES III survey).[5]

12.3 Pathophysiology of periodontitis

Periodontitis is a chronic inflammatory condition of the supporting struc-tures of the teeth (gingiva, periodontal ligament, alveolar bone). The inflammation is induced by bacteria in the subgingival biofilm (i.e. plaque in the periodontal pocket). In response to the antigenic challenge, an immune inflammatory response develops in the gingival tissues, leading to the visible signs of erythema, oedema and increased tendency to bleed. The inflammation is characterized by upregulated production of proin-flammatory cytokines (including, but not limited to, interleukin [IL]-1β, IL-6, tumour necrosis factor [TNF]-α), prostanoids (such as prostaglandin [PG] E_2) and destructive enzymes including the matrix metalloproteinases (MMPs), notably MMP-8 and MMP-9 (derived primarily from infiltrating neutrophils). A dense cellular infiltrate develops (Figure 12.1), leading to collagen breakdown and collagen-depleted zones in the gingival tissues, and proliferation of the epithelium in an apical direction (i.e. along the tooth surface in the direction of the root) in an attempt to maintain an intact epithelial barrier. This results in the pocket becoming fractionally deeper, and creates an environmental niche that is favoured by more pathogenic species in the subgingival biofilm which exacerbate and per-petuate the inflammation in the tissues.

Neutrophils, macrophages and lymphocytes infiltrate into the tissues in an attempt to eradicate the bacterial challenge, but are never completely successful in this role because the bacteria persist in the periodontal pocket. A chronic cycle is established in which the long-term presence of the

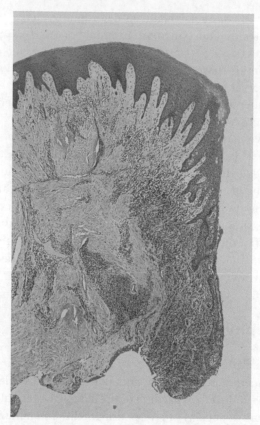

Figure 12.1 Histology of periodontal inflammation. In this section of inflamed gingiva, the tooth would be at the right edge of the slide, contacting the soft tissues. Note the infiltration of connective tissues by numerous (dark-staining) defence cells, leading to breakdown of collagen. The epithelium is proliferating into collagen-depleted areas to maintain an intact epithelial barrier. Blood vessels are dilated, there is vascular proliferation and the gingival tissues are swollen.

subgingival biofilm drives the inflammatory response, characterized by infiltration by defence cells and upregulation of inflammatory mediators and destructive enzymes, leading to the tissue damage observed in periodontitis. As the pocket deepens, the inflammation spreads to affect the periodontal ligament, resulting in the breakdown of collagen fibres and loss of attachment between the tooth and its supporting apparatus. Osteoclastic activity is enhanced, resulting in resorption of alveolar bone. Ultimately, the teeth start to become mobile, which for many patients is the first sign of disease.

Susceptible patients are those for whom a given bacterial challenge results in a dysregulated or inappropriate inflammatory response. All people have bacteria in their mouths, and most have plaque on their teeth.

Yet, not all people have periodontitis. Although the condition is *initiated* by the bacterial challenge, it is *caused* by the inflammation that subsequently develops in the periodontal tissues. Periodontitis is a chronic inflammatory disease that develops in susceptible individuals, and is not just a condition associated with poor self-care or poor oral hygiene. Susceptible patients have been shown to have upregulated inflammatory responses to bacterial challenge, resulting in more tissue damage for a given plaque challenge. Dentists now realize that successful management of this disease is as much about managing inflammation as it is about improving oral hygiene.

The mechanisms by which diabetes increases the risk for periodontitis are similar to those that are involved in the classic macro- and microvascular complications of diabetes.[3] There is no strong evidence to suggest that the subgingival microflora is any different in individuals with diabetes compared with those without, supporting that the increased risk for periodontitis in diabetes is due to altered immune-inflammatory responses. Hyperglycaemia alters tissue homeostasis and the balance of inflammatory networks in the periodontium, leading to upregulation of inflammatory responses and increased tissue damage.[6] A number of mechanisms have been identified that are likely to link the pathogenesis of diabetes and periodontitis, including:

- Diabetes results in impaired neutrophil function (adherence, chemotaxis, phagocytosis) and delayed apoptosis, leading to persistence of neutrophils in the inflamed tissues, with more opportunity for release of destructive enzymes and mediators, leading to increased tissue damage.
- Patients with diabetes may have a hyper-responsive monocyte/macrophage phenotype, leading to significantly increased production of proinflammatory cytokines and mediators.
- Formation of advanced glycation end-products (AGEs) occurs in the periodontium as it does elsewhere in the body of patients with diabetes, leading to activation of macrophages via their receptor for AGEs and subsequent release of proinflammatory mediators.
- Production of MMPs increases in diabetes.
- Patients with diabetes who are obese have higher circulating levels of adipokines, notably leptin, which is proinflammatory and could contribute to elevated tissue damage.

12.4 Management of periodontitis

Diagnosis and clinical investigation

Diagnosis of periodontitis is made after detailed assessment of the extent of tissue damage. This involves careful probing (measuring) of the pockets at six sites around every tooth, supplemented with radiographic investigation of alveolar bone destruction. These assessments are routinely performed by dentists and dental hygienists, and are clearly not part of the day-to-day work of medical practitioners. Nevertheless, there is much that the medical practitioner can do to assess the periodontal health of their patients with diabetes.

History

Ask patients about their oral health. Do they realize that diabetes increases their risk for periodontitis? If not, inform them. Do they have access to dental care? Do they have any pain? Do they have bleeding gums or mobile teeth? Does their bite feel different (e.g. as a result of loose teeth)? Do they have bad taste/bad breath (indicating plaque and/or suppuration)? Do they have any other oral problems?

Look in the mouth

A tongue spatula and pen torch are certainly sufficient for a quick visual inspection of the oral cavity. Look at the gums as well as the teeth. Look for evidence of redness and swelling affecting the gingival tissues, because these are signs of gingivitis (Plate 12.1). Look for gum recession and mobile teeth (signs of periodontitis). Despite the fact that periodontitis is usually painless, the signs of disease can be easy to spot in a brief examination, and patients may have long been aware of problems with their gums but have chosen to ignore them. Plate 12.2 shows the appearance of a 22-year-old patient with type 1 diabetes and severe periodontitis (also discussed as the Case study). The radiographic appearance of another patient with periodontitis, demonstrating extensive alveolar bone loss, is shown in Figure 12.2.

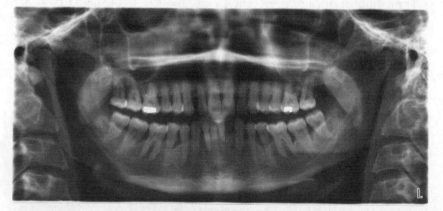

Figure 12.2 Periodontitis (radiographic appearance): 29-year-old patient with diabetes and extensive alveolar bone loss (generally 50–75% of the root length) affecting the entire dentition. The lower left lateral incisor has already spontaneously exfoliated (note the gap).

There are no specific laboratory tests for periodontitis. The diagnosis is made based on signs and symptoms (with detailed classification made after consideration of factors such as age, rate of progression and presence of risk factors). The medical practitioner will be unlikely to make a specific periodontal diagnosis, but should be able to identify gingivitis and periodontitis in most cases after visual inspection alone.

Treatment of periodontitis

Periodontal treatment is multifaceted and led by the dental team. However, the medical practitioner continues to have a vital role to play, particularly for patients with diabetes. Management of periodontitis includes the following.

Patient education, motivation and empowering

Patients have a major responsibility for managing *their* periodontitis (similar to how they have a major responsibility for managing *their* diabetes). Dentists and dental hygienists expend considerable energy in patient education, to optimize compliance and oral hygiene.

Oral hygiene instruction

The subgingival plaque bacteria perpetuate the inflammation in the periodontal tissues. Therefore, reducing the bacterial challenge by improving plaque control is a cornerstone of periodontal therapy. A variety of specialized brushes are used to clean around and between teeth, and below the gum line into the subgingival environment.

Root surface debridement (RSD)

This is a technical procedure, typically using ultrasonic instruments (Figure 12.3) to disrupt the subgingival biofilm and remove plaque and calculus. Most patients require episodes of instrumentation on a regular basis for life, interspersed by periods of maintenance care (e.g. appointments every 3 months for repeated instrumentation).

Inflammation management

Periodontitis is an inflammatory disease, and systemic pharmaceuticals are being developed to reduce inflammation in the periodontal tissues. One drug has been licensed to date, low-dose doxycycline (20 mg twice daily for 12 weeks) as an adjunct to RSD to exploit the inhibitory effect of doxycycline on MMPs without exerting antibiotic effects or leading to development of antibiotic resistance.[7] Low-dose doxycycline is not a monotherapy and must be used as an adjunct to RSD to derive clinical benefit. (Non-steroidal anti-inflammatory drugs [NSAIDs] are not indicated in the management of periodontitis due to the risk of unwanted effects and the requirement to take these agents for many years for only slight benefit.)

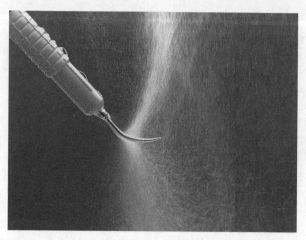

Figure 12.3 Ultrasonic scaler: the tip of this instrument vibrates at ultrasonic frequencies (30–50 kHz) and is moved across the root surface to disrupt the subgingival biofilm and remove calculus. Water spray keeps the tip cool.

Risk factor management

Smoking is the other major risk factor for periodontitis (besides diabetes). Smoking cessation forms a central component of management for all patients with periodontitis, and particularly those with diabetes. Smokers are at increased risk for development and progression of periodontitis, and treatment outcomes are impaired in those who continue to smoke. The relative risk for periodontitis in smokers varies from 1.4 to 5.0 in different research studies, with the median being 2.0.[8] The patient with diabetes who also smokes is therefore at hugely increased risk for periodontitis.

Periodontal surgery

This is not a routine treatment for periodontitis, but may be indicated in specific cases, e.g. to improve access to root surfaces for cleaning, or techniques attempting to regenerate lost bone in specific clinical situations.

It should be noted that systemic antibiotics are rarely indicated in the management of periodontitis (notwithstanding the use of low-dose doxycycline as an MMP inhibitor rather than having antibiotic efficacy at this dose). The use of systemic antibiotics in the treatment of chronic periodontitis provides no clear benefits, and runs the risk of adverse drug reactions and selection of antibiotic-resistant organisms. A large number of bacterial species (typically >300) can be found in the mouth of patients with periodontitis, and key pathogens include *Porphyromonas gingivalis, Aggregatibacter actinomycetemcomitans, Treponema denticola, Fusobacterium nucleatum, Prevotella intermedia, Tannerella forsythia,* to name but a few. It is not possible to do culture and sensitivity testing for periodontal bacteria because many of the implicated pathogens cannot be cultured. Systemic antibiotics are indicated only in specific clinical situations (e.g. necrotizing ulcerative gingivitis, necrotizing ulcerative periodontitis, some presentations of aggressive periodontitis) and should be used only together with RSD.

Prevention of periodontitis is much better than treating the disease once it has developed. The condition can be prevented from developing, and this requires the patient to commit to regular dental attendance for monitoring and professional tooth cleaning as well as maintaining excellent oral hygiene. The condition is usually painless, and most patients present late, by which time significant destruction of the periodontal tissues may have already occurred. For this reason, all patients diagnosed with diabetes should be warned about their increased risk for periodontitis. If all newly diagnosed patients with diabetes received prompt dental assessment, there is no doubt that much of the periodontitis that subsequently might develop could be prevented. Patients with diabetes should therefore be asked about their dental health, briefly examined, informed about their increased risk for periodontitis and referred for assessment by the dental team.

The potential benefits of treating periodontitis in the patient with diabetes

The impact of periodontal treatment on glycaemic control continues to be investigated by research groups around the world. A meta-analysis conducted by the Cochrane Collaboration in 2010 identified that the mean reduction in HbA1c in patients with diabetes 3–4 months after conventional periodontal treatment (i.e. RSD + oral hygiene instruction) versus no treatment was 0.40 per cent (95% CI: 0.01, 0.78).[9] However, it was noted that there are few studies available, and individual studies lacked the power to detect a significant effect. Another meta-analysis of 9 studies involving 485 patients with diabetes after periodontal treatment identified a similar standardized mean reduction in HbA1c of 0.46 per cent (95% CI: 0.11, 0.82).[10] Treatment of periodontal disease could also reduce the risk of other diabetes complications, e.g. it has been shown in a population with a high prevalence of diabetes and periodontal disease that periodontitis was a significant predictor of development of both nephropathy (2.6 times the incidence of macroalbuminuria in patients with severe periodontitis compared with control individuals) and end-stage renal disease (ESRD) (4.9 times the incidence of ESRD compared with control individuals).[11]

12.5 Other common oral complications of diabetes

A number of other oral conditions are commonly found in patients with diabetes, including xerostomia and salivary gland dysfunction, dental caries, oral candidiasis and dental abscesses.

Xerostomia and salivary gland dysfunction

Dry mouth and salivary hypofunction are common complaints for patients with diabetes. This may be due to dehydration as a result of polyuria, or in long-standing cases to microvascular damage and neuropathy affecting the major salivary glands. The problems of dry mouth can be compounded by medications that further contribute to reduced salivary flow (antihypertensives, diuretics, antidepressants, anxiolytics). Saliva is immensely important for protection against oral diseases and, when the normal environment of the oral cavity is altered because of decreased salivary flow and/or composition, the patient becomes particularly susceptible to increased plaque accumulation, fungal infections and dental caries. Soft-tissue manifestations of xerostomia include dry, atrophic and cracked mucosa, mucositis, ulcers and desquamation. Impaired masticatory function may develop, and may contribute to impaired nutritional intake. Taste impairment can particularly affect the sweet taste sensation, leading patients to favour sweet, sugary foods. Swallowing is more difficult in patients with xerostomia, and breakdown of carbohydrates in the oral cavity is impaired due to lack of availability of salivary amylase.

Patients with diabetes may occasionally present with sialosis (or sialadenosis), a non-neoplastic, non-inflammatory, recurrent, bilateral swelling of salivary glands. Usually, the parotid glands are affected, and the condition is commonly asymptomatic. Salivary flow may be reduced and autonomic innervation may be disrupted. Sialosis is associated with diabetes, malnutrition, liver cirrhosis, alcoholism, bulimia and HIV infection. Treatment focuses on controlling the underlying systemic disease as a means of minimizing gland enlargement.

There are numerous treatment options for dry mouth, including simple remedies (being well hydrated, taking frequent sips of water, sucking ice cubes, chewing sugar-free gum, using a humidifier next to the bed, not smoking, avoiding alcohol), artificial salivas and systemic treatments (i.e. pilocarpine, a cholinergic stimulant, which is indicated for xerostomia after irradiation or Sjögren's syndrome, but is not normally indicated in patients with diabetes). For all patients with dry mouth, fluoride is essential to reduce the risk of dental caries (the topical action of fluoride on enamel is more important than the systemic effect). Duraphat toothpaste contains 2800 or 5000 ppm (parts per million) fluoride (compared with around 1000 ppm in most fluoridated toothpastes) and can be prescribed, as can FluoriGard gel (0.4% stannous fluoride). Both are useful in patients with xerostomia. Sodium lauryl sulphate (SLS), a constituent of many toothpastes, can contribute to a sensation of dryness of the mucosa, so SLS-free pastes (e.g. Pronamel, Biotene Dry Mouth toothpaste and some Sensodyne formulations) can be helpful.

Prescribing an artificial saliva is a complex task. As can be seen from Table 12.1, there are a variety of preparations available. In broad terms, they can be divided into those that are based on mucin (typically porcine gastric mucin) and those that are based on carboxymethylcellulose. Patient acceptability is a key factor, and many patients may not want to use a mucin-based product. There is no clear consensus about which product is best for a given clinical situation, and patients may need to try a number of products before settling on one that works for them. For patients with remaining natural teeth, artificial salivas with an acidic pH lower than that required for enamel demineralization (pH 5.5) or dentine demineralization (pH 6.0–6.5) are contraindicated, because these would increase the risk for tooth decay. Unfortunately, information on the pH of many products is not readily available. Ideally, a saliva substitute should enhance remineralization and inhibit demineralization, and should therefore have a neutral rather than an acidic pH, contain fluoride and be supersaturated with calcium and phosphate.[12] Given the complexities of artificial saliva formulations and their indications in different clinical situations, liaising with the dental team is essential.

Dental caries

Dental caries is not a specific complication of diabetes, but dry mouth greatly increases the risk for caries as a result of loss of the remineralizing and buffering properties of saliva and increased plaque accumulation. Root caries (as opposed to enamel caries) is common in patients with xerostomia, and patients who were caries free for much of their life may present with widespread devastating caries lesions (Figure 12.4). Dental caries has been reported to be a particular problem in older patients with poorly controlled diabetes. Prevention is essential, and patients with diabetes should be using topical fluoride treatment (mouth rinses, gels, pastes) on a daily basis. The medical practitioner has a key role in advising patients with dry mouth about their increased risk for caries and recommending use of over-the-counter (OTC) products containing fluoride as well as referral for dental management.

Oral candidiasis

Oral candidiasis is an opportunistic infection that is often associated with hyperglycaemia and is commonly found in patients with poorly controlled diabetes. The causative organism is typically *Candida albicans*, a commensal resident of the oral cavity that overgrows in situations of reduced salivary flow and compromised immune responses. In broad terms, treatment of oral candidiasis includes improving oral hygiene and denture hygiene, removing local risk factors (e.g. leaving dentures out at night or constructing new dentures) and antifungals.

Table 12.1 Summary of artificial saliva products available in the UK

Product	Formulations	Constituents	pH neutral?	Fluoride containing?	Use
AS Saliva Orthana	Oral spray	Spray: porcine gastric mucin, xylitol, NaF	Y	Y	Spray on to oral mucosa as required
	Lozenges	Lozenges: porcine gastric mucin, xylitol	Y	N	Lozenges: suck one as required
Biotene Oralbalance	Gel	Lactoperoxidase, lactoferrin, lysozyme, glucose oxidase, xylitol	Y	N	Apply to oral mucosa as required
BioXtra	Gel	Lactoperoxidase, lactoferrin, lysozyme, whey colostrum, xylitol	Y	N	Apply to oral mucosa as required
Glandosane[a]	Aerosol spray	Carmellose sodium,[b] sorbitol, KCl, NaCl, MgCl$_2$, CaCl$_2$, dipotassium hydrogen phosphate	N	N	Spray on to oral mucosa as required
Luborant	Oral spray	Carmellose sodium, sorbitol, dibasic potassium phosphate, KCl, CaCl$_2$, MgCl$_2$, NaF	Y	Y	Spray on to oral mucosa as required
Salinum	Liquid	Linseed extract with dipotassium phosphate buffer (sugar free)	Y	N	Rinse approx. 2 ml around mouth and swallow as required
Saliveze	Oral spray	Carmellose sodium, CaCl$_2$, MgCl$_2$, KCl, NaCl, dibasic sodium phosphate	Y	N	Spray on to oral mucosa as required
Salivix[a]	Pastilles	Acacia, malic acid (sugar-free)	N	N	Suck one pastille as required
SST[b] (saliva-stimulating tablets)	Tablets	Citric acid, malic acid, sorbitol (sugar free)	N	N	Dissolve one tablet in mouth as required
Xerotin	Oral spray	Carmellose, sorbitol, KCl, NaCl, MgCl$_2$, CaCl$_2$, potassium phosphate	Y	N	Spray on to oral mucosa as required

[a]Not indicated in dentate patients because product is acidic.
[b]Sodium carboxymethylcellulose.
Source: *British National Formulary.*

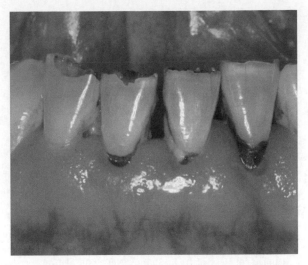

Figure 12.4 Root caries and xerostomia: 57-year-old patient with diabetes and xerostomia and root caries. Note the dry appearance of the ventral surface of the tongue (visible behind the teeth), abundant plaque deposits, gingival recession affecting three of the four lower incisors, and the dark appearance of root caries in the recession defects. There is also tooth wear (attrition) and caries affecting the incisal edges of the teeth. (Image courtesy of Professor AWG Walls, Newcastle, UK.)

The most easily recognized form is acute pseudomembranous candidiasis (thrush – Figure 12.5). This presents as diffuse white plaques that can be easily wiped off, leaving a red, raw surface, and usually affects the tongue, buccal mucosa and soft palate. Diagnosis is usually made based on clinical findings alone, although microbiological testing can be used to confirm. It should be noted, however, that a positive swab for *Candida albicans* in the absence of clinical signs does not indicate infection. Topical antifungals such as nystatin are usually sufficient to achieve resolution (100 000 units four times daily, continued for 2 weeks after resolution of signs and symptoms). In severe cases, systemic antifungals may be indicated (e.g. fluconazole 7–14 days, 50 mg/day). Chlorhexidine rinse (0.2%) is also effective against *Candida* spp. and helps control plaque and gingivitis.

Other common presentations include angular cheilitis and denture stomatitis (often occurring together). Angular cheilitis is a painful condition affecting the commissures of the lips, which appear red, fissured and sometimes ulcerated, with discomfort limiting mouth opening. It is predisposed by nutritional deficiency, over-closing of the mouth as a result of worn-down denture teeth (new dentures are usually indicated) and high sucrose intake. Denture stomatitis (chronic atrophic candidiasis) is the most common form of chronic candidiasis, and is caused by *Candida*

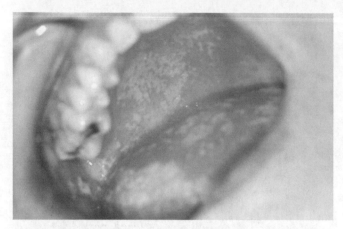

Figure 12.5 Acute pseudomembranous candidiasis: distinctive white plaques (easily removable with gauze) affecting the hard and soft palate, dorsum of tongue and buccal mucosa. (Image courtesy of Dr K. Staines, Newcastle, UK.)

spp. located on the fitting surface of dentures, particularly when the dentures are worn at night and/or are ill-fitting. Presentation ranges from pinpoint areas of erythema in the hard palate at the openings of the minor salivary glands to diffuse erythema of the entire denture-bearing area. Antifungal treatment of both the tissues and the denture base can help, but usually dentures need to be re-made to correct the problem.

Chronic hyperplastic candidiasis is another presentation of candidal infection, and represents chronic mucosal infection by *Candida* spp. Poor oral hygiene, trauma (e.g. smoking, denture wearing) and xerostomia are predisposing factors, and lesions are typically located at the commissures of the buccal mucosa. The lesions present with a raised red border and a whitish pebbly surface, and cannot be peeled off (unlike acute pseudomembranous candidiasis). Biopsy is required for diagnosis. Systemic antifungals and correction of local factors may solve the problem. Patients should be carefully monitored because this condition is considered potentially malignant.

Dental abscesses

Individuals with diabetes are more susceptible to infections in general, including those in the oral cavity. Dental abscesses may be a presenting finding in patients with underlying untreated dental disease. It is important to distinguish between localized dental abscesses that can be easily managed with routine dental procedures, and rapidly spreading infections with evidence of cellulitis and tissue necrosis. The latter can be very serious, with spread into the tissue spaces in the neck and compromised airway. Patients are typically pyrexial and seriously ill. In a patient with diabetes, this can be of particular concern due to increased risk of hypogly-caemia and ketosis. Sadly, there are a small number of deaths each year in the UK associated with rapidly spreading infections of dental origin, and rapid admission and aggressive management with intravenous antibiotics is required.

The two most common forms of localized dental abscesses are periodon-tal and periapical abscesses. Periodontal abscesses most commonly occur in patients with untreated periodontitis, and present as a fluctuant swell-ing in the gingival tissues, often with suppuration from the gingival margin. There is well-localized pain that is intensified if the overlying tissues are compressed or pressure is applied to the tooth. Treatment should focus on drainage (ideally through the periodontal pocket rather than an incision over the swelling), localized periodontal therapy and improved plaque control. Antibiotics are usually not required unless drainage cannot be achieved and/or there is evidence of pyrexia or lym-phadenopathy. In such cases, amoxicillin 250 mg three times daily for 5 days is indicated or, alternatively, metronidazole 400 mg three times daily for 5 days.

Periapical abscesses are usually a late presentation of dental caries that has extended to involve the pulp of the tooth, or are a consequence of loss of vitality (i.e. pulp necrosis). Symptoms include acute pain that is made worse by biting on the affected tooth, and a sinus tract may develop with a sinus opening in the alveolar mucosa. Treatment is usually a choice between extraction and root filling (root canal treatment). Systemic anti-biotics are not usually indicated because local management (extraction or commencing endodontic treatment) almost always eliminates the symp-toms, but, if treatment cannot be started, then systemic antibiotics can be prescribed as above.

12.6 Impact of periodontitis on other systemic diseases

Associations have been identified between periodontitis and a number of systemic diseases in addition to diabetes, including adverse pregnancy outcomes, cardiovascular disease and stroke, and pulmonary disease.[13]

Adverse pregnancy outcomes
Data in the literature either support or refute associations between adverse pregnancy outcomes (preterm, low-birthweight babies) and maternal peri-odontitis. The proposed mechanism is that bacteria in the subgingival biofilm gain access to the systemic circulation via the inflamed epithelial pocket lining, and/or inflammatory mediators produced in the periodontal

tissues (cytokines, prostaglandins) enter the systemic circulation and trigger an inflammatory cascade in the uterus, leading to premature delivery. More research is needed in this area. Periodontal treatment is safe in pregnant mothers, and those with signs of periodontal disease should be referred for dental management.

Cardiovascular disease and stroke

Atherosclerosis is an inflammatory condition, and periodontitis is associated with upregulated systemic inflammation, with evidence of elevated C-reactive protein (CRP), fibrinogen and serum cytokines in patients with periodontal disease. Periodontal bacteria have been identified in atherosclerotic plaques, and may induce inflammation in the vessel walls. A number of early reports indicated strong associations between periodontal disease and cardiovascular disease, but many of these studies failed to adequately account for shared risk factors, primarily smoking. Recent studies have identified more modest associations, and current estimates suggest that the increased risk of cardiovascular disease associated with periodontal disease is of the order of 20 per cent.[13] More research is needed, but medical practitioners should be alert to the signs and symptoms of periodontal disease in patients with cardiovascular disease.

Pulmonary disease

Studies have reported associations between respiratory infections (e.g. pneumonia) and periodontal disease, and these appear to be particularly likely in institutionalized elderly patients. Respiratory pathogens can colonize the oral cavity, residing in dental plaque. These may be aspirated to cause respiratory infections. A number of studies have identified that improving oral hygiene by brushing or using antibacterial mouth rinses can be effective in reducing the rate of respiratory infections in institutionalized patients.[13]

12.7 The role of the medical practitioner in managing oral conditions

Dealing with patients' questions about oral health and looking in the mouth can seem a daunting prospect for busy medical practitioners. But, patient-centred care dictates that oral health should be considered an integral part of general health care, particularly in patients at increased risk for oral diseases. In 2000, the US Surgeon General stated that 'oral health is essential to general health and well-being' and described the mouth as (1) a mirror of health or disease, (2) an early warning system,

> **Box 12.1 Key aspects of oral management of patients with diabetes for medical practitioners**
>
> - Ask patients about oral health, specifically the warning signs for periodontitis (bleeding gums, gum recession, mobile teeth, loss of teeth)
> - Inspect the mouth (tongue spatula and pen torch). Look for gingival inflammation, plaque and calculus, tooth mobility, dental caries and oral candidiasis
> - Explain to patients about the importance of good oral health as integral to good general health
> - Explain that treating periodontal disease is a key component of diabetes management, and that patients should comply with self-care/oral hygiene instruction
> - Liaise early with the dental health-care team, and refer for diagnosis and treatment
> - Provide smoking cessation support
> - Ensure that patients with diabetes are reminded to attend for regular dental check-ups
> - Provide the dental team with routine reports of patients' HbA1c values and information about other diabetes complications

(3) an accessible model for studying other tissues and organs and (4) a potential source of pathology affecting other systems.[14]

Box 12.1 lists some of the important aspects of care that medical practitioners can easily provide for their patients with diabetes. It is important for the medic to be aware of the oral complications of diabetes, and to liaise with the dental team. The medical practitioner has a vital role to play including the following:

- Asking the right questions and looking in the mouth (to identify signs of periodontitis, xerostomia, candidiasis, dental caries)
- Recognizing oral pathology and oral complications of diabetes
- Making patients with diabetes aware of their increased risk for oral complications
- Liaising with and referring to the dental team for joint management of patients
- Emphasizing to patients the importance of good oral health as part of the overall management of their diabetes
- Working with the patient to achieve optimal glycaemic control (to reduce the risk of all complications)
- Supporting the patient in attempts to quit smoking.

The medical practitioner should refer patients for dental assessment if they are concerned about their oral or dental status, or there is evidence of periodontal diseases, dental caries, denture problems, mucosal pathology or xerostomia. It would be very helpful to the dental team if details of the patient's diabetes management, compliance, glycaemic control and presence of other complications are included in the referral. The dental

Table 12.2 When to refer patients for dental management

Condition necessitating referral	Who to refer to
Localized dental abscess: painful fluctuant swellings, suppuration, pain on biting	General dental practitioner (GDP)
Periodontal disease: bleeding gums, mobile teeth, loss of teeth, gingival recession, tooth sensitivity, suppuration from the gingival margin	GDP
Dental caries: requiring fluoride therapy and restorative dental procedures	GDP
Oral candidiasis, e.g. denture stomatitis or angular cheilitis associated with defective dentures	GDP (for denture remake)
Oral candidiasis, e.g. recalcitrant forms of thrush, chronic hyperplastic candidiasis	Hospital specialist (oral medicine consultant)
Xerostomia	GDP (for dental management and fluoride), hospital specialist (oral medicine or restorative dentistry consultant) if severe
Painful acute gingival or periodontal conditions: extremely painful, inflamed gingiva, halitosis, exposed alveolar bone (necrotizing gingivitis and periodontitis)	Hospital specialist (periodontist or restorative dentistry consultant)
Spreading dental abscess: pyrexia, fat face, neck spread	Hospital specialist (maxillofacial consultant)

team would also welcome advice from the medical practitioner about patient management (e.g. in relation to scheduling of appointments) if lengthy dental procedures are required. Indications for referral are shown in Table 12.2.

12.8 Conclusions

A variety of oral conditions are associated with diabetes, the most significant being periodontal disease. This is a very common condition, with significantly increased prevalence in the diabetic population. A bidirectional relationship between periodontal disease and diabetes has been reported; patients with diabetes are at increased risk for periodontal disease, and periodontal disease has a negative impact on glycaemic control. Key therapeutic strategies include educating patients about shared risk for both conditions, optimizing glycaemic control, optimizing oral hygiene, reducing inflammation, smoking cessation, and empowering patients to take a leading role in managing both their diabetes and their periodontitis. Other common oral complications include xerostomia, dental caries and candidiasis. Medical health-care teams are ideally placed to inform patients with diabetes about their increased risk for oral diseases, to inspect the mouth for signs of problems, and to manage their patients jointly with dental health-care teams to provide a truly patient-centred management approach.

Case study

A 22-year-old man was referred by his GP for assessment of his oral health. The patient had an 8-year history of poorly controlled type 1 diabetes with glycated haemoglobin (HbA1c) values in the range 9.6–12.4 per cent despite intensive support from the diabetes team. There was no other relevant medical history and the patient had never smoked. The family history revealed maternal diabetes and also periodontal disease. His main complaint was that his girlfriend refused to kiss him due to bad breath. Further discussion revealed concerns about bleeding gums and mobility of teeth, and worries about losing his teeth.

Examination revealed very inflamed gingival tissues (see Plate 12.2) and gingival recession affecting many teeth, in particular the mandibular anterior teeth. Pockets of 6–9 mm were present around most of the dentition with generalized gingival bleeding and suppuration. Many of the teeth were mobile. Radiographic examination revealed generalized alveolar bone destruction affecting more than 50 per cent of the root length throughout the dentition. The diagnosis is advanced aggressive periodontitis.

Treatment involved education about the importance of oral hygiene and the links between periodontal disease and diabetes. Individually tailored oral hygiene instruction was provided using a variety of specialized brushes to clean between the teeth and around difficult areas. Ultrasonic root surface debridement was provided on multiple occasions together with adjunctive low-dose doxycycline (20 mg twice daily for 12 weeks). Gingival inflammation improved, gingival bleeding and probing depths reduced, and halitosis decreased. Compliance with diabetes management also improved, with HbA1c scores improving to 7–8 per cent.

References

1. Kelly M, Steele J, Nuttall N, et al. The condition of supporting structures. In: Walker A, Cooper I (eds), *Adult Dental Health Survey Oral health in the United Kingdom 1998*. London: The Stationery Office, 2000: 123–146.
2. O'Dowd LK, Durham J, McCracken GI, Preshaw PM. Patients' experiences of the impact of periodontal disease. *J Clin Periodontol.* 2010;**37**:334–339.

3. Mealey BL, Ocampo GL. Diabetes mellitus and periodontal disease. *Periodontology 2000* 2007;**44**:127–153.

4. Tsai C, Hayes C, Taylor GW. Glycemic control of type 2 diabetes and severe periodontal disease in the US adult population. *Community Dent Oral Epidemiol* 2002;**30**: 182–192.

5. Soskolne WA, Klinger A. The relationship between periodontal diseases and diabetes: an overview. *Ann Periodontol* 2001;**6**:91–98.

6. Preshaw PM, Foster N, Taylor JJ. Cross-susceptibility between periodontal disease and type 2 diabetes mellitus: an immunobiological perspective. *Periodontology 2000* 2007;**45**:138–157.

7. Preshaw PM. Host response modulation in periodontics. *Periodontology 2000* 2008; **48**:92–110.

8. Warnakulasuriya S, Dietrich T, Bornstein MM, et al. Oral health risks of tobacco use and effects of cessation. *Int Dent J* 2010;**60**:7–30.

9. Simpson TC, Needleman I, Wild SH, Moles DR, Mills EJ. Treatment of periodontal disease for glycaemic control in people with diabetes. *Cochrane Database Syst Rev* 2010;(5):CD004714.

10. Darre L, Vergnes JN, Gourdy P, Sixou M. Efficacy of periodontal treatment on glycaemic control in diabetic patients: A meta-analysis of interventional studies. *Diabet Metab* 2008;**34**:497–506.

11. Shultis WA, Weil EJ, Looker HC, et al. Effect of periodontitis on overt nephropathy and end-stage renal disease in type 2 diabetes. *Diabet Care* 2007;**30**:306–311.

12. Hahnel S, Behr M, Handel G, Burgers R. Saliva substitutes for the treatment of radiation-induced xerostomia-a review. *Support Care Cancer* 2009;**17**:1331–1343.

13. Pihlstrom BL, Michalowicz BS, Johnson NW. Periodontal diseases. *Lancet* 2005; **366**:1809–1820.

14. US Department of Health and Human Services. *Oral Health in America: A Report of the Surgeon General*. Rockville, MD: US Department of Health and Human Services, National Institute of Dental and Craniofacial Research, National Institutes of Health, 2000.

CHAPTER 13
Diabetes and the Skin

Hywel L Cooper, Amita Bansal and Adam E Haworth
Department of Dermatology, St Mary's Hospital, Portsmouth, UK

 Key points

- Patients with diabetes are more susceptible to bacterial infections than the general population, the most common sites being the foot and decubitus ulcers leading to leg cellulitis. Staphylococcus aureus is still the most common pathogen; however, a patient with diabetes is also at a 30-fold increase risk for group B streptococcal infections, with a significant mortality rate, despite treatment.

- Necrobiosis lipoidica is a necrobiotic granulomatous disorder that commonly affects the shins and clinically presents as atrophic yellowish-red plaques with prominent telangiectasias. In 15 per cent of patients it precedes the onset of diabetes.

- Granuloma annulare is another of the necrobiotic disorders that has long been linked with diabetes. The most common annular form is often misdiagnosed and treated as ringworm (fungal infection).

- Eruptive xanthomas, which appear as multiple reddish-yellow papules, are associated with hypertriglyceridaemia and may be the first indication of uncontrolled diabetes.

- Diabetic dermopathy is characterized by reddish-brown, round, scaly patches on the shins. Their importance is their link to other diabetic complications such as retinopathy, neuropathy and nephropathy.

 Therapeutic key points

- Bilateral leg cellulitis is exceptionally rare, and symmetrical lower limb erythema without symptoms or signs of infection is usually due to stasis, eczema, psoriasis or vasodilatory drugs such as calcium antagonists.

- People with diabetes are at much higher risk of necrotizing fasciitis. If clinically suspected cellulitis is not responding to appropriate antibiotics at appropriate doses, exclude this diagnosis.

- Athletes' foot and fungal nail infections, which in people who do not have diabetes may simply be a cosmetic rather than a medical concern, are a significant portal of entry for infection in the diabetic population and warrant treatment. If the nails are involved oral agents are required.

Diabetes: Chronic Complications, Third Edition. Edited by Kenneth M. Shaw,
Michael H. Cummings.
© 2012 John Wiley & Sons, Ltd. Published 2012 by John Wiley & Sons, Ltd.

- Necrobiosis lipoidica and granuloma annulare often have a significant psychological effect on patients because they can be cosmetically prominent. Treatment options are limited and only variably effective. Do not raise that false hope that treatments may be very effective, especially once necrobiosis causes scarring. Although their link to diabetic control is controversial, their presence is an additional manifestation of diabetes that can help in planning with the patient for the best diabetic control possible.

- The development of eruptive xanthomas or diabetic dermopathy is an indirect marker that additional treatment of dyslipidaemia or end-organ damage may be required in a patient with poorly controlled diabetes.

13.1 Introduction

Up to a third of people with diabetes will have a skin disorder associated with or accentuated by their diabetes. Fortunately for most patients with diabetes, skin disease is rarely life threatening; however, it often causes significant distress due to its appearance and symptomatology. It can also act as an important marker of complications in other organ systems. As with diabetic complications in other organs, many of the pathological changes are due to microangiopathy and also the non-enzymatic glycation (NEG) of proteins, in particular collagen.

Cutaneous manifestations of diabetes can be classified into four categories:[1]

1. Infections – both bacterial and fungal, patients with diabetes are at much higher risk
2. Skin lesions with strong-to-weak association with diabetes – necrobiosis lipoidica, granuloma annulare, eruptive xanthomas, acanthosis nigricans, diabetic dermopathy, diabetic bullae, yellow skin, perforating disorders, oral leukoplakia, lichen planus
3. Cutaneous manifestations of diabetic complications – microangiopathy, macroangiopathy, neuropathy
4. Skin reactions to diabetic treatment (e.g. sulfonylureas and insulin).

This chapter discusses these various dermatological disorders that can affect a patient with diabetes, associated complications and possible treatments. To aid the reader the most commonly used dermatological terms that are used in this chapter are briefly discussed at the start and the most frequently used treatments described in more depth at the end.

13.2 Dermatological definitions

Before discussing the specific disorders, it is useful to familiarize oneself with the commonly used dermatological terms. These are not simply used to baffle and confuse but when used properly aid the process of rash description and pattern recognition vital in arriving at a diagnosis. They also aid clear communication between medical professionals. The most commonly used terms are as follows:

Papules: raised area <5 mm in diameter.

Plaques: a flat-topped raised area >5 mm in diameter.

Macules: an area of altered colour or texture that is not raised and generally <5 mm in diameter.

Patch: a flat coloured area >5 mm.

Pedunculated: a papule with a narrow neck where it joins the skin.

Vesicle: a fluid filled blister <5 mm in diameter.

Bullae: a blister >5 mm in diameter.

Ulcer: an area of skin that has lost the epidermal layer below the basement membrane and as such will usually heal with scarring

Erosion: superficial epidermal loss above the epidermis which will therefore usually heal without scarring.

Hyperkeratosis: thickening of the skin due to accumulation of keratin

Crusting: lightly adherent material on the skin surface, usually an inflammatory/infectious exudate or dried blood.

Telangiectasia: permanent dilatation of small blood vessels visible to the naked eye.

Erythema: blanchable redness of the skin due to vasodilatation.

Pigmentation: brown discoloration of skin that can be due to either melanin from melanocytes or haemosiderin (digested blood leaking from blood vessels).

Violaceous: purple discoloration of skin.

Xanthochromia: yellow discoloration of skin.

Annular: in a ring.

Linear: in a line.

13.3 Infections

Patients with diabetes are at greater risk of infections and of increased severity of infection.

Bacterial infections

Staphylococcus aureus, as in people who do not have diabetes, is still the most common microbe causing skin infections. In the last few years, a rise in methicillin-resistant *Staphylococcus aureus* (MRSA) has begun to be increasingly important in the diabetic group.[2] Streptococcal infections are also more frequent in patients with diabetes with one study showing a 30-fold increase risk for group B streptococcal infections,[3] and an associated significant mortality rate of up to 20 per cent, despite treatment. The most common sites of infection are the leg, foot and decubitus ulcers. The risk for group A streptococcal infections is also increased at 3.7 times that of a non-diabetic population.[4]

Necrotizing fasciitis is also more common in patients with diabetes with about two-thirds of diagnosed cases being in the diabetic population. It is a potentially polymicrobial infection, most commonly seen in the legs, perineum and abdomen at sites of trauma, tissue breakdown and importantly surgical intervention. Streptococci are the most common cause with associated high anti-DNAase B and hyaluronidase antibodies (if available diagnostically). However, *Staph. aureus*, *Escherichia coli*, and *Bacteroides* and *Clostridium* spp. may also be cultured. The infection spreads along fascial planes and the patient presents with induration, erythema, necrosis and bullae formation. Pain is often severe and the patient is more toxic than would be expected from the clinical signs. Surgical debridement is urgently required and appropriate antibiotics; however, these will not work alone due to the thrombosis, and blockage seen in affected tissue prevents their action where most required.

Malignant otitis externa is an infection of the external auditory meatus, usually caused by *Pseudomonas* spp., which is potentially very invasive and can cause cranial osteomyelitis and intracranial involvement. Most patients have diabetes and the reported mortality rate is between 20 and 40 per cent. Patients complain of painful, unilateral, facial swelling with aural discharge and hearing loss.

Fungal infections
Candidal infections are more common in diabetes including intertrigo, genital, and oral and nail infections. Dermatophyte infections are also more common, with toenail onychomycosis nearly three times more prevalent. Given the risk of cellulitis in this group, it is important to treat this potential portal of infection.

Treatment
Topical treatment can be effective but oral terbinafine, despite rare hepatitis, has a risk–benefit ratio that is heavily in favour of treatment. Three months of treatment are necessary to treat a toenail infection adequately.

13.4 Necrobiotic disorders

Necrobiosis lipoidica
Necrobiosis lipoidica (NL) is considered a disorder of collagen degeneration resulting in an exaggerated granulomatous response, blood vessel wall

thickening and increased fatty deposition. The exact cause is unclear although diabetic microangiopathy is suspected, with glycoprotein deposition seen in vessel walls similar to that found in renal and eye disease. In addition there is the formation of abnormal collagen. It is well established that abnormal and defective collagen fibrils cause diabetic end-organ damage and accelerated ageing. Raised lysyl oxidase levels seen in patients with diabetes can result in increased collagen cross-linking and it is postulated that this increased collagen cross-linking precipitates the basement membrane thickening of NL.

Necrobiosis lipoidica has been reported in all races with a male:female ratio of 1:3. Although it is described as occurring at all ages, the average age of onset is in the fourth decade, with a trend to earlier disease in patients with diabetes. It has been described in about 0.3 per cent of patients with diabetes, preceding the diagnosis of diabetes in 15 per cent of patients, whereas 60 per cent of patients have the diagnosis of diabetes before its onset. Twenty-five per cent of patients had lesions that appeared with the onset of diabetes. Contrary to previous suspicions, the presence and severity of NL do not seem to correlate with a patient's glycaemic control or the duration of the disease.

Clinically, NL presents classically as asymptomatic single or multiple red–brown papules or plaques on the shins. Usually over months these expand, with the central area becoming atrophic (depressed) with prominent telangiectasia and a yellow, xanthochromic appearance due to the underlying fat being visible through the thinned dermis. The overlying skin texture is shiny and often finely wrinkled to give an appearance similar to cigarette paper (Figure 13.1). Other sites can be involved, especially the feet and elsewhere on the lower leg. Involvement of the upper limbs, trunk and face occurs in up to 15 per cent of patients.[5] Ulceration at the site of trauma and subsequent infection are occasional complications of NL (Figure 13.2). The lesions are usually painless due to associated cutaneous nerve damage in 75 per cent of the cases; however, in 25 per cent of the cases the pain can be severe. The disease is most often chronic and the plaques will continue to expand for some years before they become 'burnt out', when the active inflammatory red–brown edge disappears, leaving the central xanthochromic atrophy and macular brown post-inflammatory hyperpigmentation.

Treatment

The patient's main complaint is usually about the unsightly cosmetic appearance of the lesions. The patient should be made aware from the outset that the aim of the treatment is to settle active disease (with by no means universal success) with unfortunately no effect expected on the existing atrophy. Cosmetic camouflage techniques with long-lasting

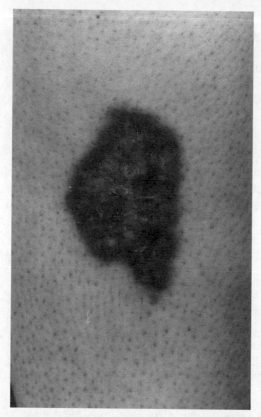

Figure 13.1 Typical necrobiosis lipoidica, here seen on the shin of a young girl with diabetes.

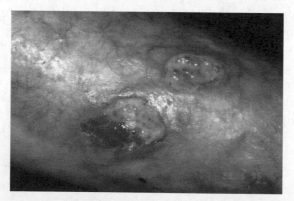

Figure 13.2 Ulcerated necrobiosis lipoidica. (Courtesy of Dr Richard Ashton, Haslar Hospital, Gosport.)

makeup formulations (including waterproofing) can be very useful in boosting patient's confidence in dealing with chronic scarring once it has occurred. In the UK the Red Cross provide an excellent service in education in these techniques.

Various treatments have been tried for active disease, with none of them being universally successful. Potent topical steroids (with or without occlusion under dressings or Clingfilm) and intralesional steroids can reduce the inflammation of early active lesions and the active borders of enlarging lesions, but have little beneficial effect on burnt-out atrophic lesions. In fact steroid use may accentuate the atrophy in already atrophic lesions. Studies report successful treatment with 0.1 per cent topical tacrolimus ointment, which is a calcineurin inhibitor with a mechanism of action similar to ciclosporin, i.e. preventing T-cell activation.[6]

Less frequently these further therapies can be tried. Owing to suspicions of a microvascular aetiology, a combination of aspirin and dipyridamole has been tried with variable results.[7] Nicotinamide has shown small benefit in reducing redness and pain.[8] Pentoxifylline,[9] intravenous prostaglandin, hyperbaric oxygen and hydroxychloroquine[10] have all been reported as helpful. Successful treatment by excision and skin graft has been described, but recurrence can occur in the graft and poor surgical wound healing on the shin is common even in patients who are not diabetic due to the poor cutaneous vasculature and thinner subepidermal planes at this site. The persistent telangiectasia can be treated with pulsed dye laser.[11] Topical tretinoin has been used with some effect to diminish the atrophy.[12]

Once ulcerated, and if topical treatments are not helping, then oral steroids up to 60 mg prednisolone daily or admitting the patient for pulsed intravenous steroids with methylprednisolone may be helpful despite the risk of significant worsening of their diabetic control. Topical PUVA (psoralen + UVA)[13], ciclosporin,[14] mycophenolate mofetil,[15] granulocyte–macrophage colony-stimulating factor (GM-CSF)[16] and infliximab[17] have all been reported as beneficial in small case series and reports.

There are several reports of squamous cell carcinoma arising in NL (similar to reports in other chronic cutaneous inflammatory conditions and scars) and hence this should always be considered in patients who develop expansile nodules or where ulceration progresses with induration or thickening at its margins.[18]

Granuloma annulare

Granuloma annulare (GA) typically presents with annular plaques made up of skin-coloured to red–purple papules, most commonly occurring on the hands and feet overlying the dorsal aspects of joints. They are usually asymptomatic but can occasionally itch. Most cases will resolve spontaneously and need no treatment, but the main morbidity comes from it being visible on the hands. There are five variants, the most common being the annular or localized form; generalized GA is rarer but seems to be more closely related to diabetes. Papular, umbilicated, linear and deep or subcutaneous GA is very rare.

Granuloma annulare has been associated primarily with type 1 diabetes, but rarely with type 2 diabetes and thyroid disease, based on an increased numbers in some small case series.[19] The frequency of GA in the general population is unknown. It does not seem to favour a particular race, ethnic group or geographical area. However, it affects females twice as often as males. GA may present at any age but the localized form is more common in young adults whereas generalized GA is more likely to present later in life. The localized form most commonly affects dorsal surfaces of the feet, hands and fingers, and extensor aspects of arms and legs, whereas the generalized forms more extensively involve the trunk (Figure 13.3 and 13.4).

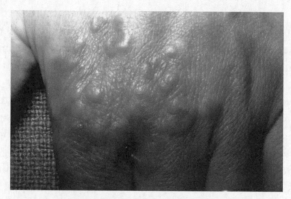

Figure 13.3 Localized granuloma annulare with typical dermal papules over the knuckles. Note that the skin markings are maintained and there is no scale. (Courtesy of Dr Richard Ashton, Haslar Hospital, Gosport.)

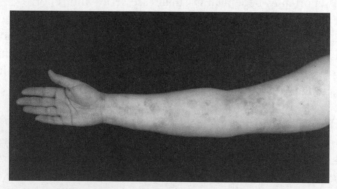

Figure 13.4 Generalized granuloma annulare with multiple, less well-defined annular plaques. There is widespread distribution including the trunk.

In the common annular form, GA is often mistaken for and treated as a fungal infection. However, being a dermal process there is no disruption of the epidermis, so GA has no scale and the fine skin markings can clearly be seen over the ring of papules. The epithelial involvement in tinea corporis (ringworm) gives the annular plaques a peripheral scale over the advancing edge. In the event of diagnostic uncertainty, an ellipse biopsy through the most palpable part of the annular edge or a group of the most prominent papules in the generalized form should be done.

Treatment

Treatment is first reassurance as to the nature of the disease and the likelihood of spontaneous resolution. Where localized GA is disabling due to itch or disfigurement, then first-line treatment is potent topical steroids. These should be applied once daily to the advancing edge. Intralesional steroids injected into the advancing edge may be effective if topical steroids are not working, but run a greater risk of steroid-induced atrophy and the procedure is painful. Where a biopsy has been taken, the disease can resolve and other destructive and scarring insults such as cryotherapy can produce a similar result, with up to 80 per cent success rate reported, but you are trading one process that will probably resolve completely with a scar. For generalized GA, if treatment is needed it must be systemic and PUVA or other light treatments are the treatment of choice. Other systemics have been reported as helpful including dapsone, hydroxychloroquine, acitretin, ciclosporin and potassium iodide. More recently topical tacrolimus has been used with some benefit.

13.5 Eruptive xanthomas

Hyperlipidaemias are clinically associated with characteristic skin lesions known as xanthomas. Phenotypically several forms of xanthoma have been described based on clinical appearance and the underlying dyslipidaemia.

Histologically xanthomas are the result of macrophage accumulation of excess lipids in the skin; clinically these manifest as yellow, orange to reddish or brown macules, papules, plaques or nodules.

The dyslipidaemia most frequently associated with diabetes is hypertriglyceridaemia, usually occurring in young people with insulin-resistant diabetes due to insulin's requirement to facilitate lipoprotein lipase clearing of triglycerides. So-called eruptive xanthomas appear rapidly as 'showers' or crops of red, orange to yellow papules. Though they can occur anywhere on the body most commonly they are seen on the extensor surfaces of the buttocks and limbs (Figure 13.5). The papules are initially

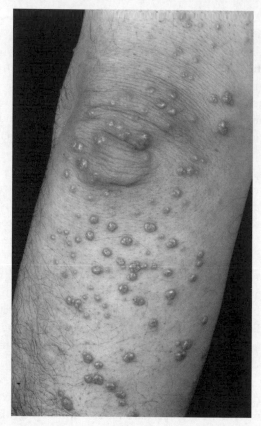

Figure 13.5 Eruptive xanthomas with multiple xanthochromic papules on the extensor surfaces.

dome shaped but often coalesce to form nodules and plaques – so-called tuboeruptive xanthomas occurring mainly over the elbows.

Recognizing eruptive xanthomas as associated with hypertriglyceridaemia at dangerous levels can help avoid such consequences as acute pancreatitis and worsening ischaemic heart disease.

Eruptive xanthomas may be the first clinical presentation and indicator of underlying uncontrolled diabetes, though familial hyperlipidaemias should also be considered.

Treatment

With strict diabetic control as required and appropriate treatment of dyslipidaemia, eruptive xanthomas resolve relatively quickly because triglycerides are more easily mobilized than cholesterol from cells.

13.6 Acanthosis nigricans

Acanthosis nigricans is a group of conditions that show pigmented, hyperkeratotic skin, usually in the flexures that are associated with hyperinsulinaemia.

Six types of acanthosis nigricans are recognized. The most common is pseudoacanthosis nigricans, which occurs with obesity and hyperinsulinaemia. It shows a strong racial disposition to dark skins. The other five are the malignancy-associated form, a drug-induced, hereditary benign form, a very rare naevoid form and a benign form that is associated with other endocrinopathies such as HAIR-AN (**h**yperandrogenism, **i**nsulin **r**esistance, **a**canthosis **n**igricans) syndrome.

The classic presentation is of warty, pigmented, poorly defined plaques that occur in the axillae, groin and neck, and have a velvety feel to them due to being made up from multiple tiny papules (Figure 13.6). The neck changes have been described as 'dirty neck'. The onset is gradual, starting in childhood if weight is more than 200 per cent of ideal and increasing at puberty. As the disease progresses and the plaques thicken, the papules may become larger and form multiple skin tags.

The malignancy-associated variant usually shows a sudden onset and tends to be more severe than its benign counterparts. The palms are almost always affected – tripe palms – and the mucous membranes show similar warty hyperkeratosis. Various tumours have been linked, including carcinoma of the bronchus, kidney, oesophagus and rectum. Hence, in a patient presenting with a sudden-onset severe acanthosis nigricans, it is important to search for any underlying malignancy, which is guided by the other associated symptoms.

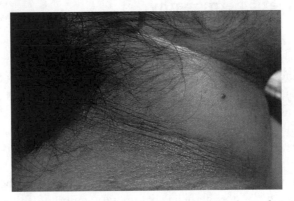

Figure 13.6 Acanthosis nigricans: typical hyperpigmented, velvety plaques occurring in the flexures in pigmented skin. (Courtesy of Dr Richard Ashton, Haslar Hospital, Gosport.)

Acanthosis nigricans is the result of epidermal keratinocyte and dermal fibroblast proliferation. In the benign forms of acanthosis nigricans, insulin at high concentrations exerts pro-proliferative effects by binding to insulin-like growth factor (IGF-I) receptors. In addition, free IGF-I levels are elevated in obese patients with hyperinsulinaemia, resulting in accelerated epidermal cell growth and differentiation. Other mediators may also be involved, including epidermal growth factor and fibroblast growth factor acting via tyrosine kinase receptors. It is hypothesized that epidermal friction may also play a contributory role, hence the predilection of acanthosis nigricans for body folds, similar to the effect of constant skin rubbing and scratching – thickening the skin in conditions such as eczema (lichenification) and lichen simplex chronicus (thickened skin as a result of scratching habit).

In malignant acanthosis nigricans, the stimulating factor is probably secreted by the underlying tumour or as a response to it. Transforming growth factor (TGF)-α is structurally similar to epidermal growth factor (EGF), potentially inducing similar epidermal responses.

Insulin injections themselves may induce a localized acanthosis nigricans especially at the injection site due to activation of IGF receptors.

Treatment
The mainstay of treatment is reduction of insulin resistance by weight reduction, but vitamin D analogues and oral and topical retinoids have all been tried with limited success. HAIR-AN syndrome patients may be treated with oral contraceptives and metformin. The troublesome skin tags can be removed by cryotherapy, shave excision or simple cautery.

13.7 Diabetic dermopathy

Diabetic dermopathy (Figure 13.7) presents as asymptomatic, pigmented, scaly papules and plaques on the shins, hence the alias 'shin spots'. It is common and occurs in 24 per cent of patients with diabetes and 40 per cent over 50 years. Their importance is their link to other diabetic complications such as retinopathy, neuropathy and nephropathy. They start as multiple small brown macules that develop fine scale and, over a period of a few years, will fade to leave subtle atrophic scars. At this stage they are difficult to see, but as they are continually being produced it seems to the patient as if they do not go away. They are thought to be related to microangiopathy and endothelial basement membrane thickening with glycosylated collagen, although a recent laser Doppler study demonstrated increased blood flow in the macules; this does not, of course, exclude a prior vascular insult. They are more common as the duration of diabetes

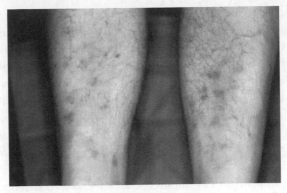

Figure 13.7 Diabetic dermopathy. (Courtesy of Dr Richard Ashton, Haslar Hospital, Gosport.)

increases. Since their first naming in 1965 they have been described in normal individuals.

Treatment

Treatment is unnecessary because they are harmless in themselves and will usually resolve with time; moisturization may help if they are unusually symptomatic.

13.8 Diabetic bullae (bullosis diabeticorum)

Bullosis diabeticorum is rare, 44 cases being reported since its first description in 1967. It is now likely that more cases go unreported and the real importance of awareness of this condition is to prevent erroneous treatments of other blistering disorders. The bullae are of sudden onset, almost universally on the feet, although bullae on the hands have been reported in one case; typically they are several centimetres in diameter, although there are reports of smaller vesicles. They are filled with clear yellow fluid and the base of the blister is quiet, i.e. there is no inflammation around the blister. An important diagnostic sign is that they are not itchy. They heal with no scarring over a few weeks. There is some support for them being fragility based in that suction blisters can be produced more easily in the skin of someone with diabetes.

The main differential diagnosis is bullous pemphigoid, in which intensely itchy large bullae occur on the lower leg, arm and occasionally the trunk, of elderly patients (>65 years) with surrounding erythema and urticaria. A biopsy should be taken for normal histology and a sample sent for immunofluorescence. This will demonstrate the immunobullous nature of pemphigoid with a band of IgG and C3 demonstrable at the dermoepidermal junction. Routine histology in bullosis diabeticorum shows a blister split between the dermis and epidermis, with very little reaction in the surrounding skin, hence the thick-walled tense blister in a quiet background. Bullous pemphigoid shows a split at a similar level, giving the same blister, but the surrounding skin shows an intense infiltrate with many eosinophils, which is clinically seen with an inflammatory base to the blisters and surrounding urticaria. Most laboratories can also demonstrate the relevant skin autoantibody on serum. As pemphigoid is much more common than bullosis diabeticorum and needs high-dose oral steroid treatment, differentiating these two conditions is vital. Porphyria cutanea tarda can present with blistering of the hands in a light-exposed distribution and may be seen in a diabetic population due to the link with haemochromatosis, so porphyrins should be measured in patients with more prominent involvement on the upper limbs. Other causes of thick-walled tense blisters are drug induced, e.g. barbiturates, and thermal or chemical burns. As the condition is self-limiting, no specific treatment is necessary.

13.9 Diabetic stiff skin

In the skin diabetes simulates a premature ageing syndrome. Collagen's age can be determined by its resistance to enzymatic degradation and Hamlin et al.[20] showed that young patients who had died of their diabetes had tendon collagen that degraded similarly to that of normal individuals 60 years their senior. The glycosylation of collagen within the dermis and blood vessel endothelium underlies much of the pathology in this condition and in the skin produces a group of conditions that are described separately but really are part of a spectrum of disorders. Diabetic thick skin includes the conditions of limited joint mobility, scleroderma-like syndrome and scleroedema diabeticorum.

Limited joint mobility

This condition is why all patients at diabetic review are asked to make a prayer sign. Thickening of the collagen within the skin and connective tissue around joints produces reduced mobility and thickened waxy skin. The little finger is the first affected and the disease progresses laterally to affect all digits. As the joint itself is uninvolved, the synonym 'cheiroarthropathy' is misleading. Detection is by the prayer sign where affected individuals are unable to oppose their palms when asked. The true importance of this condition is that it is closely related to retinopathy and nephropathy, and is the earliest marker for these complications. The use of this condition as a marker seems to decrease as patients become chronologically older, and is more significant in children and young patients with diabetes. Thirty-five per cent of adolescent patients with type 1 diabetes have limited joint mobility,[21] more commonly in the subtalar joint than in those of the hands. The proportion of patients with type 2 diabetics affected is reported to range from 10 per cent to 85 per cent. Poor diabetic control is a risk factor for development of the condition, with a 46 per cent increased risk of the disease for every raised unit of HbA1c, and tight control will gradually reduce the stiffness. Pleasingly, Infante et al. showed a fourfold reduction in the prevalence of limited joint mobility in children between 1976 and 1998, ascribing this to the improved glycaemic control over this period.[22]

Scleroderma-like syndrome

Often associated with limited joint mobility, scleroderma-like syndrome presents with thickened waxy skin over the dorsa of the hands and feet. Around the knuckles there may be tiny papules. It is reported in 5–25 per cent of patients with diabetes and is linked to the duration of the disease.

Treatment

Treatment is with improved glycaemic control.

Diabetic scleroedema

Scleroedema is a localized induration and thickening of the skin that can be either post-infective, associated with blood dyscrasias, or associated with diabetes. It should not be confused with the rather similar sounding condition scleroderma, which for those of us with dyslexia has always been a difficult distinction. Onset is gradual and usually involves the neck, upper back and face. The face can become expressionless. Involvement of the shoulders, upper limbs and trunk can then follow. Truncal and lower limb involvement is rare but reported. The skin develops a hard, woody, thickened feel. There may be restriction of joint movements, and pharyngeal involvement with dysphagia has been reported. It is described as rare but probably represents under-reporting, with one study finding the condition in 14 per cent of patients with diabetes.[23] Scleroedema is most common in obese patients with type 2 diabetes who are often difficult to control and go on to need insulin; however, it is not associated with an increased risk of other diabetic complications, although this has not been universally found. Investigation should include an anti-streptolysin O (ASO) titre and a screen for a paraproteinaemia to exclude other causes of the scleroedema.

Treatment

Treatment has been attempted with methotrexate and prostaglandin E_1, but the most promising treatment is radiotherapy.

13.10 Perforating disorders

This is a rare group of disorders in which altered dermal collagen and elastin are extruded through the epidermis, so-called 'transepidermal elimination'. Four variants are recognized: Kyrle's disease, perforating folliculitis, reactive perforating collagenosis and perforating serpiginous elastosis. These rare entities are most commonly seen in association with renal failure and diabetes. It is often difficult to differentiate among these historically defined entities because the differences can be very subtle.

Clinically they present as itchy papules on the limbs and trunk with a keratotic centre. These grow over a few weeks and then settle to leave hypopigmentation or hyperpigmentation and scarring. If suspected, a skin biopsy should be taken from a fresh papule that has not been excoriated. Classic changes include altered collagen being extruded within a cup of thickened epidermis surrounded by a mild lymphocytic infiltrate.

Treatment

Treatment is not universally successful and patients often continue to develop new lesions. Strong topical steroids have been reported as useful, as have topical retinoids, UVB and PUVA, TENS (transcutaneous electrical nerve stimulation) for itching and allopurinol.

13.11 Skin reactions to diabetic treatments

Insulin

Patients occasionally experience local erythema, oedema and pruritus at the insulin injection site. This condition is usually self-limiting. This may be related to factors other than insulin, such as irritants in the skin-cleansing agent, preservatives or trace quantities of latex in pre-filled syringes.[24] Insulin subcutaneously can result in lipoatrophy (depression in the skin) or lipohypertrophy (enlargement or thickening of tissue).

Sulfonylureas

Skin reactions to sulfonylureas may be part of a generalized hypersensitivity with phenotype from mild erythema, itching and photosensitivity to life-threatening condition such as Steven–Johnson syndrome and toxic epidermal necrolysis.[25]

13.12 Dermatological therapeutics

Topical treatments

These come in either cream or ointment form. Ointments are in a Vaseline-like (petrolatum) base and are thick and greasy. They are preferred over creams because they have a significant additional moisturizing effect. They contain no preservatives unlike creams. Creams are milky and are preferred by patients because they absorb into the skin more easily. They have a higher concentration of water than ointments and so may be a reservoir for bacteria; thus they need preservatives that are a potential cause of allergic contact dermatitis.

Topical steroids are useful for treating various conditions such as granuloma annulare, necrobiosis lipoidica and perforating disorders. They come in four potencies: mild, moderate, potent and very potent. Mild steroids include hydrocortisone and can be applied without risk of side effects such as skin thinning. They are safe for long-term use on the face and available over the counter in the UK. Moderate potency steroids include clobetasol butyrate (Eumovate). They are safe for long-term use on the body and short-term use on the face (1–2 weeks). Examples of potent topical steroids are betamethasone valerate (Betnovate) and mometasone furoate (Elocon), which can be used short term on the body; they should be avoided on the face except under expert supervision and should be used with extreme care in the flexures. Clobetasol propionate (Dermovate) is a very potent topical steroid and should be used with care. In conditions such as granuloma annulare and necrobiosis lipoidica it can be used under occlusion to increase its penetration. There is a severe risk of atrophy with this if it is not undertaken correctly.

Side effects are usually related to the potency of the cream. Skin atrophy and striae are those most feared but, if used appropriately for short duration of time, are rarely seen nowadays. Cutaneous infections, particularly staphylococcal, can be worsened by treatment with topical steroids, but the addition of either a topical or an oral antibiotic will be adequate where the steroid treatment needs to be continued. Cataracts have been reported with long-term use of potent or very potent creams on the eyelids, but not with mild alternatives. They may precipitate acne or perioral dermatitis (multiple papules, pustules and vesicles occurring around the mouth with a clear border around the lips) and should then be discontinued.

Topical retinoids are useful for treating the perforating disorders and acanthosis nigricans and are supplied in cream or gel form. They are vitamin A derivatives and can irritate the skin. Adapalene 0.1 per cent is probably the least irritant and is hence preferred where it is needed. They should be applied once daily. They can make the skin more susceptible to sunburn and so ultraviolet avoidance or good sun protection may be needed.

Vitamin D analogues are most commonly prescribed for psoriasis but have been used in treatment of acanthosis nigricans. Calcipotriol (Dovonex), calcitriol (Silkis) and tacalcitol (Curatoderm) are the three products available. They bind to the steroid family of nuclear super receptors and reduce cell turnover and therefore hyperkeratosis. Side effects are usually local, with redness and irritation being the most common. Overuse can theoretically cause hypercalcaemia and care should be taken in renal failure or dysfunction. Calcipotriol should be limited to 100 g/week and calcitriol to less than 35 per cent of body surface area.

Tacrolimus is an immunomodulator that is a ciclosporin analogue, and is available for topical treatment. It has been used to treat both granuloma annulare and necrobiosis lipoidica and works by suppressing antigen-specific T-cell activation and inhibiting inflammatory cytokine release. It acts similarly to a topical steroid but does not have the skin-thinning side effects. It is an ointment that is used twice daily and patients must be warned that it is likely to sting for the first few applications. This is due to local release of substance P from nerve endings which are then depleted of this chemical, allowing the side effect to subside. Other side effects include worsening or precipitation of skin infections, particularly herpes simplex, and some patients flush if they concurrently drink alcohol. There is a theoretical risk that the reduction in skin immune surveillance could increase skin cancer risk and so UV light exposure should be minimized.

Imiquimod is licensed for the treatment of genital warts and superficial skin cancers but has also been used for treating granuloma annulare. It is a toll-like receptor 7 analogue that increases interferon-α, TNF and IL-12. It is applied from a sachet, usually three times a week, and causes a localized inflammatory reaction.

Cryotherapy

Cryotherapy is the application of liquid nitrogen to the skin to cause a controlled cold injury. It can be used to treat granuloma annulare and necrobiosis lipoidica. The liquid is sprayed on with a gun; the required area is frozen to achieve an ice ball and then maintained at that temperature for the given time, usually 10–30 s. It is painful and will often produce blistering followed by an eschar. This settles to leave some element of scaring and often post-inflammatory hypopigmentation.

Phototherapy

There are three types of UV treatment, broadband UVB, narrowband UVB and PUVA. In all cases the patient stands in a UV cabinet with the relevant area exposed. Face shields, clothes or sun block can protect areas not to be treated. The first treatments are often only for 10–15 s, but over a period of 8–10 weeks they can build up to 5–10 min exposure. The exposure time depends on a patient's skin type, and test doses are shone on to the patient's arm to gauge the starting time. Ten weeks is the average duration of treatment.

UVB penetrates less deeply than UVA and hence has potentially fewer side effects; however, this also means lower efficacy. UVB is given three times weekly and so the patient must be able to attend this frequently and also be able to stand in the cabinet for the necessary exposure. Side effects are mainly the risk of burning. Narrow-band UVB is a relatively newer modality where the UV rays are concentrated around 311 nm. This seems to be more effective than broadband UVB, which uses a wide mix of wavelengths in the UVB spectrum. It has been shown to be as effective as PUVA in the treatment of psoriasis.

PUVA is the combination of a photosensitizer (psoralens) and UVA. It can be given in three ways – topical, bath or oral – and is a twice-a-week regimen, compared with three times a week necessary for UVB. With topical PUVA, a gel psoralen is applied to a limited area, in bath treatment the patient lies in a bath with the psoralen in the water for 15 min and in oral treatment they take a psoralen tablet 2 h before treatment. The skin becomes sensitive to UVA and they are then exposed in a similar way to the UVB regimen. Side effects are more common, including irritation and burning, photosensitivity of the treated area for 24 h (including the lens of the eye with oral PUVA), nausea with the oral regimen and, in all modalities, a definite increased risk in squamous cell carcinoma if more than 250 treatments are undertaken.

Case study

A 35-year-old woman with recently well controlled type 1 diabetes of 20 years duration presented with a slowly enlarging, asymptomatic, 'red patch' on her left shin. It was now 20 mm in diameter and she was mortified that it would get larger, spread to her body and face, and stop her wearing her beloved knee-length skirts.

On examination she had an annular erythematous plaque with central atrophy, yellow discoloration and prominent telangiectasia unilaterally, directly over the midpoint of the shin. There was no ulceration.

What is the likely diagnosis and how would you manage this patient?

This is a classic description of necrobiosis lipoidica diabeticorum. It is associated with diabetes but causal association with poor diabetic control is now less established than once argued. Counselling about the natural history of the disease (slow progression, ulceration but potential for activity to diminish and burn out to occur) is important but, once atrophy has been established, this is not going to recover. Treatment is difficult, response is highly variable and unrealistic targets should be avoided. Potent topical steroids (particularly to the active edge to avoid further central atrophy) or, if less active, topical tacrolimus 0.1% can be applied once daily. Injecting low-strength triamcinalone (10 mg/ml, maximum 2 ml) around the active edge can prevent ulceration if it appears incipient. This is preferable to the potential side effects of oral or pulsed intravenous steroids and their effects on diabetic control. If new adjacent or distant patches (opposite shine most often) appear UV therapy (typically PUVA) can be tried, and again has the benefit of being a skin-directed therapy without many systemic side effects. At all points when therapies with additional side effects and only limited reports of benefits are discussed, realistic expectation is the key. Atrophy and scarring will not be reversed but additional ulceration and activity (new lesions) could be prevented. If cosmesis is the main concern and disease activity is low or burnt out, camouflage has much better results and can give patients very pleasing outcome because they are educated to do it themselves. This is very important because case reports and series have carried out trials with variable success of a combination of aspirin and dipyridamole, nicotinamide, pentoxifylline, intravenous prostaglandin, hyperbaric oxygen, hydroxychloroquine, ciclosporin, mycophenolate mofetil, GM-CSF (granulocyte–macrophage colony-stimulating factor) and infliximab, some of which have obvious and very significant risks in themselves.

Do not underestimate the psychological effects of visible manifestations of disease, which are often far more debilitating to patients than associated conditions with far more serious consequences. It is often the reason patients won't leave the house or partake in the exercise that they may need.

References

1. Romano G, Moretti G, Di Benedetto A, et al. Skin lesions in diabetes mellitus: Prevalence and clinical correlations. *Diabet Res Clin Pract* 1998;**39**:101–106.
2. Dang CN, Prasad YD, Boulton AJ, Jude EB. Methicillin-resistant *Staphylococcus aureus* in the diabetic foot clinic: a worsening problem. *Diabet Med* 2003;**20**:159–161.
3. Farley MM, Harvey RC, Stull T, et al. A population-based assessment of invasive disease due to group B Streptococcus in nonpregnant adults. *N Engl J Med* 1993; **328**:1807–1811.
4. Davies HD, McGeer A, Schwartz B, et al. Invasive group A streptococcal infections in Ontario, Canada. Ontario Group A Streptococcal Study Group. *N Engl J Med* 1996;**335**:547–554.
5. Kavanagh GM, Novelli M, Hartog M, Kennedy CT. Necrobiosis lipoidica – involvement of atypical sites. *Clin Exp Dermatol* 1993;**18**:543–544.
6. Clayton TH, Harrison PV. Successful treatment of chronic ulcerated necrobiosis lipoidica with 0.1% topical tacrolimus ointment. *Br J Dermatol* 2005;**152**:581–582.

7. Statham B, Finlay AY, Marks R. A randomized double blind comparison of an aspirin dipyridamole combination versus a placebo in the treatment of necrobiosis lipoidica. *Acta Dermatol Venereol* 1981;**61**:270–271.

8. Handfield-Jones S, Jones S, Peachey R. High dose nicotinamide in the treatment of necrobiosis lipoidica. *Br J Dermatol* 1988;**118**:693–696.

9. Basaria S, Braga-Basaria M. Necrobiosis lipoidica diabeticorum: response to pentoxiphylline. *J Endocrinol Invest* 2003;**26**:1037–1040.

10. Nguyen K, Washenik K, Shupack J. Necrobiosis lipoidica diabeticorum treated with chloroquine. *J Am Acad Dermatol* 2002;**46**(2 suppl):S34–36.

11. Currie CL, Monk BE. Pulsed dye laser treatment of necrobiosis lipoidica: report of a case. *J Cutan Laser Ther* 1999;**1**:239–241.

12. Heymann WR. Necrobiosis lipoidica treated with topical tretinoin. *Cutis* 1996; **58**:53–54.

13. De Rie MA, Sommer A, Hoekzema R, Neumann HA. Treatment of necrobiosis lipoidica with topical psoralen plus ultraviolet A. *Br J Dermatol* 2002;**147**:743–747.

14. Stanway A, Rademaker M, Newman P. Healing of severe ulcerative necrobiosis lipoidica with cyclosporin. *Australas J Dermatol* 2004;**45**:119–122.

15. Reinhard G, Lohmann F, Uerlich M, Bauer R, Bieber T. Successful treatment of ulcerated necrobiosis lipoidica with mycophenolate mofetil. *Acta Dermatol Venereol* 2000;**80**:312–313.

16. Evans AV, Atherton DJ. Recalcitrant ulcers in necrobiosis lipoidica diabeticorum healed by topical granulocyte-macrophage colony-stimulating factor. *Br J Dermatol* 2002;**147**:1023–1025.

17. Kolde G, Muche JM, Schulze P, Fischer P, Lichey J. Infliximab: a promising new treatment option for ulcerated necrobiosis lipoidica. *Dermatology* 2003;**206**: 180–181.

18. Santos-Juanes J, Galache C, Curto JR, Carrasco MP, Ribas A, Sanchez del Rio J. Squamous cell carcinoma arising in long-standing necrobiosis lipoidica. *J Eur Acad Dermatol Venereol* 2004;**18**:199–200.

19. Kakourou T, Psychou F, Voutetakis A, Xaidara A, Stefanaki K, Dacou-Voutetakis C. Low serum insulin values in children with multiple lesions of granuloma annulare: a prospective study. *J Eur Acad Dermatol Venereol* 2005;**19**:30–34.

20. Hamlin CR, Kohn RR, Luschin JH. Apparent accelerated aging of human collagen in diabetes mellitus. *Diabetes* 1975;**24**:902–904.

21. Duffin AC, Donaghue KC, Potter M, et al. Limited joint mobility in the hands and feet of adolescents with type 1 diabetes mellitus. *Diabet Med* 1999;**16**:125–130.

22. Infante JR, Rosenbloom AL, Silverstein JH, Garzarella L, Pollock BH. Changes in frequency and severity of limited joint mobility in children with type 1 diabetes mellitus between 1976–78 and 1998. *J Pediatr* 2001;**138**:33–37.

23. Sattar MA, Diab S, Sugathan TN, Sivanandasingham P, Fenech FF. Scleroedema diabeticorum: a minor but often unrecognized complication of diabetes mellitus. *Diabet Med* 1988;**5**:465–468.

24. Roest MAB, Shaw S, Orton DI. Insulin-injection-site reactions associated with type i latex allergy. *N Engl J Med* 2003;**348**:265–266.

25. Duncan C, Sommerfield AJ, Nawroz I, Campbell IW. Stevens–Johnson syndrome with visceral arteritis due to sulphonylurea therapy. *Pract Diabet Int* 2004;**21**: 195–198.

CHAPTER 14

Diabetes and Cancer

Steven S Coughlin[1] and Edward L Giovannucci[2]

[1]Epidemiology Program, Office of Public Health, Department of Veterans Affairs, Washington, DC, and Department of Epidemiology, Rollins School of Public Health, Emory University, Atlanta, GA, USA

[2]Department of Epidemiology, Harvard School of Public Health, Boston, MA, USA

 Key points

- Several cancers have been consistently associated with diabetes including pancreatic, colorectal, endometrial and liver cancer.

- Hyperinsulinaemia may be an underlying factor in chronic conditions such as obesity, type 2 diabetes mellitus and certain forms of cancer.

- Obesity and physical inactivity are important determinants of hyperinsulinaemia and insulin resistance.

- Obesity influences the amount of free insulin-like growth factor I (IGF-I) available to cells, but is not an important determinant of total IGF-I in the blood.

- Increases in serum or plasma levels of IGF-I have been observed in several epidemiological studies of colorectal, prostate and premenopausal breast cancer.

 Therapeutic key points

- Clinicians who treat cancer patients must consider the cardiac, hepatic, renal and neurological complications that are commonly seen among people with diabetes.

- Evidence from clinical trials and population-based studies suggests that, after a cancer diagnosis and treatment, patients with diabetes experience higher mortality and cancer recurrence rates than patients without.

- Patients with hyperglycaemia or diabetes who undergo cancer treatment may be more likely to experience certain side effects than patients who do not have hyperglycaemia or diabetes.

- A growing body of evidence suggests that metformin protects against the development of certain cancers and may improve prognosis in patients with breast cancer; randomized trials are currently ongoing.

Diabetes: Chronic Complications, Third Edition. Edited by Kenneth M. Shaw, Michael H. Cummings.

© 2012 John Wiley & Sons, Ltd. Published 2012 by John Wiley & Sons, Ltd.

14.1 Introduction

Epidemiological studies have found that diabetes mellitus may alter the risk of developing several cancers.[1,2] Cancers that have been consistently associated with diabetes include pancreatic, colorectal, endometrial and liver cancer, although some earlier studies involved small numbers of people with diabetes or did not adjust for important confounding variables.

Higher insulin levels may contribute to increased tumour growth.[3] In epidemiological studies, insulin-like growth factor I (IGF-I) has been associated with increased risk of colorectal cancer. IGF-I may act as a promoter of colon tumour cell growth. Similar mechanisms may account for associations observed in epidemiological studies between diabetes and cancer of the breast and other sites. Increases in circulating levels of IGF-I have been observed in some epidemiological studies of prostate and premenopausal breast cancer.[4-6] There may be additional biological mechanisms by which diabetes mellitus increases risk of cancer at specific sites.

The evidence from epidemiological and in vitro studies of a link between diabetes and hyperinsulinaemia and risk of common cancers has generated interest in questions surrounding the possible carcinogenic effect of medications used to treat diabetes such as insulin analogues. Taken overall, results from epidemiological studies with an observational design and clinical trials that have examined an association between insulin glargine and cancer risk have been inconclusive.[7] Oral hypoglycaemic agents such as metformin have been studied as possible chemopreventive and adjuvant therapies for cancer. A growing body of evidence suggests that metformin protects against the development of certain cancers and may improve prognosis in patients with cancer.[7]

The coexistence of diabetes and cancer is likely to rise with increases in life expectancy and the prevalence of obesity.[7] Currently, about 8–18 per cent of people with cancer also have diabetes. When treating cancer patients, clinicians must consider the cardiac, hepatic, renal and neurological complications that are commonly seen among patients with diabetes.[8] For example, some chemotherapeutic agents are used at lower doses or omitted from regimens to avoid toxicity in patients with cardiovascular disease.

In this chapter we consider associations between diabetes and specific cancer sites that have been identified in epidemiological studies of cancer incidence or mortality. Associations between hyperinsulinaemia and cancer risk are also considered. We then review the associations that have been reported between IFG-I and its binding proteins, and risk of cancer of the pancreas, colon, rectum, breast and prostate. Later in this chapter, we consider studies of antidiabetic drugs and cancer as well as key issues pertaining to the treatment of cancer with diabetes.

14.2 Associations between diabetes and specific cancer sites

Pancreatic cancer

Studies have found that patients with diabetes have an increased risk of pancreatic cancer.[2,9] A meta-analysis of 17 case–control and 19 cohort or nested case–control studies of pancreatic cancer published from 1966 to 2005 yielded a summary odds ratio of 1.82 (95% confidence interval [CI] 1.66–1.89).[10] Diabetes is both a risk factor for pancreatic cancer and a potential consequence of pancreatic cancer. Although reverse causation is a potential concern, studies have shown that diabetes is a risk factor for cancer many years in advance. Other studies have shown that abnormal glucose metabolism is associated with pancreatic cancer mortality. A graded dose–response relationship has been observed between fasting glucose and pancreatic cancer in cohort studies.

Liver cancer

Several epidemiological studies have observed an increased risk of primary liver cancer.[1,11] The possible biological mechanisms are poorly understood, but alcohol consumption is a risk factor for both diabetes and liver cancer. Nevertheless, more recent studies of diabetes and liver cancer have found an association between these two conditions even after adjusting for alcohol consumption, smoking, serological markers of viral hepatitis and other important confounding factors.

Colorectal cancer

Weak associations with diabetes mellitus have been reported in case–control and cohort studies of colon cancer, although not all have adjusted for other risk factors. Diabetes was found to be predictive of mortality from colon cancer in the Cancer Prevention Study II, a prospective mortality study of 1.2 million US men and women enrolled in 1982 by more than 77 000 American Cancer Study volunteers in all 50 states, the District of Columbia and Puerto Rico.[9] A systematic review and meta-analysis of data from 15 studies found that diabetes was associated with a 30 per cent excess risk of colorectal cancer (relative risk [RR] 1.30, 95% CI 1.20–1.40).[12] No important differences were found by gender or anatomical subsite (colon vs rectum). The biological plausibility of an association between diabetes mellitus and colon cancer relates to slower bowel transit in people with diabetes (with increased exposure to toxic substances), increased production of carcinogenic bile acids and higher insulin levels.

Breast cancer

Diabetes has also been associated with the development of breast cancer in women. In the Nurses' Health Study, diabetes was associated with a modest increase in the risk of developing breast cancer after adjusting for possible confounding factors.[13] However, an association between diabetes mellitus and breast cancer risk in women has not been established by studies carried out to date. Although results of studies conducted so far have been inconsistent, the hypothesized association is biologically plausible. Breast cancer has been related to cell proliferation in response to sex hormones and growth factors such as IGF-I.[14] Hyperinsulinaemia with insulin resistance has been reported to be an independent risk factor for breast cancer in case–control studies. However, four prospective studies have examined insulin or C-peptide and risk of breast cancer, and no association was observed with overall or premenopausal or postmenopausal breast cancer. A meta-analysis showed excess risk of breast cancer with high circulating C-peptide or insulin, which was, however, entirely driven by case–control studies.[15]

Prostate cancer

Men with diabetes have been reported to have lower risks of prostate cancer incidence[1,6] and mortality.[9] For example, diabetes was associated with reduced risk of prostate cancer in the Cancer Prevention Study II (RR 0.63, 95% CI 0.56–0.71) but only after 4 or more years following diagnosis of diabetes.[16] A pattern of increased prostate cancer risk shortly after diabetes diagnosis and lower risk with longer duration of the disease was observed for both aggressive and non-aggressive prostate cancer.[16] A meta-analysis of 19 studies found an inverse association between diabetes mellitus and prostate cancer (RR 0.84, 95% CI 0.76–0.9).[17] The plasma concentration of total and free testosterone, which may be involved in prostate cancer carcinogenesis or progression of the disease, is lower in men with diabetes mellitus.[1] However, higher testosterone levels have not been consistently associated with prostate cancer risk.

Other cancer sites

A positive association with diabetes (RR 2.10, 95% CI 1.75–2.53) was reported in a recent meta-analysis involving 16 studies of endometrial cancer.[18] Other types of cancer associated with diabetes mellitus in some studies include ovarian cancer, cancer of the biliary tract, kidney cancer and non-Hodgkin's lymphoma.

14.3 Hyperinsulinaemia and cancer risk

Individuals with diabetes mellitus initially experience hyperglycaemia and hyperinsulinaemia, although insulin concentrations eventually decrease due to pancreatic β-cell depletion.[19] Hyperinsulinaemia has been hypothesized to be an underlying factor in chronic conditions such as obesity, type 2 diabetes mellitus and certain forms of cancer. Obesity and physical inactivity are important determinants of hyperinsulinaemia and insulin resistance.[19] Several metabolic disturbances including hyperglycaemia and hypertriglyceridaemia are associated with hyperinsulinaemia and insulin resistance. In the discussion that follows, results from epidemiological studies of hyperinsulinaemia and risk of cancer of the pancreas, colon, prostate and other sites are discussed in relation to possible biological mechanisms for observed associations.

Pancreatic cancer

The biological mechanism by which diabetes leads to pancreatic cancer may relate to hyperinsulinaemia. Insulin levels are higher in patients with diabetes and in obese people, and obesity has been associated with pancreatic cancer in cohort studies. Insulin concentrations in pancreatic ductal cells are 20-fold higher than in the systemic circulation.[20] Experimental studies have shown that insulin promotes growth in human pancreatic cell lines. Peripheral insulin resistance is associated with increased cell turnover of pancreatic islet cells, and stimulation of islet cell proliferation may enhance pancreatic carcinogenesis. Epidemiological studies of elevated insulin levels and pancreatic cancer risk have assessed hyperinsulinaemia and insulin secretion in various ways (e.g. fasting or non-fasting insulin or C-peptide levels).

Colorectal cancer

In the Physicians' Health Study, which involved 15 000 male doctors, levels of C-peptide were associated with the risk of developing colorectal cancer among people who did not have diabetes.[3] Men with C-peptide in the top versus the bottom quintile had a 2.7-fold increased risk of colorectal cancer with adjustment for body mass index and exercise.[3] These observations are consistent with the hypothesis that hyperinsulinaemia is an important factor in the development of colon cancer. Elevated insulin levels may occur early in the natural history of diabetes mellitus as the result of insulin resistance and decline over time among patients with diabetes as the result of damage to β cells. Although hyperinsulinaemia appears to be a marker for increased colon cancer risk, it remains unclear whether this is due to a direct effect of insulin on tumour growth or to other changes such as an increase in IGF-I.[19]

Prostate cancer

Several epidemiological studies have examined plasma glucose and insulin levels in relation to prostate cancer risk. Hyperglycaemia, which is associated with hyperinsulinaemia, was associated with a statistically non-significant increased risk of prostate cancer in the Chicago Heart Association

Detection Project cohort, although not all studies have observed an association between insulin or glucose levels and prostate cancer risk. Despite the inconsistency of results across studies, elevated insulin levels may increase risk of prostate cancer progression.[19]

14.4 IGF-I and its binding proteins and risk of cancer

IGF-I and its binding proteins are regulatory peptides that influence cell growth and survival. Hyperinsulinaemia increases IGF-I activity in colorectal, prostatic and other tissues. IGF-I is involved in cell proliferation and differentiation. It may promote tumour development by stimulating cell proliferation and inhibiting apoptosis. Serum levels of IGF-I vary widely between individuals. Both IGF-I and IGF-II are primarily produced in the liver. A large variety of cells express IGF-I and IGF-II receptors. IGF-binding protein 3 (IGFBP-3) is the main carrier protein for IGF-I in the blood. Several high-affinity IGF-I binding proteins have been identified, including IGFBP-1, IGFBP-2 and IGFBP-3. The tissue activity of IGF-I, which binds to the IGF-I receptor on the target cell surface, is determined by free IGF-I that is not bound to binding proteins.[20] Obesity influences the amount of free IGF-I available to cells, but is not an important determinant of total circulating IGF-I levels.[19] Insulin inhibits the synthesis of IGFBP-1 in the liver and other tissues, and thereby increases circulating levels of free IGF-I. In contrast to IGF-I, IGF-II and IGFBP-3, plasma levels of IGFBP-1 are altered acutely by recent food intake and regulated by several hormones involved in glucose and energy homeostasis.[21]

IGF-I, IGF-II and IGFBP-1, and risk of pancreatic cancer

Wolpin et al.[21] conducted a nested case–control study of IGFBP-1 and colorectal cancer risk among men and women who had been enrolled in the Health Professionals Follow-up Study, the Nurses' Health Study, the Physicians' Health Study and the Women's Health Initiative. A total of 144 incident cases of pancreatic cancer were identified along with 429 matched control individuals. Prediagnostic plasma levels of IGFBP-1 were inversely associated with pancreatic cancer risk. When compared with participants in the three highest quartiles of plasma IGFBP-1, those in the lowest quartile had a relative risk of pancreatic cancer of 2.07 (95% CI 1.26–3.39), after adjusting for IGF-I, C-peptide and other risk factors. Among a somewhat larger sample of participants from these four US cohort studies (212 incident cases of pancreatic cancer and 635 matched controls), no associations were observed between plasma levels of IGF-I, IGF-II or IFGBP-3 and pancreatic cancer.[20] Prior studies in small samples of pancreatic cancer cases from Finland and Japan provide little or no support for a significant association between prediagnostic plasma levels of IGF-I or IGFBP-3 and pancreatic cancer risk.

IGF-I, IGFBP-1, IGFBP-2 and IGFBP-3, and risk of colorectal cancer

Epidemiological studies of circulating IGF-I and colon cancer risk have generally found modest increases in risk.[19] Wei et al.[22] conducted a nested case–control study of IGF-I, IGFBP-1, IGFBP-3 and C-peptide levels and colorectal cancer risk among women who had been enrolled in the Nurses' Health Study; 182 incident cases of colorectal cancer were identified over a 10-year follow-up period and were matched to 350 control individuals. Fasting IGFBP-1 was inversely associated with risk of colon cancer (RR 0.28, 95% CI 0.11–0.75), and C-peptide levels were weakly associated with colon cancer risk (RR 1.76, 95% CI 0.85–3.63). High C-peptide levels and low IGFBP-1 levels are indictors of hyperinsulinaemia. The multicentre European Prospective Investigation into Cancer and Nutrition (EPIC) cohort study is the largest study on the topic, comprising 1121 colorectal cancer cases and 1121 control individuals.[23] Comparing the highest with the lowest quintile in IGF-I concentrations, the RR for colorectal cancer was non-significant (RR 1.07). The authors investigated the association between IGF-I and colorectal cancer stratified by dietary intake and found significant positive associations among individuals with low intake of milk and dairy calcium. The most recent meta-analysis published in 2010 by the authors of the EPIC analysis shows a moderately significantly increased risk of colorectal cancer (RR per standard deviation increase in IGF-I = 1.07), even when including the null finding from the large EPIC study.[23]

IGF-I, IGFBP-1 and IGFBP-3, and risk of breast cancer

The relationship between prediagnostic IGF-I and IGFBP-3 levels and breast cancer risk was recently examined in a meta-analysis of data from 17 prospective studies conducted in 12 countries.[24] The overall odds ratio for breast cancer for women in the highest versus the lowest quintile of IGF-I concentration was 1.28 (95% CI 1.14–1.44). The positive association with IGF-I, which was not substantially modified by IGFBP-3 or menopausal status, was limited to oestrogen-receptor-positive breast cancers. Although some studies have suggested that IGF-I is positively associated with risk of breast cancer among premenopausal women, the results of epidemiological studies have been inconsistent. Schernhammer et al.[25] conducted a nested case–control study of IGF-I, IGFBP-1 and IGFBP-3 and breast cancer risk in the Nurses' Health Study II cohort, which mainly consists of premenopausal women. Plasma levels of IGF-I and its binding proteins were measured using prediagnostic samples obtained from 317 women diagnosed with invasive or *in situ* breast cancer and 634 matched control women. Overall, plasma IGF-I, IGFBP-1 and IGFBP-3 were not associated with breast cancer risk. In order to further examine the relationships between IGF-I and breast cancer risk among premenopausal women, Rinaldi et al.[26] conducted a pooled analysis of data from three prospective studies in New York, northern Sweden and Milan, Italy. Statistically non-significant, positive associations were observed between IGF-I and IGFBP-3 and breast cancer risk among younger women.

In general, results from epidemiological studies do not support an association between IGFBP-1 and breast cancer risk. Although results from some epidemiological studies support an association between IGFBP-3 and risk of breast cancer among younger women, results to date have been inconsistent. This inconsistency across studies may be accounted for by differences in study design and lack of standardization across assays.

IGF-I and IGFBP-3, and risk of prostate cancer

IGF-I promotes cell proliferation and inhibits apoptosis in normal prostate and tumour cells *in vitro*. In most, but not all, epidemiological studies, IGF-I levels have been associated with an increased risk of prostate cancer, particularly advanced cancer.[19] In their systematic review and meta-analysis of IGF-I, IGFBP-3 and cancer risk, Renehan et al.[27] found that high concentrations of IGF-I were associated with an increased risk of prostate cancer. The summary odds ratio comparing the 75th versus the 25th percentile was 1.49 (95% CI 1.14–1.95). A recent systematic review and meta-analysis of IGF-I and its binding proteins and risk of prostate cancer confirmed that increased levels of IGF-I are positively associated with prostate cancer.[28] There was weak evidence that the associations of IGF-I and IGFBP-3 with prostate cancer are stronger for advanced disease.

In a case–control study of prostate cancer nested in the European Prospective Investigation into Cancer and Nutrition cohort, the relative risk of prostate cancer was 1.35 (95% CI 0.99–1.82 for highest vs lowest tertile of IGF-I). The association between serum IGF-I concentration and risk of prostate cancer was slightly stronger for advanced-stage disease.

14.5 Diabetes treatment and cancer

Medications used to treat diabetes, as discussed elsewhere in this book, include drugs that increase insulin sensitivity and decrease hyperinsulinaemia, such as metformin and thiazolidinediones, and those that increase insulin levels such as sulfonylureas, exogenous insulin and insulin analogues. Given that hyperinsulinaemia has been implicated in carcinogenesis, it is plausible that drugs that act directly or indirectly on insulin exposure could influence cancer risk. However, the evidence that specific drugs affect risk is complicated by numerous methodological challenges, such as confounding by indication, and the complex and progressive nature of hyperglycaemia in patients with diabetes, which frequently leads to therapy from multiple drugs.

Insulin and secretagogues

The evidence from epidemiological and in vitro studies of a link between hyperinsulinaemia and risk of common cancers has generated questions about the possible carcinogenic effect of insulin analogues. Studies that have compared cancer risk among patients receiving different types of antidiabetic medications must be evaluated in the light of the growing body of evidence that suggests that metformin protects against cancer. As Nicolucci[7] put it, 'it is not clear whether secretagogues increase cancer risk or simply metformin lowers the average risk in those who are taking this drug'. Epidemiological studies of this long-acting insulin analogue, including observational studies conducted in Germany, Sweden, Scotland and the UK, were followed by a meta-analysis of 31 clinical trials. Results from the meta-analysis did not show an association between insulin glargine and increased cancer risk, although duration of use may not have been sufficiently long and the number of individual cancers were low. Taken overall, results to date do not consistently support an association between insulin glargine and cancer risk, but further more definitive work is warranted.

Metformin

Oral hypoglycaemic agents such as metformin have been studied as possible chemopreventive and adjuvant therapies for cancer. Evidence to date suggests that metformin protects against the development of certain cancers and may improve prognosis in patients with cancer.[7] For example, in a cohort study in the Netherlands, in which 1353 people with diabetes were followed for a median of 9.6 years, patients taking metformin had a reduced risk of cancer mortality compared with patients not taking metformin at baseline (hazard ratio 0.43, 95% CI 0.23–0.80). Randomized trials are currently ongoing to test the possible cancer chemopreventive effect of metformin and to examine its effectiveness as an adjuvant therapy for breast cancer.

14.6 Treatment of cancer among diabetics

Although this review has primarily focused on the development of cancer of the colon, rectum, pancreas, prostate, breast and other sites among people with diabetes, hypoglycaemia or elevated insulin or IGF-I levels, the co-occurrence of diabetes and cancer raises important issues for clinicians who treat cancer patients. As noted above, about 8–18 per cent of people with cancer also have diabetes. The coexistence of the two conditions varies by cancer site.[7] Clinicians who treat diabetic cancer patients must consider the cardiac, hepatic, renal and neurological complications that are commonly seen among patients with diabetes.[8] Richardson and Pollack[8] noted that some chemotherapeutic agents (e.g. anthracyclines) are used at lower doses or omitted from regimens to avoid cardiotoxicity in patients with pre-existing cardiovascular disease, such as coronary heart disease or congestive heart failure associated with diabetes. As a further example, chemotherapeutic agents that cause or exacerbate renal insufficiency (e.g. cisplatin) must be avoided or used cautiously among patients with decreased renal function.[8] Many cancer chemotherapeutic agents are excreted by the kidney and may worsen pre-existing renal insufficiency due to diabetic nephropathy or other conditions.

Taken overall, evidence from clinical trials and population-based studies indicate that, after cancer diagnosis and treatment, patients with diabetes experience higher mortality and cancer recurrence rates than non-diabetic patients, although more clinical research on this topic is needed.[8] Reported studies have indicated that patients with hyperglycaemia or diabetes who undergo cancer treatment may be more likely to experience certain side effects (e.g. infections leading to sepsis) than patients who do not have hyperglycaemia or diabetes. Serious side effects have been described among head and neck cancer patients with diabetes who were treated with certain drug regimens. Based on current knowledge, the speculated but unsubstantiated role of some diabetes drugs in affecting cancer risk should not be a major factor in choosing among therapies for the average patient.

14.7 Conclusions

As highlighted in this chapter, diabetes mellitus and associated conditions such as hyperglycaemia and hyperinsulinaemia have been associated with the risk of several cancers including pancreatic, colorectal, endometrial and liver cancer. Associations identified with other cancer sites in epidemiological studies are suggestive. It is unknown whether the association between diabetes and some cancers is largely due to shared factors such as obesity and inactivity, or whether the specific metabolic derangements associated with diabetes such as hyperinsulinaemia and hyperglycaemia directly increase cancer risk. Nevertheless, because obesity and physical inactivity are the main determinants of insulin resistance and hyperinsulinaemia, the public health importance of these findings is clear. Evidence-based interventions that increase physical activity and reduce obesity in clinical settings and in communities are likely to have beneficial effects on risk of diabetes and several common cancers. Of particular interest for aetiological research are the studies that have shown that the IGF-I axis is related to cancer risk. Increases in circulating levels of IGF-I have been observed in several epidemiological studies of colorectal, prostate and breast cancer.

Clinicians who treat cancer patients must consider the cardiac, hepatic, renal and neurological complications that are commonly seen among patients with diabetes. Evidence has been found in clinical trials and population-based studies to suggest that, after a cancer diagnosis and treatment, patients with diabetes experience higher mortality and cancer recurrence rates than non-diabetic patients. In addition, patients with hyperglycaemia or diabetes undergoing cancer treatment may be more likely to experience certain side effects than patients who do not have hyperglycaemia or diabetes. A growing body of evidence suggests that metformin protects against the development of certain cancers and may improve prognosis in patients with breast cancer. Randomized trials to test these hypotheses are currently ongoing.

References

1. Adami HO, McLaughlin J, Ekbom A, et al. Cancer risk in patients with diabetes mellitus. *Cancer Causes Control* 1991;**2**:307–314.
2. Calle EE, Murphy TK, Rodriguez C, et al. Diabetes mellitus and pancreatic cancer mortality in a prospective cohort of United States adults. *Cancer Causes Control* 1998;**9**:403–410.
3. Ma J, Pollak MN, Giovannucci E, et al. Prospective study of colorectal cancer risk in men and plasma levels of insulin-like growth factor (IGF)-1 and IGF-binding protein-3. *J Natl Cancer Instit* 1999;**91**:620–625.
4. Hankinson SE, Willett WC, Colditz GA, et al. Circulating concentrations of insulin-like growth factor-I and risk of breast cancer. *Lancet* 1998;**351**:1393–1396.
5. Wolk A, Mantzoros CS, Anderson SO, et al. Insulin-like growth factor 1 and prostate cancer risk: a population-based, case-control study. *J Natl Cancer Instit* 1998;**90**: 911–915.
6. Giovannucci E, Rimm EB, Stampfer MJ, et al. Diabetes mellitus and risk of prostate cancer. *Cancer Causes Control* 1998;**9**:3–9.
7. Nicolucci A. Epidemiological aspects of neoplasms in diabetes. *Acta Diabetol* 2010;**47**:87–95.
8. Richardson LC, Pollack LA. Therapy insight: influence of type 2 diabetes on the development, treatment and outcomes of cancer. *Natl Clin Pract Oncol* 2005;**2**: 48–53.
9. Coughlin SS, Calle EE, Teras LR, et al. Diabetes mellitus as a predictor of cancer mortality in a large cohort of US adults. *Am J Epidemiol* 2004;**159**:1160–1167.
10. Huxley R, Ansary-Moghaddam A, Berrington de Gonzalez A, Woodward M. Type-II diabetes and pancreatic cancer: a meta-analysis of 36 studies. *Br J Cancer* 2005; **92**:2076–2083.

11. La Vecchia C, Negri E, D'Avanzo B, et al. Medical history and primary liver cancer. *Cancer Res* 1990;**50**:6274–6277.

12. Larsson SC, Orsini N, Wolk A. Diabetes mellitus and risk of colorectal cancer: a meta-analysis. *J Natl Cancer Instit* 2005;**97**:1679–1687.

13. Michels KB, Solomon CG, Hu FB, et al. Nurses' Health Study. Type 2 diabetes and subsequent incidence of breast cancer. *Diabet Care* 2003;**26**:1752–1758.

14. Talamini R, Franceschi S, Favero A, et al. Selected medical conditions and risk of breast cancer. *Br J Cancer* 1997;**75**:1699–1703.

15. Pisani, P. Hyper-insulinaemia and cancer, meta-analyses of epidemiological studies. *Arch Physiol Biochem* 2008;**114**:63–70.

16. Rodriguez C, Patel AV, Mondul AM, et al. Diabetes and risk of prostate cancer in a prospective cohort of US men. *Am J Epidemiol* 2005;**161**:147–152.

17. Kasper JS, Giovannucci E. A meta-analysis of diabetes mellitus and the risk of prostate cancer. *Cancer Epidemiol Biomarkers Prev* 2006;**15**:2056–2062.

18. Friberg E, Orsini N, Mantzoros CS, Wolk A. Diabetes mellitus and risk of endometrial cancer: a meta-analysis. *Diabetologia* 2007;**50**:1365–1374.

19. Giovannucci E, Michaud D. The role of obesity and related metabolic disturbances in cancers of the colon, prostate, and pancreas. *Gastroenterology* 2007;**132**: 2208–2225.

20. Wolpin BM, Michaud DS, Giovannucci EL, et al. Circulating insulin-like growth factor axis and the risk of pancreatic cancer in four prospective cohorts. *Br J Cancer* 2007;**97**:98–104.

21. Wolpin BM, Michaud DS, Giovannucci EL, et al. Circulating insulin-like growth factor binding protein-1 and the risk of pancreatic cancer. *Cancer Res* 2007;**67**: 7923–7928.

22. Wei EK, Ma J, Pollak MN, et al. A prospective study of C-peptide, insulin-like growth factor-I, insulin-like growth factor binding protein-1, and the risk of colorectal cancer in women. *Cancer Epidemiol Biomarkers Prev* 2005;**14**:850–855.

23. Rinaldi S, Cleveland R, Norat T, et al. Serum levels of IGF-I, IGFBP-3 and colorectal cancer risk: results from the EPIC cohort, plus a meta-analysis of prospective studies. *Int J Cancer* 2010;**1**:1702–1715.

24. Endogenous Hormones and Breast Cancer Collaborative Group. Insulin-like growth factor 1 (IGF1), IGF binding protein 3 (IGFBP3), and breast cancer risk: pooled individual data analysis of 17 prospective studies. *Lancet Oncol* 2010;**11**:530–542.

25. Schernhammer ES, Holly JM, Hunter DJ, et al. Insulin-like growth factor-I, its binding proteins (IGFBP-1 and IFGBP-3), and growth hormone and breast cancer risk in The Nurses Health Study II. *Endocrine-Related Cancer* 2006;**13**:583–592.

26. Rinaldi S, Peeters PH, Berrino F, et al. IGF-I, IGFBP-3 and breast cancer risk in women: the European Prospective Investigation into Cancer and Nutrition (EPIC). *Endocrine-Related Cancer* 2006;**13**:593–605.

27. Renehan AG, Zwahlen M, Minder C, et al. Insulin-like growth factor (IGF)-I, IGF binding protein-3, and cancer risk: systematic review and meta-regression analysis. *Lancet* 2004;**363**:1346–1353.

28. Rowlands M-A, Gunnell D, Harris R, et al. Circulating insulin-like growth factor (IGF) peptides and prostate cancer risk: a systematic review and meta-analysis. *Int J Cancer* 2009;**124**:2416–2429.

Multiple Choice Questions

Chapter 1

1. What percentage of people with type 1 diabetes can be expected to have diabetic retinopathy at diagnosis?
   A 85–100 per cent
   B 37–84 per cent
   C 20–37 per cent
   D 2–19 per cent
   E <2 per cent

2. What percentage of people with type 2 diabetes can be expected to have diabetic retinopathy present at the time of diagnosis of diabetes?
   A 85–100 per cent
   B 37–84 per cent
   C 20–37 per cent
   D 2–19 per cent
   E <2 per cent

3. Which of these statements about treating diabetic eye disease is false?
   A The use of angiotensin-converting enzyme Inhibitors is contraindicated.
   B Laser therapy can usually be performed as an outpatient procedure.
   C Laser therapy gives a better result in proliferative eye disease than in maculopathy.
   D Worsening maculopathy is a risk of cataract extraction.
   E Panretinal photocoagulation can affect ability to drive.

Diabetes: Chronic Complications, Third Edition. Edited by Kenneth M. Shaw, Michael H. Cummings.
© 2012 John Wiley & Sons, Ltd. Published 2012 by John Wiley & Sons, Ltd.

4. Which of these is not a feature of R1M0/background diabetic retinopathy?
   A Hard exudates
   B Microaneurysms
   C Venous beading
   D 'Dot' haemorrhages
   E 'Blot' haemorrhages

Chapter 2

1. Which one of the following medications does not require a dose reduction in the setting of reduced GFR and/or is contraindicated if GFR <60 ml/min per $1.73\,m^2$?
   A Sitagliptin
   B Fenofibrate
   C Metformin
   D Atorvastatin
   E Exenatide

2. Which of the following is not true with regard to statin use in people with diabetic CKD?
   A Statins reduce cardiovascular events in people with diabetes and CKD stages I–IV.
   B Statins in combination with ezetrol are not contraindicated in people with CKD.
   C Statins reduce CV events in people with end-stage renal disease (ESRD).
   D People with microalbuminuria should generally be on a statin.
   E The combination of a statin and a fibrate is not contraindicated in people with reduced GFR.

3. With regard to microalbuminuria, which one of the following statements is false?
   A Lack of microalbuminuria does not exclude renal disease.
   B Microalbuminuria is a marker of increased risk for cardiovascular disease.
   C All patients with microalbuminuria will progress to more advanced stages of CKD.
   D Microalbuminuria may remit to normoalbuminuria without any specific intervention.
   E Microalbuminuria refers to detectable but low concentrations of albumin in urine.

4. With regard to blood pressure control in people with diabetes and CKD, which of the following is not true?
   A ACE inhibitors and angiotensin receptor blockers (ARBs) are equally effective in reducing albuminuria.
   B The combination of an ACE inhibitor and an ARB confers renal protection over and above the use of each agent alone.
   C The general blood pressure target for people with diabetic CKD and proteinuria is <125/75 mmHg.
   D The optimal BP target for preventing progression of CKD is not established.
   E In patients treated with ARBs, implementing salt restriction confers further benefits in terms of BP reduction.

5. With regard to assessment of renal function in people with diabetes, which of the following is true?
   A An eGFR derived from an MDRD formula significantly underestimates GFR in the normal range.
   B A decline in GFR is always preceded by a rise in albuminuria.
   C Cystatin C is not a more accurate measure of renal function than creatinine for people with GFR levels in the normal range.
   D Albuminuria can be accurately estimated from one spot ACR measurement.
   E Acute hyperglycaemia has no effect on albuminuria.

Chapter 3

1. NAFLD confers a higher risk of all of the following except:
   A Hepatocellular carcinoma
   B Cardiovascular disease
   C Advanced liver disease
   D Autoimmune hepatitis

2. The gold standard for assessing the extent of steatohepatitis and cirrhosis in patients with suspected fatty liver disease is:
   A Fibroscan
   B Laboratory values
   C Liver biopsy
   D Abdominal MRI

3. Aggressive weight loss via dietary modifications or bariatric surgery is recommended for all patients with NAFLD.
   A True
   B False

Chapter 4

1. A 57-year-old man presents for evaluation of long-standing diabetes. He has had type 2 diabetes mellitus for 25 years. He has developed severe peripheral neuropathy and has a difficult time keeping his blood sugar <250 mg/dl. Over the last 2 years he has had continuous diarrhoea and has lost 18 kg (40 lb). He has frequent bouts of faecal incontinence. His 48-hour stool collection yielded a faecal fat output of 20 g/24 h. Probable causes for this picture include all of the following EXCEPT:
   A Diabetic neuropathy
   B Excessive sorbitol ingestion
   C Small bowel bacterial overgrowth
   D Coeliac disease
   E Pancreatic exocrine insufficiency

2. A 35-year-old woman with a 15-year history of diabetes presents with nausea, vomiting, early satiety and weight loss of 9 kg (20 lb) in the past year. She reports often vomiting food eaten 1 or 2 days previously. She has hyperglycaemia (glucose 238 mg/dl), glycated Hb 8.5%, proteinuria (4 g/24 h), and serum albumin 2.4 g/dl, total cholesterol 445 mg/dl and creatinine 1.7 mg/dl. The most likely diagnosis is:
   A Emesis secondary to uraemia.
   B Diabetic gastroparesis with malnutrition
   C Diabetic gastroparesis with nephrotic syndrome
   D Chronic pancreatitis and malnutrition secondary to hyperlipidaemia
   E *H. pylori* infection without ulceration

3. In the patient described in question 2, upper gastrointestinal endoscopy shows the presence of retained undigested food, and no evidence of ulceration, or pyloric obstruction. A CLO test on a gastric mucosal sample is positive. The most appropriate test to assess the cause of the vomiting is:
   A No tests, but eradication of *H. pylori* and review after 6 weeks
   B Gastric emptying test for solids or solids and liquids
   C Brain MRI including special 'cuts' to visualize vagal nuclei
   D CCK-secretin-stimulated measurement of pancreatic exocrine function
   E Antropyloroduodenal manometry or, if unavailable, autonomic function test and surface electrogastrography

4. A 48-year-old man with a 17-year history of diabetes presents with a 2-year history of chronic diarrhoea: watery to loose, occasionally nocturnal, no blood, no mucus, rarely floats or contains undigested food. His diarrhoea did not improve when he was given a broad-spectrum antibiotic for a chest infection. He noted no difference when on a gluten-free diet. Quantitative faecal fat output is within normal limits. Abdominal and rectal exams are normal. His chart includes his HLA haplotype (A1B8). What is his most likely diagnosis?

   A Coeliac disease
   B Chronic pancreatic insufficiency
   C Diabetic diarrhoea
   D Bacterial overgrowth
   E Pudendal neuropathy secondary to longstanding diabetes

Chapter 5

1. How common is foot ulceration in the diabetic population?
   A Between 1 and 2 per cent
   B Between 5 and 7.4 per cent
   C Between 10 and 20 per cent
   D Less than 1 per cent

2. What is a common precipitating factor for tissue damage in the ischaemic foot?
   A Bony fractures
   B Minor trauma, e.g. from ill-fitting footwear
   C Arterial embolism
   D Raised cholesterol

3. In a patient with diabetes and neuropathy with a warm red mid-foot, the most important condition to consider is:
   A Gout
   B Septic arthritis
   C Fungal infection
   D Acute Charcot disease

4. The following symptoms suggest neuropathic pain:
   A Pain predominantly at night worsened by contact with bedsheets
   B Burning sensations in the feet punctuated by sharp electric-shock pains
   C Continuous pain or discomfort not relieved by traditional analgesics
   D All of the above

Chapter 6

1. A diagnosis of diabetic autonomic neuropathy can be confirmed by:
   A Abnormal heart rate response to Valsalva's manoeuvre
   B Abnormal expired to inspired heart rate ratio
   C Abnormal blood pressure response to standing
   D Evidence of delayed gastric emptying
   E None of the above

2. The following test predominantly parasympathetic nerve function:
   A Abnormal heart rate response to Valsalva's manoeuvre
   B Abnormal expired:inspired heart rate ratio
   C Abnormal blood pressure response to standing
   D Dark-adapted pupil diameter
   E Low frequency heart rate variability

3. The following are typical features of diabetic diarrhoea:
   A Painful symptoms
   B More troublesome during the day
   C Often associated with faecal incontinence
   D Ameliorated by therapy with metformin
   E May alternate with periods of constipation

4. Treatment of gastroparesis includes:
   A Domperidone
   B Propantheline bromide
   C GLP-1 analogues
   D Antiemetics such as prochlorperazine
   E Loperamide

Chapter 7

1. Which of the following is not involved in tumescence?
   A The sympathetic nervous system
   B The corpus cavernosum
   C The helicine artery
   D Cyclic GMP
   E Dopamine

2. Oral phosphodiesterase type 5 (PDE-5) inhibitors should be avoided in patients taking
   A An angiotensin II receptor blocker
   B A potassium channel activator

    C A β blocker

    D A α_1 blocker

    E A thiazide diuretic

3. In patients who develop priapism after intracavernosal injection therapy, which option would you not recommend in trying to achieve detumescence?

    A Aspiration of blood from the corpus cavernosum

    B Using an exercise bike

    C The application of ice packs around the penis

    D α_1 Blockers

    E Surgical shunt procedures

4. Which of the following statements is true?

    A A therapeutic trial of testosterone can be used in any patient with erectile dysfunction and decreased libido.

    B The effects of oral PDE-5 inhibitors are enhanced by alcohol consumption.

    C Patients with angina should not be treated for erectile dysfunction.

    D Penile Doppler studies are a useful test in most cases of erectile dysfunction.

    E Enhancement of cyclic AMP availability is a pharmacological pathway that is used for the treatment of erectile dysfunction.

Chapter 8

1. In type 2 diabetes, heart failure:

    A Presents more commonly in men

    B Is best treated by coronary revascularization

    C Occurs independently of hypertension and coronary artery disease

    D Is improved with glitazone therapy

2. Hypertension and diabetes:

    A Is more common with type 1 than type 2 diabetes

    B Is greater when microalbuminuria is detected

    C Blood pressure treatment does not reduce risk of developing future microvascular complications

    D β Blockers are first-line treatment

3. Insulin deficiency is associated with:

    A Increased triglycerides

    B Increased lipoprotein lipase activity

    C Reduced LDL-cholesterol susceptibility to oxidation

    D Improved lipid status with nephropathy

4. Glycaemic control and diabetes:
   A Intensified blood glucose control improves life expectancy
   B Hyperglycaemia occurs in more than one in four patients with acute coronary syndrome
   C Insulin is the first choice of glucose-lowering therapy in heart failure
   D Is the top priority in multifactorial intervention

Chapter 9

1. Cognitive function impairment as a result of acute hypoglycaemia:
   A Occurs only when symptoms of hypoglycaemia are present
   B Occurs in everyone at approximately 3 mmol/l
   C Does not occur in those patients with a recurrent hypoglycaemic experience
   D Generally only returns to normal 30–40 minutes after the return of euglycaemia

2. The following are recognized risk factors for stroke in diabetes:
   A Atrial fibrillation
   B Hypertension or hyperlipidaemia
   C Recurrent hypoglycaemia
   D Type 2 rather than type 1 diabetes

3. Which of the following statements are true?
   A Type 1 diabetes is a risk factor in the development of haemorrhagic stroke.
   B Avoidance of treatment-associated hypoglycaemia necessarily increases an individual's exposure to hyperglycaemia and thus increased long-term risk.
   C Children under the age of 5 years are less at risk of long-term risks from hypoglycaemia because of the increased brain plasticity of youth.
   D Blood glucose levels measured at admission to hospital in patients with cerebrovascular disease have no impact on the outcome of the admission.

Chapter 10

1. Which of the following may be used to assess depression in a person with diabetes?
   A HADS rating score
   B PANSS rating score

    C PHQ-9 questionnaire
    D Diagnostic interview
    E Serum cortisol

2. Which of the following statements about the relationship between diabetes and depression are TRUE?
    A The risk of diabetes is increased two- to threefold in people with depression.
    B The risk of depression is decreased in people receiving insulin compared with people treated with oral hypoglycaemic agents.
    C Painful neuropathy increases the risk of depression.
    D Antidepressants improve mild depression in people with diabetes.
    E Psychotherapy is associated with improved glycaemic control as well as improvements in depressive symptoms in people with diabetes and depression.

3. Which of the following factors explains the increase in diabetes in people with schizophrenia?
    A Genetics
    B High birthweight
    C Poor nutrition
    D Antipsychotic medication
    E Physical inactivity

4. Which of the following is true about screening for cardiovascular risk factors in people with severe mental illness?
    A The rate of undiagnosed diabetes is the same as the general population.
    B Screening should be undertaken before the initiation of antipsychotic medication.
    C Screening is more likely to occur in people with severe mental illness compared with the general population.
    D Screening should be undertaken only in people over the age of 40 years as for the rest of the population.
    E Cardiovascular risk tables have been validated in people with severe mental illness.

Chapter 11

1. What is the most likely explanation for the arthritis of the patient in case study 1?
    A Scleroderma
    B Adult-onset Still's disease

C Haemochromatosis

D Gout

2. The most likely explanation of the right hand symptoms of the patient in case study 2 is:

   A Diabetic polyneuropathy

   B Overuse/repetitive-strain syndrome

   C Carpal tunnel syndrome

   D Alcoholic neuropathy

   E None of the above

3. What is the next step in the management of the symptoms of the patient in case study 3?

   A Shoulder immobilization

   B Aggressive physical therapy to regain range of motion

   C Manipulation of his shoulder under anaesthesia

   D Pain control

   E Intra-articular injection with steroids

Chapter 12

1. What percentage of the general UK adult population has advanced periodontitis?

   A 0–5 per cent

   B Approximately 10 per cent

   C Approximately 30 per cent

   D >50 per cent

2. What magnitude of reduction in mean HbA1c has been reported in meta-analyses of studies that investigated the impact of periodontal treatment on glycaemic control?

   A <0.1 per cent

   B 0.4 per cent

   C 1.0 per cent

   D 1.4 per cent

3. What systemic medication has been licensed as an adjunctive treatment for the management of periodontitis?

   A Aspirin 75 mg once daily indefinitely

   B Amoxicillin 250 mg three times daily for 7 days

   C Doxycycline 20 mg twice daily for 12 weeks

   D Metronidazole 400 mg three times daily for 7 days

Chapter 13

1. A 28-year-old woman with type 1 diabetes has a 1-year history of an erythematous to yellow, asymptomatic, non-scaly, slightly atrophic plaque on her shin. What is the most likely diagnosis?
   A Eczema
   B Psoriasis
   C Necrobiosis lipoidica
   D Lichen planus
   E Actinic porokeratosis

2. A 60-year-old man with insulin-treated type 2 diabetes and known hypertension and ischaemic heart disease keeps getting recurrent bilateral lower leg erythema on a basis of persistently swollen ankles. Though his legs are itchy he feels well in himself. What could be contributing to his condition?
   A His calcium antagonist medication for his blood pressure
   B Bilateral cellulitis
   C Eczema
   D Psoriasis
   E Lipodermatosclerosis

3. A 35-year-old man presents feeling tired with nocturia and a rapid onset of yellow papules clustered over his elbows and buttocks. What could be contributing to his presentation?
   A New-onset diabetes
   B Hypertriglyceridaemia
   C If he had a familial defective apolipoprotein B-100
   D His known apolipoprotein CII deficiency
   E His familial combined hypercholesterolaemia
   F The fact that he lives on crisps and non-diet cola drinks and multivitamins.

Chapter 14

1. Which of the following has not been consistently associated with diabetes in epidemiological studies?
   A Pancreatic cancer
   B Colorectal cancer
   C Leukaemia
   D Liver cancer
   E Endometrial cancer

2. Which of the following is true about insulin-like growth factor I?
   A IGF-I is a binding protein that influences cell growth and survival.
   B IGF-I is involved in cell proliferation and differentiation.
   C IGF-I is primarily produced in the liver.
   D Serum levels of IGF-I vary widely between individuals.
   E All of the above.

3. Which of the following is true about the treatment of cancer patients with comorbid diabetes?
   A Serious side effects have been described among head and neck cancer patients treated with certain drug regimens.
   B Cancer chemotherapeutic agents may worsen pre-existing renal insufficiency due to diabetic nephropathy.
   C Patients with diabetes or hyperglycaemic who undergo cancer treatment may be more likely to experience infections leading to sepsis.
   D All of the above.
   E None of the above.

Answers

Chapter 1

1: E
2: C
3: A
4: C

Chapter 2

1: D
2: C
3: C
4: B
5: A

Chapter 3

1: D
2: C
3: B

Chapter 4

1: B
Patients with long-standing type 1 diabetes frequently develop diabetic neuropathy which can affect both peripheral and autonomic nerves. Diarrhoea is a frequent complication occurring in upwards of 20 per cent of these patients. The key distinction to make in assessing such patients is to distinguish patients with steatorrhoea from those without it. Small bowel bacterial overgrowth, coeliac disease and pancreatic exocrine insufficiency occur with greater frequency in people with

Diabetes: Chronic Complications, Third Edition. Edited by Kenneth M. Shaw, Michael H. Cummings.
© 2012 John Wiley & Sons, Ltd. Published 2012 by John Wiley & Sons, Ltd.

diabetes than in the general population and should be sought with appropriate tests in people with diabetes and steatorrhoea. People with diabetes but no steatorrhoea may have a secretory diarrhoea that seems to be due to reduction in adrenergic input to the enterocytes, probably as a result of diabetic autonomic neuropathy. Other problems such as ingestion of excess sorbitol, a sweetener used in many dietetic products, produce an osmotic diarrhoea without steatorrhoea. In this patient steatorrhoea is present, making answers C, D and E likely and answer B unlikely. Answer A, diabetic autonomic neuropathy, is probably the explanation for his faecal incontinence. Incontinence is not just a manifestation of 'severe' diarrhoea, but instead usually represents a problem with the neuromuscular apparatus preserving continence. Defects in patients with diabetes and faecal incontinence include impaired sensation and decreased anal sphincter strength, both probably due to neuropathy.

Folwaczny C, Riepl R, Tschop M, Landgraf R. Gastrointestinal involvement in patients with diabetes mellitus: Part I (first of two parts). Epidemiology, pathophysiology, clinical findings. *Z Gastroenterol* 1999;**37**:803–815.

Ziegler D. Diagnosis and treatment of diabetic autonomic neuropathy. *Curr Diab Rep* 2001;**1**:216–227.

2: C

The patient has the classic symptoms of gastroparesis with a long-standing history of diabetes and related complications, such as nephrotic syndrome. Several clinical series document the association of retinopathy, nephropathy and neuropathy with diabetic gastroparesis. However, delayed gastric emptying also occurs with type 2 diabetes. Associated risk factors include vagal neuropathy, hyperglycaemia, and effects of medications including exenetide used for postprandial hyperglycaemia.

3: B

Pancreatic function and brain imaging are not indicated based on the clinical history. Autonomic reflex screen and EGG would provide corroborative evidence of a disturbance in neural control of gastric function. Manometry is invasive and only available at specialized centres; it provides detailed physiological data, but does not necessarily assess severity of the gastroparesis or change a patient's management. *H. pylori* gastritis will not cause delayed stomach emptying and hence eradication of *H. pylori* will not be helpful. Gastric emptying measurement appraises the severity of the gastric stasis and helps guide nutritional and pharmacological management.

Park M-I, Camilleri M. Gastroparesis: clinical update. *Am J Gastroenterol* 2006;**101**: 1129–1139.

4: C

The most likely is diarrhoea due to diabetes, with no associated complications such as coeliac sprue, bacterial overgrowth or pancreatic insufficiency. A large proportion of patients with type 1 diabetes and coeliac disease have HLA-1B8 haplotype.

Valdovinos MA, Camilleri M, Zimmerman BR. Chronic diarrhea in diabetes mellitus: mechanisms and an approach to diagnosis and treatment. *Mayo Clin Proc* 1993;**68**: 691–702.

Chapter 5

1: B
2: B
3: D
4: D

Chapter 6

1: E
2: A, B
3: C, E
4: A, D

Chapter 7

1: A

It is the parasympathetic nervous system that facilitates erections. The sympathetic nervous system facilitates ejaculation and detumescence. Cyclic GMP is a mediator of penile smooth muscle relaxation, stimulated by nitric oxide. Dopamine is one of the chemical messengers within the hypothalamus that is stimulated by the presence of testosterone and is part of the neuronal pathway leading to tumescence.

2: B

Nicorandil because it is a nitric oxide donor.

3: D

α_1 Blockers would induce vasodilatation and further worsen the problem. A selective α_1-adrenergic agent (usually phenylephrine) is used to promote penile vasoconstriction. All other options are also aimed at reducing penile blood flow.

4: E

This pathway forms the basis of treatment with prostaglandin E_1 therapies (intraurethral pellets or intracavernosal injections) that increase cAMP availability and penile smooth muscle relaxation. Testosterone is indicated only for proven hypogonadism. Alcohol reduces the efficacy of PDE-5 inhibitors (sildenafil and vardenafil) or has no effect (tadalafil). Stable angina does not preclude an active sex life and penile Doppler studies nearly always demonstrate reduced penile blood flow in ED, but does not usually alter patient management.

Chapter 8

1: C
Heart failure occurs more commonly in women with diabetes than men; it is not significantly improved by revascularization. Both hypertension and coronary disease may contribute to pathogenesis, but a 'cardiomyopathy' as a direct metabolic consequence is recognized.

2: B
Hypertension, frequently part of the metabolic syndrome, is more commonly observed with type 2 diabetes. Early nephropathy, as indicated by positive microalbuminuria status, is associated with higher blood pressure levels. Several randomized controlled trials (RCTs) have confirmed the benefit of blood pressure reduction in the prevention of microangiopathic complications. β Blockers can impair insulin secretion and may be linked to new or aggravated diabetes.

3: A
Hypertriglyceridaemia is increased in diabetes, particularly type 2, and with poor glycaemic control. Lipoprotein lipase activity is reduced whereas LDL-cholesterol oxidation is increased. Renal impairment is associated with increasing dyslipidaemia.

4: B
Recent RCTs of intensified glycaemic therapy have failed to demonstrate a clear improvement in life expectancy and some (e.g. ACCORD) have been associated with increased mortality. Hyperglycaemia is a very common finding with acute coronary syndromes. Insulin has not been shown to have any additional benefit in heart failure over other glucose-lowering agents. Although reduction of hyperglycaemia is beneficial, tight control of lipids and blood pressure is associated with greater dividends, particularly in cardiovascular protection.

Chapter 9

1: B, D
It is important to recognize that neither symptoms nor past experience is a good guide to the presence or absence of hypoglycaemia that may

impact on cerebral function. In most individuals cognitive function is measurably reduced as the blood glucose levels drop between 3 and 2.8 mmol/L, and this occurs independent of the previous degree of hypoglycaemic exposure or symptomatic awareness. Following an episode of hypoglycaemia with cognitive impairment, it is particularly important to educate patients who drive that, even if they feel better and their re-tested blood glucose level is now >5, cognitive function (and thus reaction times) take 30–40 minutes to return to normal so any driving should be delayed at least this long.

2: A, B, D
The majority of stroke disease in diabetes is associated with type 2 rather than type 1 and adds to the presence of other established risk factors. Although there is perhaps some plausibility to the suggestion that recurrent hypoglycaemia might increase risk through recurrent adrenergic episodes, this has in fact never been described in surveys and is far outweighed by the atheromatous burden associated with poor glycaemic control.

3: none
Neither type 1 nor type 2 diabetes is associated with increased haemorrhagic stroke risk. The avoidance of hypoglycaemic can be achieved (with care and attention to required insulin changes) without impact on overall glycaemia, and indeed in many cases will actually improve the overall level of control by reduction of post-hypoglycaemic hyperglycaemia, which can often last for hours as a result of counter-regulatory insulin resistance. Children under 5 are most likely to be at the highest risk of hypoglycaemia-induced long-term change, with studies suggesting that those experiencing such episodes under the age of 5 may suffer a 5- to 7-point reduction in their IQ scores at age 11. Admission glucose levels for many clinical circumstances (including in particular stroke disease) have a profound impact on the likely outcome – the challenge of clinical research projects thus far has been to show that control of these levels is safely achievable and reduces adverse outcome.

Chapter 10

1: A, C, D
2: A, C, E
3: A, C, D, E
4: B

Chapter 11

1: C

The clinical and radiological features are those of haemochromatosis ('bronze diabetes'). The metacarpophalangeal arthritis with hook-like osteophytes is the hallmark sign of haemochromatosis arthritis. This, accompanied by the high ferritin level, diabetes and transaminitis, makes haemochromatosis the most likely diagnosis. The radiological findings are not those of gout ('rat-bite' lesions at articular areas) or pseudogout (chondrocalcinosis in the fibrocartilage); the indolent, rather than episodic and violent, arthritis is unusual for crystal-induced synovitis. Still's disease is possible, but generally would have certain other rheumatic symptoms and high inflammatory markers. Scleroderma patients can have an inflammatory arthritis as well, but the patient's presentation is not typical of that entity.

3: D

The patient has 'adhesive capsulitis'. This can develop spontaneously in people with diabetes. The condition is characterized by three distinct phases: painful, adhesive and resolution phases. The problem can last for months. There is no role for shoulder immobilization because this can further worsen the already limited range of motion. Aggressive physical therapy typically does not provide much benefit and may worsen patients' symptoms. As the condition is self-limited, initial treatment should be conservative and focus on pain control. Shoulder manipulation under anaesthesia is reserved for refractory cases. The role of intra-articular steroid injection is controversial.

2: C

Although the patient had poorly controlled diabetes with symptoms of diabetic neuropathy in her toes, she had unilateral paraesthesias in her right hand. This is more consistent with a local entrapment syndrome such as carpal tunnel syndrome. The nerve conduction study confirmed the diagnosis. Furthermore, her work as a baker required repetitive motions which place her at risk for this syndrome. She consumed more alcohol than would be preferred for a patient with diabetes; it doubtless contributed to her poor glucose control, but the quantity imbibed and nerve conduction findings were inconsistent with alcoholic neuropathy.

Chapter 12

1: B
2: B
3: C

Chapter 13

1: C

Although all are conditions that can be seen on the shin, eczema, psoriasis and porokeratosis are usually scaly, eczema and lichen planus usually itchy and actinic porokeratosi usually, on the basis of chronic sun damage, a rarity in even the most tanned sunbed-loving individuals at age 28. Necrobiosis lipoidica diabeticorum, to give its full name, is most often associated with diabetes (rarely not) and is classically as described above. It is quite stubborn to treat but topical as well as intralesional streroids, UV therapy and topical calcineurin inhibitors can be tried. Go and read the chapter to find out more.

2: A, C, D, E

This is really a question of what it isn't. Bilateral cellulitis is really a misnomer, a bit like triple pneumonia. The likelihood of a patient developing a staphylococcal or streptococcal cellulitis simultaneously in two non-consanguineous areas of skin (the proximity of feet to each other doesn't count) is extremely unlikely, unless it was a very big dog bite that caught both legs at the same time, or they caused a penetrating injury to both feet with the same non-sterile podiatry tool, or they stuck both feet in a festering puddle (unlikely but possible). Although people with diabetes are at higher risk of cellulitis, particularly from portals of entry such as tinea pedis and neuropathic ulcers, and have a reduced ability to fend off infection, the problem is almost exclusively unilateral.

   All the other conditions and medication can cause bilateral leg rashes or swelling far more commonly and should be treated appropriately. If you don't know the underlying cause of a patient's bilateral swollen 'rashy' legs then call someone who may and don't resort to empirical unnecessary antibiotics unless there is clinical evidence of infection.

3: A, B, D, E, F

What is being described dermatologically is eruptive xanthoma. This is associated with hypertriglyceridaemia, which is in turn associated with new-onset diabetes, particularly with low insulin levels or resistance to the actions necessary for lipoprotein lipase to effectively clear triglyceride from the blood. Apolipoprotein CII is also required for lipoprotein lipase to clear triglycerides (hence a genetic defect causes hypertriglyceridaemia), whereas B-100 defects result in high cholesterol and more classically tendinous pattern xanthomas. This question is based on a patient that the author saw 6 months ago; his poor diet was certainly not helping matters, but he did have undiagnosed familial combined hyperlipidaemia and new-onset type 2 diabetes.

Chapter 14

1: C
All of the cancers listed except for leukaemia have been associated with diabetes in epidemiological studies.
2: E
3: D

Index

Figures and Tables are indicated by *italic page numbers.*

Diabetes: Chronic Complications, Third Edition. Edited by Kenneth M. Shaw,
Michael H. Cummings.
© 2012 John Wiley & Sons, Ltd. Published 2012 by John Wiley & Sons, Ltd.